DOCTORS on TRIAL

For David, lost

DOCTORS on TRIAL

With an Introduction by Ivan Illich

Dr. John S. Bradshaw

PADDINGTON
PRESS LTD
NEW YORK & LONDON

Library of Congress Cataloging in Publication Data
Bradshaw, John, 1918–
    Doctors on trial.

    Bibliography: p.
    Inclues index.
    1. Physicians—Miscellanea. 2. Medicine—
Miscellanea. I. Title.
R707.B84   610.69'52   78–8947
ISBN 0 448 22070 9 (U.S. and Canada only)

Filmset in England by SX Composing Ltd, Rayleigh, Essex.
Printed and bound in the United States.
Designed by Patricia Pillay

IN THE UNITED STATES
PADDINGTON PRESS
Distributed by
GROSSET & DUNLAP

IN THE UNITED KINGDOM
PADDINGTON PRESS

IN CANADA
Distributed by
RANDOM HOUSE OF CANADA LTD.

IN SOUTHERN AFRICA
Distributed by
ERNEST STANTON (PUBLISHERS) (PTY.) LTD.

CONTENTS

PART I
WHAT DOCTORS DO

PART II
WHAT DOCTORS ARE

PART III
WHAT DOCTORS MIGHT BE

FOREWORD

THIS BOOK HAS BEEN written to be read and understood by ordinary men and women. It is not primarily intended for doctors or other experts although I hope that many of them will read it also, and with profit.

Three points should be made. First, the book's genesis: for years I have collected references and other items relevant to my special interests in medicine. Many doctors do the same. This accumulation helped in prompting me to write this book and gave me most of the material for it; but it was only as the book developed that it became obvious there had been an unconscious method to my magpie years – the collected material formed a pattern, which is more or less the pattern of this book. The book, in other words, has been gestating for many years.

Next, the format: facts are sometimes dry, and there were thousands of them to be presented. To make them interesting and digestible I chose the format of a purported court of enquiry. The doctor witnesses and the personnel of the court of enquiry had their origin, therefore, only in my imagination. The only other fictional elements occur where some statements of medical fact or reactions to them are, to provide authenticity, given the coloring of emotion, judgment, emphasis, and so on, that is normal in speech.

Third, and most important, the facts: all quotations in the book are real, and their sources are given. Nearly all apparent statements of fact in the book would be accepted as such by any well-informed doctor. Most are verifiable in standard lay or medical texts. When a statement is especially important and/or surprising, and may not be accepted or verifiable, I have provided a reference to a supporting source; and in most cases a purely medical source seemed appropriate.

Wherever possible I have culled the references from recent issues of medical journals rather than from books. This is because in books doctors do not usually reveal their errors, their hopes, their doubts, or their fears as readily as they do in the pages of medical journals, and because the subject matter is altering rapidly and books on medical topics are usually two or three years out-of-date when published. (I have tried to make this book an exception in that respect.)

In the event the references are largely taken from what most doctors would accept are the four most important, general-purpose medical journals in the English-speaking world (indeed, in the world as a whole): the *Journal of the American Medical Association*, the *New England Journal of Medicine*, the *Lancet*, and the *British Medical Journal*, the first two being American journals and the last two British. Because their titles appear so often in the lists of references I have used the following abbreviations for three of these journal titles:

   BMJ   — *British Medical Journal*,
   JAMA — *Journal of the American Medical Association*, and
   NEJM — *New England Journal of Medicine*.

Lancet needs no abbreviation. I am aware that these are not among the various official abbreviations; but I am also aware that they are very easy to associate with the full titles, and are, certainly as regards the first two of the trio, the abbreviations for those titles that are commonly used by doctors in their ordinary writings and conversation.

I have so set out the references as to remove one impediment to ready lay access to them – contrary to the usual practice, I have given dates of publication of journal issues, rather than volume numbers.

Where there has been a choice of appropriate references open to me I have used a combination of criteria: the reference most recently published, the one most readily comprehensible by the lay reader, the one that provides the greatest spread of information and of further references; and, I confess, the one on which I could most easily lay my hands. This in part explains why not all the references are to the original source. I do not think the ordinary reader would thank me for meticulousness in this respect, if indeed I had had the time to be capable of it: most of the western medical scene was to be surveyed, and there are some 800 references in all.

Most references are in support of specific statements, but some are given under a particular topic heading; and this is done either when a session's specific references (even if studied in their entirety, as most of them should be, and not just in relation to the point they document) are insufficient to provide needed background information; or when the material for all or a part of one topic has been drawn from a number of sources and blended together.

Lastly, the fact that this book is critical of many aspects of modern western medicine does not mean that any individual doctor is criticized, let alone that the value of doctors is totally decried. As is repeatedly made clear in the book, there are many occasions on which it is essential to consult the best doctor one can find, and many others on which it is highly desirable to do so. Those lay people who read this book will be more knowledgeable about doctors and what they can and cannot do. That knowledge should prove of mutual benefit in their future encounters with members of the profession, while doctor readers may gain some insight into themselves, hopefully beneficial.

JSB

Galway
June 1978

ACKNOWLEDGMENTS

My grateful thanks are due to a number of individuals and organizations for permission to quote or otherwise make use of copyright material. I wish then to thank: Professor Cairns Aitken, Dr Charles D. Aring, Mr Humphrey Arthur, CBE, Dr Glin Bennet, Dr Donnell W. Boardman, Mrs Rosalind Calland, Professor A. G. M. Campbell, Dr Raymond S. Duff, Dr George Dunea, Dr Peter M. Dunn, Dr Leon Eisenberg, Dr J. R. Ellis, MBE, Dr H. Friebel, Dr J. Warren Harthorne, Dr Hershel Jick, Professor Marshal H. Klaus, Dr Jim Lawless, Dr I. S. L. Loudon, Mr R. J. Maxwell, Professor John J. McNamara, Professor Harold C. Neu, Mr K. Norcross, Lord Platt, Dr D. Noel Raine, Dr Eliot Slater, Professor Anne R. Somers, Professor Howard M. Spiro, and Dr Gillian Strube.

I should like to thank also: Dr Stephen Lock, editor of the British Medical Journal; *Dr Ian Munro, editor of the* Lancet; *Dr Franz Ingelfinger, ex-editor of the* New England Journal of Medicine; *and Mr Robert Blyth, editor of the* Pharmaceutical Journal *(London).*

I should like to thank, in addition: the American Medical Association, the British Journal of Obstetrics and Gynaecology, *Her Majesty's Stationery Office, McKinsey and Co. Inc., the* Medical Research Council, *the* New Scientist, *the honorary editors of the* Proceedings of the Royal Society of Medicine, *the Royal College of Physicians of London,* Science, The Times, *the Tobacco Research Council, and the World Health Organization.*

INTRODUCTION
by Ivan Illich

With this book, Dr. Bradshaw closes a decade of social analysis on the effectiveness of modern medicine. In simple language and with a fine ear for grammar, he sums up the public indictment of today's medical system. What some of us have argued, what we have raved about with pathos or with petulance, what we have tried to demonstrate with statistical graphs or with rhetorical devices, John Bradshaw lays before a court of public opinion.

No argument in this book was foreign to me. No quotation, direct or indirect, could not have been documented from my own readings as a layman in medicine or by statements from eminent physicians. And yet, I too was gripped and surprised by the quiet and inexorable proceedings in John Bradshaw's court.

Arguments have come from René Dubos, Archibald Cochrane, Thomas McKeown, John Powles. These arguments were given official shape in government reports such as Lalonde's on the health of Canadians, The Shrivastava commission on health care in India, and also in the studies on "Health and People" produced under the guidance of Dr. Halfdan Mahler by WHO (World Health Organization) . As a result, the health professions were forced to set for themselves new goals. Medicalized prevention, bureaucratic environmentalism, professionalized self-care from birth to death, competed during the early seventies for that popular prestige which only recently had been lost by the generals who conducted the "war" against cancer and malaria. In 1979 this kind of new illusion could become more iatrogenic than the previous trust in hospital-centered medicine. Dr. Bradshaw convinces his readers that it would be folly to seek public health in any such transmogrification of biocracy.

In Session Eighteen of his court proceedings, John Bradshaw sums up his verdict: "We must look for hope, not to doctors, but to those, whether or not they are medically qualified, who see the need to create a new society, of which health will be an integral part (as ill-health is of ours)".

IVAN ILLICH
Cuernavaca, Mexico
July 1978

PART I
What Doctors Do

i

MISTAKES DOCTORS HAVE MADE

JUDGE: It is a privilege for me, a recently retired British judge, to have been invited to sit in public in this very old New York court-room to preside over a Court of Inquiry convened, 'To determine whether western doctors today are more productive of ill-health than of health'. I am pleased to see the court crowded with members of the general public for it is they and those who will subsequently read the court proceedings who are most affected by the issues at stake, and who in the end constitute a kind of jury.

Let me explain that about a year ago some consumer organizations in the United States were considering, with various American medical organizations, the widespread dissatisfaction with modern medicine that has of recent years been felt by many ordinary Americans. In the end they approached the corresponding parties in the United Kingdom who were, they knew, concerned about a similar phenomenon in Britain; and after discussions it was agreed to hold a joint Anglo-American inquiry, which I was invited to conduct with the aid of an English barrister, or attorney as you would call him here. The American venue and the British legal personnel would, it was felt, provide a nice balance.

The inquiry is to consist of an examination by the court of a number of medical witnesses, chosen by the medical, and acceptable to the consumer, organizations; and the bulk of it will comprise a cross-examination of the witnesses by my attorney colleague, Mr James Hunter here; though I myself am, of course, free to ask questions of the witnesses, who in turn are free to make their own separate statements. The medical organizations declined to have what one might call a 'defense' attorney on the grounds that the doctors were all experts, best able to present the medical case by themselves.

The ordinary rules of legal procedure common to our two countries will apply. I would emphasize that this is a most serious inquiry into the state of medicine in the western world; and it will fall to me after the last of the sessions to sum up and to give a judgment. I should add that I am Mr Justice Raeburn, until recently a judge of the English High Court. As we are in the United States, and in what used to be one of your courtrooms, I shall be addressed as 'Judge', and not, in the English manner, as 'My Lord'. For the same reason the proceedings of the court will be transcribed in American, rather than English, spelling.

Each session will be taken up with the examination of one witness; and the topics for the various sessions have been agreed by the consumer and medical organizations on both sides of the Atlantic as being representative of those giving rise to concern. Similarly, the doctor witnesses, though very knowledgeable on their various topics – and told in advance on what aspects they are to be questioned – are meant to be representative of the profession rather than being merely supreme experts in particular narrow fields. Something less than half of them come from the United States, the same proportion from the United Kingdom, and the remainder from other countries. Let us have our first witness.

Enter Professor Thomas Mead

HUNTER (*rising*): You are Professor Thomas Mead, now a Professor of Medical History here in the USA, and formerly an internist – or general physician, as we say in England? (*Pause*) Is masturbation harmful, professor?

MEAD: The modern view is that it is harmful only in those who feel guilty about it, and then the harm is purely mental.

HUNTER: Masturbation is normal in young people, and probably always has been? One should even be worried perhaps over an adolescent who does *not* masturbate?

MEAD: I would hardly say 'worried'.

HUNTER: At least you would not carry any concern to the point of thinking that masturbation might lead to insanity, blindness, impotence, and sterility? (*Pause*) You realize that doctors in the United States, in England and other western countries used commonly to believe it had such effects?

MEAD: In the last century perhaps. We are wiser now.

HUNTER: You are sure? (*Mead nods*) It is a published fact[1] that in 1959 half the students in a group of Philadelphia medical schools believed masturbation to be a frequent cause of mental illness. Did you know doctors used also to believe that the practice of birth control was liable to lead to nymphomania, serious mental disorders, and even suicide?

MEAD: All that sort of nonsense was jettisoned a long time back, Mr Hunter.

HUNTER: And some modern medical judgments will not be?

MEAD: They may be changed in detail, but not often, I think, in principle.

HUNTER: A substantial number of doctors in the last century believed infectious diseases were spread by noxious substances in the air, miasmata, vapors – by bad smells, to use a lay expression.

MEAD: That is true.

HUNTER: And did the belief not persist after Pasteur and others had shown that germs were the cause, at least the immediate cause, of those diseases?

MEAD: The belief had been abandoned by the end of the nineteenth century.

HUNTER: Will you accept that in *this* century some orthodox medical men were putting forward the miasmatic theory in books for the general public? Or do I have to table some of the books to convince you?

MEAD: I am surprised, but I guess superstitions always linger on—

HUNTER: So orthodox medical men in the last century and in this were superstitious? Is it possible that doctors today are ever superstitious?

MEAD: It is extremely unlikely. In the last fifty years medicine has become scientific. We have reliable methods now for determining whether a medical theory is true or false. I doubt that any eminent doctor in this century has believed for very long in a totally mistaken theory concerning disease.

HUNTER: You have heard of Sir William Arbuthnot Lane, who died in 1943? He practised as a surgeon in England in this century? (*Mead nods*) And he was orthodox and eminent?

MEAD: Yes, technically he was a brilliant surgeon, I believe.

HUNTER: Among his operations was there not one in which he removed or 'bypassed' a part of a patient's large bowel on the ground that, as a result of chronic constipation, poisons were entering the blood stream from the waste material in the bowel and were causing disease? (*Mead nods*) A theory that is now wholly discredited? – There are no poisons coming from the bowel? There *are* none in the bowel?

MEAD: None in Lane's sense, that is true.

HUNTER: And yet the operation was performed many times by him, and he held the theory tenaciously for a very long time? (*Mead nods*) What was the term applied to the offending section of bowel? – I mean the innocent section.

MEAD: It was called – er – Lane's 'kink'. But for every doctor who has held a theory later shown to be false there were a hundred who didn't.

JUDGE: Many doctors must have shared Lane's view, professor, or else they would not have sent patients to him.

MEAD: Yes, judge. I was referring to modern doctors pioneering new theories.

HUNTER: Most doctors simply accept what the pioneers of the profession are teaching? (*Mead nods*) *Currently* teaching? Let us look at some more twentieth-century pioneer theories then. Will you explain to the court what 'focal sepsis' means?

MEAD: That there is a so-called 'septic' area in one localized part of the body – a septic 'focus'. In other words, a collection of harmful bacteria, perhaps throwing off toxins; in or near the teeth, say, or in the tonsils or sinuses, or the appendix or gall bladder.

HUNTER: And was not focal sepsis once invoked by eminent medical men as the cause of many diseases? (*Mead nods*) In the 1920s and 1930s? In your lifetime and mine? What diseases?

MEAD: A lot of mental illness particularly, and arthritis, and various other conditions whose cause was unknown.

HUNTER: And in the case of mental illness, for example, what treatment would be carried out?

MEAD: Teeth and tonsils, supposedly infected were removed; sinuses were washed out. . . .

HUNTER: With what effect on the mental illness in question?

MEAD: None at all, of course.

HUNTER: People remained as mad as before but had no teeth? Did some doctors not claim, however, to observe an improvement on occasion as a result of the treatment? (*Mead nods*) So that again in this century a lot of orthodox, eminent doctors believed in another piece of superstitious nonsense?

MEAD: I guess you could put it like that.

HUNTER: You are acquainted with the condition known as schizophrenia, professor? It is a serious and common mental condition, particularly affecting younger people? An incurable condition, though it sometimes clears up spontaneously, and nowadays can at least be controlled?

MEAD: That is true.

HUNTER: And insulin is a substance produced by the pancreatic gland that lowers the level of the blood sugar, and in big doses puts a person into a coma in consequence? – A state of deep unconsciousness?

MEAD: Correct.

HUNTER: A coma is a serious, even life-threatening state? (*Mead nods*) In the 1930s, forties and fifties was it not common practice in mental hospitals in your country and other western countries to treat schizophrenic patients by giving them a big injection of insulin every day for weeks on end so that each day they went into a state of coma – from which after a time they were revived by the giving of glucose in large amounts? And did not some patients, so treated, die?

MEAD: Some. Very, very few.

HUNTER: And was insulin coma of the least benefit in schizophrenia.

MEAD: A majority of psychiatrists today would say it was valueless.

HUNTER: The *great* majority? So that yet again in this century orthodox eminent medical men held a view – and acted on it – that was later shown to be untenable? (*Pause*) When was convulsion therapy introduced?

MEAD: Round about the mid-1930s.

HUNTER: For?

MEAD: For schizophrenia. It was believed that epilepsy and schizophrenia never coexisted in one person. It was argued that perhaps the fits – the convulsions – that occur in epilepsy protected in some way against schizophrenia.

HUNTER: Did the giving of convulsive treatment to schizophrenics who were not epileptic cure or improve them?

MEAD: Regrettably it did not. However, it was found that it *did* relieve depression. This was long before the anti-depressant drugs appeared.

HUNTER: Whether or not, and to what degree, electrical convulsive treatment does relieve depression has been a matter of dispute among experts?

MEAD: Yes, but the majority is in favour of it.

HUNTER: Was it eventually found that epilepsy and schizophrenia *could* coexist in the same patient? (*Mead nods*) So that here is a treatment, introduced for one condition for what turned out to be a mistaken reason, that is alleged to be good for another condition – though some doctors dispute its value – and that does, I believe, carry certain risks and drawbacks?

MEAD: That is one way of putting the matter.

HUNTER: Will you tell us, professor, about the operation of prefrontal lobotomy, which was often performed, I believe, in the 1930s, forties, and fifties?

MEAD: It commonly meant the making of openings in the skull – trepanning – and then an extensive cutting across of the front part of the brain on each side. The object, briefly, was to divide certain connecting nerve channels. In Britain the term 'leucotomy' was used, but that is now reserved for a more modern, much less radical operation.

HUNTER: The exact function of those channels you mention and of the forward part of the brain to which they go is not completely known? And for what mental diseases was this lobotomy operation used?

MEAD: For severe cases of depression and of what is known as obsessive-compulsive neurosis, for certain personality disorders, for severe anxiety states, for severe hypochondriasis, for—

HUNTER: Perhaps my question should have been 'For what mental diseases was it not used?' Well now, what effect did it have on the patient's personality?

MEAD: In general, it made the patients less anxious, rather placid, without much thought for others or for the future, and perhaps rather shallow.

HUNTER: Human cabbages? (*Mead nods*) Did it cure or improve the mental disorders for which it was performed?

MEAD: To be truthful – no, not really, not in most cases. It masked some of their features, that was all.

HUNTER: It deprived the patient of the capacity to suffer at the price of losing the capacity for joy?

MEAD: In a sense.

HUNTER: My question had only one sense, professor. That type of operation is now largely discredited?

MEAD: Yes, but the technique of leucotomy – the new operation – has been greatly refined in recent years with much better results.

HUNTER: None the less the crude operation was performed quite commonly less than 25 years ago in America, in the United Kingdom, and elsewhere?

MEAD: We all make mistakes, Mr Hunter, and some of us try to learn from them, as I have indicated.

HUNTER: The public learns too, does it not? – The more recent operations of psychosurgery, as it is called, have aroused very great controversy in the United States? Yes? There have been demonstrations against them? – Particularly those intended to influence people's behavior.

MEAD: Regrettably, yes.

HUNTER: You do not think the lay public should take an interest in what surgeons may be proposing to do to their brains? (*Pause*) Before we leave the subject may I just ask if skulls found by archeologists have not shown that trepanning, the operation of boring holes in people's skulls, was performed in prehistoric times as well as in the twentieth century? – To let out evil spirits? Or so it is believed.

MEAD: That is true, sir.

HUNTER: And with as much benefit as produced by trepanning plus lobotomy?

MEAD: I would not like to say with what benefit.

HUNTER: Your loyalty to your prehistoric colleagues is in the best medical tradition, professor.

JUDGE: And you are provoking the witness, Mr Hunter. Be so good as to stop.

HUNTER: Yes, judge. Tell me, professor: at the time you were a student was it not routine practice, when a doctor was faced with what is called an iron-deficiency anemia, apart from his looking for any serious cause, for the doctor to treat the anemia with iron-containing medicines?

MEAD: That is certainly so.

HUNTER: And once the iron-containing pigment in the blood – the hemoglobin, as it is called – reached the so-called normal level again all concerned felt very pleased with themselves? (*Pause*) Has it not been shown more recently[2] that such treatment does not, in fact, relieve most of the symptoms traditionally taught as being due to such anemia? And that, in fact, a mild-to-moderate degree of such anemia may even, if anything, have a slightly beneficial effect on health, certainly on the possibility of a person developing heart disease?[3]

MEAD: Yes, scientific investigation has discovered that.

HUNTER: So the older but quite recent teaching was wrong? Was it not also the custom, when you were a medical student, to keep a patient in bed for two or three weeks after almost any abdominal operation? And is it not the custom today to keep most such patients in bed for only a day or two?

MEAD: There are excellent reasons, as we now appreciate, for getting them up much earlier than we used to.

HUNTER: There *seem* to be excellent reasons, surely? I mean, 30 years ago there *seemed* to be excellent reasons for *not* getting them up earlier. Despite all the examples I have quoted do you really think, professor, that doctors in this century, indeed in the last decade or two, have been guided only by scientifically established truth?

MEAD: On the whole, yes. There are a few exceptions.

HUNTER: Such as freezing of the stomach for peptic ulceration,[4] which was practised quite recently, was it not? (*Mead nods*) Or removal of the large bowel for epilepsy?[4] Or of the adrenal glands for high blood pressure?[4] Or cutting of the sympathetic nervous ganglia for high blood pressure or for asthma?[4] – To mention just a few more of the useless and discredited procedures that have been practised routinely, some of them in the last 20 years.

MEAD: No one is infallible, Mr Hunter.

HUNTER: And, in fact, doctors are as fallible as the next man, but their faults can have more serious consequences? (*Pause*) You are a professor of medical history? Is it normal practice in medical schools for the students to be told about the mistaken theories that have been held by doctors, the useless procedures they have praised and practiced, the therapeutic miseries they have inflicted upon patients?

MEAD: Such matters are certainly mentioned.

HUNTER: With as much emphasis as is given to the so-called

triumphs and certainties of medicine?

MEAD: Naturally not. One cannot be wholly negative. One must not instil cynicism into young minds.

HUNTER: Or a love of truth? Or any element of doubt that the *current* teaching might be mistaken? Is there a single book, written by a doctor for medical students, with any such title as *Mistakes Doctors Have Made?*

MEAD: To the best of my knowledge, no.

HUNTER: A multi-volume work might be required, might it not? Thank you, professor. (*Sits*)

JUDGE: You must not provoke the witnesses, Mr Hunter. You might provoke me too. Should you, Professor Mead, care to mention for us, as an antidote to Mr Hunter's catalogue, a few of the successes of modern medicine? – Bearing in mind that he is listening?

MEAD: Most certainly, judge. There is the completion of the conquest of infectious diseases, which was begun in the last century and continued even more successfully in the present century with the help of vaccines and sulfa drugs and antibiotics, and, of course, of further improvements in hygiene, sanitation, nutrition, and housing. There have been enormous improvements in anesthesia, and in surgical techniques so that people who would certainly have died in 1900 are now cured or relieved and given a further span of useful, happy life. There have been improvements in methods of diagnosis, and in almost every aspect of treatment. Above all, underlying this there has been a striking development in the scientific basis of medicine with corresponding benefits for humanity. In brief, mankind has more life and has it more abundantly – thanks to modern medicine.

JUDGE: Mr Hunter's abundance seems to be of doubts, I fear.

HUNTER (*rising*): Professor Mead, the examples of doctor error that I gave you were all concrete individual instances?

MEAD: Yes.

HUNTER: And you have given us a host of sweeping generalities, which in fact pre-empt judgments on the very topics into which this court is to inquire?

MEAD: I could give you dozens of concrete instances of the kind of thing to which I was referring.

HUNTER: Then give me one, please.

MEAD: I would call your attention, Mr Hunter, to malaria, a disease that not very long ago was killing more people than any other single disease; but that in this century, particularly in the last 30 years, has been brought under control thanks to a whole range of anti-malarial drugs, to the use of insecticides, to drainage schemes, and the treatment of stagnant water; to all of which we may before too long be able to add an anti-malarial vaccine. A triumph for medical science – indisputable, magnificent. Hundreds of millions of lives have certainly been saved.

HUNTER (*after a pause*): Hundreds of millions? Tell me, professor, you have heard of the population explosion?

MEAD: Of course.

HUNTER: In which countries in general is the population increasing most rapidly?

MEAD: In tropical or near-tropical countries.

HUNTER: In which countries was – and is – malaria most prevalent?

MEAD: In those same countries.

HUNTER: Do you think there is any connection at all between the control of malaria and overpopulation?

MEAD: Oh, that is much too simple.

HUNTER: Will you answer my simple question?

MEAD: Yes, obviously there is some connection; but if a doctor is faced with a sick person, a dying person, he must do something – he cannot start thinking in political terms.

HUNTER: You think that starving to death is a political matter, but that dying of malaria is a medical matter? That doctors should wear blinkers? Or perhaps that they invariably do? (*Pause*) And did the men who developed DDT or who invented and perfected the anti-malarial drugs or who investigated malaria in the laboratory – do you think they always had a person with them dying of malaria?

MEAD: I think your question highly objectionable.

JUDGE: It was you who raised the matter of a doctor faced with a dying person, professor; I think Mr Hunter did not mean to give any offence.

MEAD: I think those men used their imagination. And most of them were pure scientists, not doctors.

HUNTER: So any triumph was for science, not medicine? And now will you use your imagination, professor? – And think of the children saved from malaria but dying instead, later on, more slowly of starvation – due to overpopulation.

MEAD: I do not need to be told of it.

HUNTER: No, there are the advertisements by western charities in the newspapers, are there not? Did western science use its imagination and foresee that western charities would be advertising the other face of its triumphs? (*Pause*) Then tell me: do you think overpopulation is a threat to world peace?

MEAD: Yes, it obviously is – one of many.

HUNTER: A very, very prominent one? – A threat that might conceivably lead to thermonuclear war with the United States of America in the front line?

MEAD: Possibly.

HUNTER: And to the extinction of mankind?

MEAD: Oh, I am sure that will not happen.

HUNTER: You had no doubts two minutes ago about the rightness of conquering malaria. Do you really think now that the control of malaria has resulted in mankind having – what was it? – having more life and having it more abundantly?

MEAD: Are you really suggesting to me, Mr Hunter, that doctors should have sat down years ago, weighed all the pros and cons, and said 'No, we mustn't attempt to eradicate malaria because that would lead to overpopulation and a lot of other troubles'? Are you?

HUNTER: With respect, professor, it is you who are putting an over-simplified question. And I am not a witness, I am not required to answer it, though with the judge's permission I will.

JUDGE: Yes, Mr Hunter we want the truth, even at the cost of a little informality.

HUNTER: Of course, professor, those doctors could not have done what you suggest, no man could. Hardly any men possess the fore-sight, the breadth of vision, or the depth of moral courage and understanding to think and to behave in such ways. The doctors were elements in a social process enormously bigger and stronger than themselves, as we see in retrospect; and for them its par-ticular impetus was simply towards saving more lives, making people live longer, getting rid of pain and illness – then. They did not envisage the larger consequences and for what they did I do not blame them, though I do not praise them either; I have hind-sight. The nature of that larger process, what it is that motivates western doctors – indeed, modern western man – at the deepest level it is the business of this court to discover. In other words, professor, the question you put to me will really receive its answer from the deliberations of this court very gradually in the course of the next two or three weeks. Thank you, professor. (*Sits*)

JUDGE: Professor, we are most grateful to you; but before you stand down let me say a few words that may be of help to you and to all those who are attending the hearings or may read the transcript of them. We are here to try to establish the truth. No personal ani-mosity is involved. Mr Hunter's case so far goes strongly against the grain of your thinking and your medical upbringing; but I must ask you – and those others – not to jump to conclusions, to listen carefully to the arguments as they develop, and, above all, to ask yourself frequently whether some preconception on one side or the other may not be hindering your search for the truth.

I agree with Mr Hunter in one respect: the final reckoning is some time away. This court is now adjourned.

REFERENCES—SESSION ONE
1. Lief, H. I., in Brecher, R., and Brecher, E. (eds.), *An Analysis of Human Sexual Response*, p. 308, Panther Books, London, 1968.
2. Elwood, P. C., and Hughes, D., *BMJ* August 1, 1970, p. 254.
3. Rifkind, B. M., and Gale, M., *Lancet*, September 23, 1967, p. 640.
4. Hiatt, H. H., *NEJM*, July 31, 1975, p. 235.

OBESITY

Enter Dr James McGilly

HUNTER (*rising*): You are Dr James McGilly, from Australia; a doctor specializing to some extent in the management of obesity? (*McGilly nods*) I should like to establish first, doctor, how common and important obesity is, and what its causes are, so that no one may be in any doubt as to the great relevance to our inquiry of the medical approach to this condition. So now: how common is it in the western world?

McGILLY: Just how common one says it is depends on one's definition of obesity. Almost every expert would accept that at least 20 percent of people in the United States or Britain are obese; and some experts would put the figure as high as 50 percent. At any one time some 10 or 15 percent of the population in these countries is trying to slim. The position is much the same in most other developed countries.

HUNTER: And in poor countries, which are short of food?

McGILLY: It is very uncommon, although among the poor people of developed countries, such as this country or my own, it is as common as in the rich people or even commoner. That is because they eat a lot of things like sugar and fried potatoes, which are very fattening, rather than lean meat or fresh fruit and vegetables.

HUNTER: Does obesity affect the likelihood of dying of other conditions?

McGILLY: Yes: as a rule of thumb, the expectation of life is reduced by about 1 percent for every pound – or roughly every half kilogram – a person is over his ideal weight. Diabetes, heart disease, raised blood pressure, gall stones – all these are more common in the obese. And conditions like bronchitis are worse because, of course, there is more weight for the breathless bronchitic person to carry round. And arthritis, varicose veins, and flat feet, and accidents are all more common.

HUNTER: So that we are faced with a very serious condition?

McGILLY: And one that is the most common nutritional disorder in the western world.

HUNTER: And its immediate cause is?

McGILLY: Its *immediate* cause is an intake of food in excess of the body's requirements for energy purposes.

HUNTER: Eating too much?

McGILLY: Yes, although some obese people, in fact, eat less than the non-obese. If a person is *very* inactive – if, for instance, he is confined to bed over a long period for some reason – then he may become obese on a relatively small intake of food.

HUNTER: But this is a minority? And it is certainly a small minority of obese people who have some disorder of the glands that is responsible for their condition? (*McGilly nods*) What other rare causes of obesity are there, doctor?

MCGILLY: It is said sometimes to be an inherited condition; but this is not a common element, and in any case it is difficult to be sure whether parents have passed on to a child a true tendency to be fat or have merely given it in its childhood permanent eating habits that will tend to make it fat. And then there are one or two disorders of the nervous system that are occasionally responsible for obesity.

HUNTER: But the vast majority of cases is due to what? – Gluttony?

MCGILLY: No, the suggestion of some kind of fault is neither valid nor helpful. Most people who are obese have become so because of psychosocial factors. In other words, the taking of food helps to relieve tension and anxiety, and there's a lot of both in our modern western world, and very often they can be found in the obese person. As for social factors: there are various pressures in society that help to make people eat more than they need. It is in the present century and in the western world that for the first time in history there has been more than enough food for hundreds of millions of people. Previously, by and large, people ate what they could get. And then there is the advertising of food and drink, and the tempting ways in which food is presented, and the refinement of food – so that in the case of sugar, which is a highly refined substance, one can consume a great many calories in a very small bulk. Nothing but calories, no protein or minerals or vitamins or dietary fiber; and calories mean fat. And then there are the common modern habits of eating snacks at cocktail parties, of giving business lunches, of nibbling between meals, and of taking alcoholic and non-alcoholic drinks, most of the latter containing a lot of calories and, like sugar, very little in the way of needed nutrients. Alcoholic drinks too are a rich source of calories.

JUDGE: You indict our western society, doctor, in other words?

MCGILLY: I do.

HUNTER: Would you include in your catalogue the sitting in automobiles or in front of television sets that our civilization encourages?

MCGILLY: Yes, one would certainly include all those elements that in one way or another mean we do not take exercise, which uses up food calories and perhaps helps to keep our appetite-control centers in trim. All labor-saving devices are included, and modern heating, but for which we'd have to use more of our food energy in keeping ourselves warm. As for watching television, of course, we spend more time on only two things in our lives – work and sleep.

HUNTER: And what about the artificial feeding of babies and obesity?

McGILLY: That too must probably take some of the blame. Wholly breast-fed babies usually do not get fat. Bottle-fed babies who, quite apart from their bottle feeds, are usually given cereals and sugar very early in life, as well as various other fattening foods, often get fat, and are given prizes at baby shows for it. Some doctors think that the fat baby often becomes the fat child who often becomes the fat adult, though there is some debate about that. It may be also that bottle-feeding prevents the proper development of the appetite-controlling center in the brain.[1]

HUNTER: Would it be true then to say that widespread obesity is a condition due to our western way of life, indeed peculiar to it?

McGILLY: Certainly. One of the absolutely characteristic western diseases.

HUNTER: So we have a serious and very common condition, usually social and psychological in origin, which is characteristic of our civilization, and I can now ask you what doctors do about it.

McGILLY: They explain the condition in simple terms, they advise the patient on a low-calorie diet, often they will give him an appetite-reducing drug to help bolster his will power, and sometimes they will advise the taking of regular exercise, perhaps by walking or cycling, say, or on a special exercising machine or in special classes. A low-calorie diet of the usual kind means that consumption of sugar and of our highly refined white flour and of items made from them (white bread, cakes, cookies, sweets, pastry, jam, puddings, and so on) and also the consumption of very fatty foodstuffs are reduced. Whole-grain cereal products, most fresh fruit and vegetables, lean meat, fish, and poultry – these are recommended instead.

HUNTER: And how often do the doctors see the patient after the initial visit?

McGILLY: Perhaps not as often as they should.

HUNTER: And yet would you not agree, in view of your earlier remarks, that what the obese patient greatly needs is understanding and sympathy, which could be provided by the doctor at a series of follow-up visits? (*McGilly nods*) But they are often not provided? Instead the patient is given a drug? How effective are these appetite-reducing drugs?

McGILLY: Some of them can be helpful for a time in some patients.

HUNTER: But they nearly all have drawbacks of one sort or another? The amphetamine drugs, which I believe were once widely used in the UK, and still are widely used here in the USA, have a major drawback, have they not? – They are drugs of dependence? – People get hooked on them?

McGILLY: Correct. And in fact they are not of much value for reducing appetite.

HUNTER: But tens of millions of amphetamine-type tablets were or are being prescribed by American and British doctors even after wide publicity about their dangers? (*McGilly nods*) Tell me, Dr McGilly, what is refractory obesity?

McGILLY: The kind that does not respond to relatively simple measures.

HUNTER: Is it a fact that sometimes refractory obesity simply means that the patient is not sticking to his diet because the sympathy and support and explanation that are needed are not being given by the doctor?

McGILLY: Yes, that is true.

HUNTER: And that other cases are due to the patient having simply been given a prescription for a drug, and the doctor having failed even to point out the crucial importance of keeping to a low-calorie diet with or without the help of a drug? (*McGilly nods*) And that other cases are due to the fact that, having lost a lot of weight in the first few days on a diet (most of the loss being fluid), the patient becomes disappointed when the rate of loss of weight slows down, and simply gives up – again due to lack of explanation and encouragement?

McGILLY: Yes, although there are some cases of refractory obesity where the doctor is in no sense at fault.

HUNTER: Is gross refractory obesity sometimes treated by taking the patient into hospital and literally starving him?

McGILLY: Yes, but there is little hunger involved after the first day or two; this is practiced only in special units, and only for the very grossly obese.

HUNTER: The starvation sometimes has serious effects on the heart or kidney? On occasion it has resulted in sudden death from heart failure? (*McGilly nods*) Well now, is gross obesity also sometimes treated, especially here in America, by the surgical removal of large strips of fat from beneath the patient's skin, particularly from the belly?

McGILLY: That is a reasonable enough treatment if it improves the patient cosmetically.

HUNTER: But not very – er – elegant? Another form of treatment for gross or refractory obesity, again particularly popular here, is an operation either to exclude most of the stomach from the digestive tract, or to bypass a part of the intestine?

MCGILLY: Yes.

HUNTER: In the second case the patient feels distended on much less food than normal and so eats less? (*McGilly nods*) 'Bypass' is an automobile term, an engineer's term? And the automobile may help to cause obesity?

JUDGE: Dr McGilly's silence, Mr Hunter, may be construed as consent – to the obvious.

HUNTER (*to McGilly*): About 5 percent of those who have the by-pass operation die from it?[2]

MCGILLY: They are very obese people who want treatment and for whom all other forms of treatment have failed.

HUNTER: Those who survive the operation, as well as losing weight, may develop severe diarrhea, or serious disease of the liver, kidney, or pancreas, or arthritis, or mental disorder?

MCGILLY: Yes.

HUNTER: Is there not also a form of treatment for refractory obesity that involves destroying a part of the brain – one that is involved in appetite control – by means of X-rays or even actual brain surgery?

MCGILLY: That is true. It has gone out of fashion. I mean rather that it is now not widely used.

HUNTER: And is not another form of treatment to splint the person's upper and lower jaws together so that it is possible to take fluid but not to chew solid foods?[3] (*McGilly nods*) This too is not what one would call a very elegant form of treatment?

MCGILLY: Agreed, but simply to pull out an aching tooth is not very elegant, though it may be very effective.

HUNTER: For how long are the jaws kept splintered, doctor?

MCGILLY: For some months.

HUNTER: Does it take months to extract a tooth? And a majority of patients, treated by jaw splinting, put on weight again once the splinting is removed, do they not?[3] (*Pause*) You have heard of behavioral treatment of obesity?[4] Operant conditioning, as it is called. Is it effective?

MCGILLY: The results so far are quite promising.

HUNTER: This approach was devised by medical men?

MCGILLY: No, by psychologists.

HUNTER: And briefly, what does it consist of?

MCGILLY: It consists of making the patient very much more conscious of the exact place of food and of eating in his or her life –

so that he may recognize what controls his eating and make appropriate changes. The patient has to keep a careful record of the composition of all meals that he takes, when he had them, what his mood was at the time, and so on. He is to eat only in a particular room, he is to prepare his food himself, and only one portion at a time. He counts the number of mouthfuls he has. He weighs himself four times a day, and so on.

HUNTER: Anything else? I mean, is there something else to behavioral therapy, different from all that?

McGILLY: Oh, you mean the need for a trained therapist to be in charge?

HUNTER: What I really meant was someone to see the patient regularly to give him guidance and support and reward.

McGILLY: The trained therapist. Yes, positive reinforcement is certainly needed.

HUNTER: 'Support' and 'reward' are simpler terms with the same meaning, are they not? And you did not mention it spontaneously; and it is the very thing you said just now was often missing from the medical management of obesity. (*Pause*) Is there any other non-medical category, Dr McGilly, that has attempted to cope with obesity?

McGILLY: There are lay organizations, the members of which meet regularly in local groups. There is nearly always a very positive, even fervent or evangelical kind of atmosphere involved.

HUNTER: You sound as though you feel superior to that kind of thing. No? And yet that atmosphere, present in a group, provides obese people with the very support you said they need and that doctors often fail to give. Are these lay organizations more or less successful than doctors in dealing with obesity?

McGILLY: On the whole I would say more successful than doctors.

HUNTER: And would you not say that those non-medical approaches to obesity are more gentle, more acceptable than splinting the jaws or bypassing the bowel or giving drugs that may produce addiction?

McGILLY: I think you are simply saying that non-medical people have less power – well, less inclination – to interfere radically.

HUNTER: Yes, I *am* saying that. And I am saying that they are in this case more effective. And you have not denied it. (*Pause*) There are special medical societies for the study of obesity, are there not? And special meetings, some of them international, to discuss the very latest developments in connection with obesity. You are attending such a meeting here in New York at present?

McGILLY: That is true.

HUNTER: A growth industry, one might say? – Especially in its failures. (*Pause*) At these meetings do the participating doctors eat only low-calorie meals?

McGILLY: No, they do not. Anyway not usually.

HUNTER: They often eat high-calorie meals?

McGILLY: Perhaps. Sometimes.

HUNTER: They drink alcoholic, high-calorie drinks at the meetings? (*McGilly nods*) They arrive by plane or automobile? (*He nods again*) Not on the bicycles they recommend to their obese patients? (*Pause*) They watch television, they use lifts, taxis, heated conference halls and hotels? (*Pause*) Would you agree that most of the medical treatments for obesity are as mu᾽ characteristic of our western civilization as are the causes of it? They would not, they could not have been applied in any other epoch?

McGILLY: I have never thought of it like that; but yes, I think that is true.

HUNTER: Are doctors themselves conspicuously slim, compared with other people?

McGILLY: I would not say so.

HUNTER: No further questions, judge, for the moment. (*Sits*)

JUDGE: You wish to add anything, doctor?

McGILLY: Yes, judge, I do in view of what has been said or implied about doctors. We did not invent the tensions and frustrations of modern life that often help to produce obesity. Doctors did not invent refined sugar, and low-extraction white flour, and sweets and cakes and breakfast cereals, and sweet drinks and alcoholic drinks, and all the other fattening items. Or the automobile, or labor-saving appliances, or television. We are simply trying to deal with the end product of a process we did not initiate.

HUNTER (*rising*): Though not very successfully, doctor, as you've admitted. And are doctors not central figures in our western civilization?

McGILLY: In a sense. But that does not make us responsible for all its ills.

HUNTER: Not even in part? You agreed that early artificial feeding of babies might be the first step to adult obesity. Did doctors in various western countries in the earlier part of this century not play a big part in converting women to artificial feeding of babies instead of breast-feeding?

McGILLY: Some part, that is unfortunately true.

HUNTER: And are they now trying to undo that damage?

McGILLY: Some individual doctors are; but no, not the profession as a whole, I fear. Not yet.

HUNTER: When and in what country did doctors last campaign

against the widespread availability and the advertising of sweets and sugary drinks and fatty, sugary confectionery – all the items we mentioned earlier?

McGILLY: They have to my knowledge never campaigned against them.

HUNTER: But they have campaigned for more money for themselves? They are not wholly ignorant of the techniques of lobbying governments? (*Pause*) Thank you, doctor: your silence, like theirs, is very eloquent.

JUDGE: And I now declare this court adjourned – for a lunch that I take it will, in Mr Hunter's case, be almost invisible.

REFERENCES—SESSION TWO
1. Hall, B., *Lancet*, April 5, 1975, p. 779.
2. Leading Article, *BMJ*, November 27, 1976, p. 1278.
3. Rodgers, S., *et al.*, *Lancet*, June 11, 1977, p. 1221.
4. Pomerlau, O., Bass, F., and Crown, V., *NEJM*, June 12, 1975, p. 1277.

General Reading
Garrow, J. S., *Energy Balance and Obesity in Man*, Associated Scientific Publishers, Amsterdam, 1974.
Anderson, J., *BMJ*, February 26, 1972, p. 560.
Mann, G. V., *NEJM*, July 25, 1974, p. 178; and August 1, 1974, p. 226.
Bennett, J. R., and Baddeley, M., *BMJ*, October 30, 1976, p. 1052.
Select Committee on Nutrition and Human Needs, United States Senate, *Dietary Goals for the United States*, US Government Printing Office, Washington, 1977.

Obesity in Children
Editorial, *Lancet*, January 5, 1974, p. 17. (Also deals briefly with brain surgery for obesity.)
Leading Article, *BMJ*, June 28, 1975, p. 706.
Leading Article, *BMJ*, June 30, 1973, p. 727.

Surgery for Obesity
Leading Article, *BMJ*, June 15, 1974, p. 575.
Meyerowitz, B. R., Gruber, R. P., and Laub, D. R., *JAMA*, July 23, 1973, p. 408.
Moxley, R. T., III, Pozefsky, T., and Lockwood, D. H., *NEJM*, April 25, 1974, p. 921.
Editorial, *JAMA*, March 22, 1976, p. 1261.
Editorial, *NEJM*, July 1, 1976, p. 43.

CORONARY HEART DISEASE

Enter Professor David Brent

HUNTER: You are David Brent, a Professor of Cardiology here in the United States? First, how common is coronary heart disease, professor?

BRENT: It is now the most common killing disease of western man whereas 60 or 70 years ago it was almost unknown – though doctors could diagnose it then all right. It kills about 200,000 people a year in Britain, and over 650,000 in this country;[1] more than all forms of cancer combined. And the people it kills are often in the prime of life, the male victims especially: two out of five male deaths in the age group 35 to 44 in your country are due to coronary heart disease; and though it doesn't kill nearly as many younger women, it has been getting more common in them too,[2] though in general it's more usual in men.

HUNTER: And what causes this modern plague of ours?

BRENT: The background condition is a fatty deposit in the smooth lining of the arteries of the heart – the coronary arteries. Other arteries are affected by this atheroma (which literally means 'porridge'), but it produces its most serious damage in the coronary arteries. When it affects the arteries to the brain it often results in a stroke. The deposit contains various substances – in particular, as well as fats, a waxy substance called cholesterol.

HUNTER: Atheroma is a form of hardening of the arteries? Is it common?

BRENT: Yes, it's present to *some* extent in most adults in western countries. It stimulates scar tissue to form round it, so that the fully developed condition is called atherosclerosis, meaning a fatty scar. Any one affected coronary artery will commonly show a number of atherosclerotic patches which prevent it opening up properly when the heart is needing more blood because, say, the person is taking exercise. Also a clot (or thrombus) can form on one of these patches, blocking the artery altogether.

HUNTER: A coronary thrombosis?

BRENT: As it used to be called, and still is by non-medical people. A coronary. Actually the process isn't always as straightforward as that, but no matter. When a coronary artery is permanently blocked the portion of heart muscle to which it would supply blood – containing oxygen and nourishment to keep it alive – simply dies, the condition being called by doctors 'myocardial infarction', which means 'death of heart muscle'. The patient gets a sudden severe pain in the chest (or sometimes in the arm or jaw – a referred pain, as it's called), usually coming on when he's not exerting himself; and often he dies at once or very quickly. That depends on how big the artery is, how the heart responds, and so on. If he doesn't die, the pain will persist for a long time, and the heart may start beating in the wrong way, or it may fail slowly, and this again may kill the patient. Those who recover from a first coronary may succumb to a second one; but some will have a series of attacks, and a few will have one attack and then not another for years or for the rest of their lives. Also one can suffer death of a portion of the heart muscle without ever having had an obvious coronary attack.

HUNTER: And what about the other kind of coronary heart disease, angina pectoris?

BRENT: It means literally 'pain in the chest', but this pain comes on when the patient is exerting himself or is upset, and, although it is so severe that it stops the patient in his tracks, it usually passes off after a short time and probably doesn't as a rule cause any death of heart muscle. The patient has simply been asking a bit too much of his heart, and because its arteries are atherosclerotic and can't open up properly there isn't enough extra blood to supply the temporary extra needs of the heart muscle, so pain occurs. However, once the patient stops exerting himself – stops walking upstairs, say – the heart's demand gets less and in a short time it *will* be getting enough blood, and the pain will vanish. Angina may also sometimes be caused by cold making a coronary artery go into spasm.[3] The patient with angina usually has a whole series of attacks, and he can develop a coronary – just as a recovered coronary patient can develop angina. However, it's coronary thrombosis that's contributed most to the coronary epidemic.

HUNTER: And now what causes atheroma and what causes the thrombosis?

BRENT: We're not absolutely sure except that a number of factors are involved. We do know there are certain risk factors – rough-and-ready predictor factors – for coronary heart disease. If one records the characteristics of a large number of people (whether they smoke cigarettes, are overweight, and so on), it's easy enough to discover over a period of years what factors were most often present beforehand in the group who later develop coronary heart disease. That has been done here in a town called Framingham, Massachusetts. And one can compare in this way the populations of different countries, or look at what happens to populations that migrate or suffer for some other reason a big change in diet, say, as in time of war. Discover, in other words, what changes precede a big increase in coronaries.

HUNTER: Why aren't they necessarily causes, those that are found to be associated with an increase?

BRENT: Some of them may be; but some are probably just coincidental; and some may simply be related to another factor, whether suspected or not, that is itself a cause. We know that obesity, for instance, is often associated with hypertension – a raised blood pressure – which probably is one of the true 'causes'. It's one of the three major risk factors, the other two being cigarette smoking, and a raised level in the blood plasma of cholesterol and, less importantly, of certain fats called triglycerides. Increasing age is another important risk factor; so is a lack of regular vigorous exercise; and so very possibly is deficiency of dietary fiber[4] – a lack in the diet of whole cereal foods, fruit and vegetables.

HUNTER: And what about the stress that one is always hearing quoted?

BRENT: Maybe it's of some importance; and a few experts think there's a special kind of striving, time-obsessed personality that makes a person much more liable to develop coronary heart disease. Obesity and diabetes I must mention too, though they're both probably indirect in their effect. Most experts don't rate sugar intake very high as a risk factor. Hard drinking water has some limited protective effect. There's sometimes an inherited tendency to coronary heart disease. The pill increases the risk a little, particularly in older women. Among the also-rans are an excess of vitamin D, and a lack of vitamin E or of selenium. And we know a good deal, at any rate in the case of the main risk factors, about the detailed mechanisms by which they operate – or anyway could operate. The more risk factors you have, of course, the greater the danger. However, even if you can't alter your age or sex or inheritance, or your personality very much, nearly all the other risk factors are theoretically open to change.

HUNTER: You mean one can give up cigarette smoking, one can lose weight on a slimming diet, one can take regular exercise, even cut down the stress in one's life; one can see to it that one gets some dietary fiber?

BRENT: Correct. One can do all those things. In theory. And nearly all cases of high blood pressure can be controlled with modern drugs. And a raised plasma cholesterol *can* usually be lowered if one cuts down one's total intake of fats considerably. It helps cholesterol-wise and palatability-wise if one makes a relatively *small* cut in certain liquid fats (the polyunsaturated kind, as they're called – maize oil, sunflower seed oil, and so on), and a relatively much bigger cut in solid saturated fats: that is, animal fats and hardened vegetable fats. And, though it's not so important, one should probably cut one's intake of cholesterol too, which is mostly found with saturated animal fats and particularly in eggs. What this means in practice is less fatty meat, and more lean meat, fish, and poultry; less butter and dripping and lard and cream, and more soft margarine, more of the oils I mentioned, cottage cheese instead of ordinary cheese, separated or filled milk, and yoghurt; and a big cut in fried foods, cakes, biscuits, pastry, and so on – they all contain fat – and a lot more wholemeal bread, and fruit and vegetables to fill the gap left by this missing fat and to supply dietary fiber. If it's the triglyceride fats that are mostly raised, one should cut down especially on carbohydrates (sugar, refined flour) and on alcohol. One can do all these things in theory.

HUNTER: You keep saying that, professor. Why only in theory?

BRENT: Because in practice one has to be quite strong-willed to achieve them. If you think of the risk factors for coronary heart disease – too much food, especially fatty food, and sugary food and drinks, and alcohol; cigarettes; lack of exercise; stress; high blood pressure; lack of wholegrain cereals, fresh fruit and vegetables; the pill – if you think of them, they pretty well add up to an inventory of the central elements in our modern western way of life.

HUNTER: You are saying coronary heart disease is a typical western disease, due to factors special to our type of civilization?

BRENT: Right. Factors that, if you think, have mostly developed in this century: our grandparents – certainly our great-grandparents – didn't eat all the fat we eat, and they certainly got more dietary fiber-rich foods; they didn't smoke cigarettes; they didn't have automobiles and TV sets to prevent them taking exercise. Almost every single item I mentioned is a twentieth-century item, at any rate as regards its general availability. And we now have a whole complicated system with its own momentum geared to turning out those items: factories for cigarettes and automobiles, factory farms for fatty meat and for eggs and butter – we even have butter mountains – newspapers and TV stations advertising most of those risk factors, and not advertising the things we should be going for. A 1977 Committee of our own United States Senate[5] saw all this. So in the same year did a Committee of your own House of Commons.[6] And they both recommended education of the public, including use of the mass media. It's certainly been make people aware of the coronary risk factors, and make people shown that, by using the mass media extensively, you can do something about them,[7] which is fine in a way, though I think it's a bit like using the devil just to fend off the devil instead of tackling the problem more fundamentally.

HUNTER: I want to ask you about that in a minute, professor – about your own ideas on how to deal with the coronary epidemic; but as a preliminary may I ask how and with what success most doctors deal with coronary heart disease?

BRENT: They wait till it's developed, then they treat it. Anginal attacks: there are some tablets the patient can put under his tongue that will help to get rid of the pain fairly quickly; and a new kind of drug he can take regularly to help prevent attacks. And there's a whole battery of drugs that may be needed for the coronary thrombosis patient. He will often get them in a coronary care unit, of course.

HUNTER: One specially designed and equipped for intensive care of the coronary patient?

BRENT: Yes, it has a very high proportion of doctors and nurses to patients, the action of the patients' hearts is constantly watched on oscilloscopes – a kind of television screen – and other bodily functions are monitored too; and there's a variety of drugs and a lot of instruments with which to treat pain, changes in the heart's rhythm, stoppage of the heart, and so on.

HUNTER: These units represent high-technology medicine in its most advanced form, the very latest in medical thinking on coronary thrombosis treatment? (*Brent nods*) There are many of them? They cost a lot of money? (*He nods again*) And the results?

BRENT: Are not so good. You see, in a big proportion of cases nobody thinks it might be a coronary till it's too late to get the person to a hospital. None of the lay people involved, I mean. Very often there's been no previous evidence of coronary disease at all. A middle-aged man, under 50, perhaps under 40, has some pain. He and his relatives or friends think it's simply indigestion or some other innocent condition. An English doctor with a special interest in heart conditions has described how he, a doctor, fell into just that trap when he himself had a coronary.[8] By the time anyone wakes up to the real importance of the pain it may be too late: in other words, a lot of the deaths in these people are the very first recognized sign of coronary heart disease; and death, when it occurs, is often quick, probably within two hours of the first symptom in at least 50 percent of fatal coronary attacks, indeed often in a matter of minutes; and within four hours in about 70 percent – and four hours is about the average time after symptoms are first noticed for patients to get into a coronary care unit; those who do get into one. Whether we like it or not, 60 or 70 percent of coronary deaths occur outside hospital.

HUNTER: But now for those coronary patients who do survive the first few hours and so stand a good chance of getting to the coronary care unit: does getting there improve *their* chances of survival greatly?

BRENT: Not greatly, I'm afraid. You see for those patients who are going to die *after* the first few hours there's little one can do, anywhere at all, about the factors causing death. A study in Denmark[9] showed just the same death rate in coronary patients in one hospital before and after a coronary care unit was set up. These units probably do save some lives, but at a very, very high cost – because of the expensive equipment and the high staffing ratio they have. Here in the States a hospital will sometimes provide a coronary care unit simply for fear of medico-legal complications if it doesn't, even though there's one already in another hospital just down the road. That sort of duplication doesn't make for efficiency, let alone economy.[10] What's more, a lot of patients rushed into the units turn out not to have a coronary at all, they *do* just have indigestion or else are drunk; but someone has to pick up the check.

HUNTER: These units have been described as very frightening for some patients?

BRENT: Oh, they can be, yes. All the wires and machinery and noises, and the tense atmosphere can be frightening – enough literally to frighten some patients to death.[11] Most doctors, if they had a coronary, would probably choose treatment at home for themselves except in special circumstances. There was one very good trial,[12] carried out in your country, of the results of treating coronary patients at home or in a hospital, and there didn't seem to be much difference in the outcome between the two. In those cases where the heart's rhythm is badly upset, then hospital treatment *may* be best – if the patient can be got there in time. But the general value of coronary units has been questioned here,[13,14] as well as in your own country.[15,16]

HUNTER: Are there not also special coronary ambulances, mobile coronary units, that in a sense take the coronary care unit to the patient so that he may get expert treatment before or during transit to the hospital unit?

BRENT: Yes, don't we see and hear them every day? But there's often the same long delay in calling for them as there is in calling for an ordinary ambulance, and yet, to save minutes, they go so fast they've had accidents on occasion. And there are doubts about these too.[17,18] There was one study in Miami[19] of the value of this kind of ambulance in dealing with what's called ventricular fibrillation of the heart. There were 301 subjects. The heart rhythm was put right in 199. Of this number 98 died before they could be got to hospital. Of the 101 who did make it to hospital 59 died there. 42 were discharged. At the time of the report only 22 of those 42 were still alive, having survived 16.9 months on average; and five of the 42 patients who left the hospital alive had severe brain damage as a result of the heart condition.

HUNTER: You set great store by that study?

BRENT: Yes, because it followed the patients up for some time – it didn't just look at whether the heart's rhythm could be put right at once by the coronary ambulance. What's the good of doing that if a lot of the patients die soon afterwards, and others in the hospital, and more again soon after they go home? At some point we have to ask, 'Is it worth it? What else couldn't we be spending the money on?' – Prevention in younger individuals?

HUNTER: Is there not a surgical operation used for coronary patients?

BRENT: Yes, coronary bypass is the popular kind right now. It means taking a short piece from one of the patient's leg veins and using it to short-circuit the part of a coronary artery where there's a block due to atherosclerosis. It's a major operation, calling for very highly skilled personnel; and even then about 1.5 percent of patients don't survive it. It's used chiefly for angina when it won't respond to medical treatment, or in which death of heart muscle occurs without an obvious thrombosis; or when the left main coronary artery is affected. The surgeons still haven't got all that worked out exactly.

HUNTER: It is a successful operation?

BRENT: They haven't got that one worked out either. It's a lot more popular here in the States than under the National Health Service in your country, where the surgeon doesn't get any extra money for operating. Possibly it doesn't lengthen life, but it may relieve or partly relieve anginal pain in some patients and so make life more pleasant.

HUNTER: How many such doubtfully beneficial and occasionally fatal operations are now performed in the United States each year?

BRENT: Around 70,000. At roughly 12,500 dollars a time.

HUNTER: Almost a billion dollars? And do some heart surgeons not want to see the number of operations increased?

BRENT: Yes, one estimate a few years back called for operations costing altogether, with the associated investigations, over 100 billion dollars a year, which is almost the total we were spending on all medical care in the States at the time.[20]

HUNTER: Would you agree, professor, that all these forms of expensive treatment of coronary heart disease are typical of our western approach to life, peculiar to our time, peculiar to it in much the same way as the causes of coronary heart disease that we mentioned earlier? (*Brent nods*) The same television screen that makes for a lack of exercise is found in the coronary care unit? The same automobile that also makes for lack of exercise is called an ambulance when it rushes the coronary patient to hospital? The stress that helps to cause coronary disease is found in the coronary care unit itself? The excess of money that buys fatty and cholesterol-rich foodstuffs also buys a bypass operation for the angina they help to produce? And 'bypass' equals 'automobile', which means lack of exercise?

BRENT: You have a point there. I'll add that it's been suggested that in a home where there's someone who might develop fibrillation of the heart a defibrillating machine should be kept. Where? – Where would you think? – Right next to the television set was the place suggested.[21]

HUNTER: And so what conclusion do you draw from all this?

BRENT: The main lesson is that our best hope of cutting coronary deaths substantially is to try and prevent the diease ever developing.

HUNTER: And how would you do that? – I mean *you*, Professor David Brent.

BRENT: Well, my views are a bit way out. Not too far, but a bit. I believe we should do two things: we should take all the preventive measures that for years have been advised – and sometimes practiced – in this country, but we should put them across and make them easy to adopt by every single means at our disposal; and second, we should see that prevention starts, not at 25 or 40 or 50, but at birth. We should use the mass media, yes – put across the right messages, stop the wrong ones – and we should use the schools, we should use every form of health education that will work; but we should also get at the farmers to make them produce the right foods, and at the food manufacturers, and at the supermarket people; make them alter their foods by taxing this food and not taxing that one, make them label their foods with the content of cholesterol, polyunsaturates, calories, the lot; teach the housewives what foods to use and how best to cook them; get at the soft drink manufacturers, the cigarette manufacturers – yes, and the automobile manufacturers too. There are no sacred cows where coronary deaths are conerned. I want to turn everyone completely against cigarette smoking, for instance. I mean not just so that the kids don't ever start it, but so they never even think of starting it. And I want everyone to have the right kind of diet, and to take regular exercise as an ordinary part of life, and to take life more easily.

HUNTER: Is not this – or some of it – what was recommended by the Senate Committee[5] you mentioned earlier?

BRENT: That's right; but only in 1977, and I'm a bit further out again than that Committee; and I want to see action, not recommendations.

HUNTER: And why that second point, about starting with the newborn baby?

BRENT: Well, for two reasons. It's never too early to start the right habits. Mine is a whole-population approach. Second, the seeds of coronary heart disease may be sown in young babies – by artificial feeding, and early weaning. The food we provide for most of our babies is over-rich, sugarized, salty, and full of cow's milk.[22] Human milk is quite different in its fat composition from cow's milk. And fatty streaking in the arteries, which may eventually lead to atheroma, starts very, very early in life. It's been shown too that in children the blood pressure, the blood sugar and plasma cholesterol levels, and obesity are all related to one another the same way as they are in adults.[23]

HUNTER: Not all your fellow doctors would go along with your views, professor?

BRENT: No, sir. There's a whole spectrum of opinion among doctors on this issue. Some extremists think, apart from cigarette smoking, the evidence of any actual benefit from doing this or that, unless in the very exceptional case, is simply not on: they want cast-iron proof on coronary prevention before they'll budge an inch. That strikes me as unacceptable because a lot of the things I've suggested, like taking exercise or eating less fat, will almost certainly do no harm and often will obviously do some good quite apart from coronary heart disease. But you name any niggling objection to *doing* something, and these boys have raised it. I mean the scientific boys now, not those who think you're interfering with people's liberty if you try to stop them, for what you think is their own good, from smoking cigarettes[24] or eating fat.[25] I have some sympathy with *them*.

HUNTER: And after the scientific nihilists? Who's on the next step up the preventive ladder?

BRENT: Well, some doctors think we need to do a lot more research before we attempt primary prevention on a *mass* scale; they think it's difficult – it is – if not downright unwise to change the way of life of a whole population. What I say is our way of life *has* been entirely changed in this century, largely by commercial interests: hence the coronary epidemic. Anyway, what they do say is, if you should find, by screening special groups, or happen to come across, certain people, even certain children, with a very high plasma cholesterol and/or triglyceride level, for instance, then you ought to find just what metabolic type it is – what the particular faulty mechanism is – and treat it correspondingly with drugs, or a rigid diet, controlled by a doctor,[26] or even with an intestinal bypass operation, or a special kind of dialysis.[27]

HUNTER: And how do they know which people to test?

BRENT: Oh, those with a bad family history – of coronary heart disease, or of raised plasma cholesterol levels – or who are known already to have one or two coronary risk factors. And these doctors will treat other risk factors if found to be present, but only in the high-risk people. Then there are other doctors again who would do a bit more than that, or even quite a lot more, some of them.

HUNTER: And what about screening an entire population, of, say, middle-aged men for coronary risk factors, and then trying to eliminate those factors?

BRENT: Yes, this is a higher step again up the ladder, but I'm not sold on it. First, there's a lot of people to screen – because most of us are coronary risks – so the screening and the subsequent advice and follow-up would be mighty expensive. And then, while we know that a high plasma cholesterol or lack of exercise or a raised blood pressure are common, we're not sure in the case of some of the individual risk factors at just what level we should say, 'Above this point and you should do something: below it you needn't worry.' Any cigarette smoking at all is bad, we know that; but with some of the others just where do you draw the line? And we're not quite sure either, at least with most of the risk factors, that, if you do find them by screening and succeed in altering them (which isn't easy), you'll certainly affect the chance of any *particular* person getting coronary heart disease.

HUNTER: You mean they're not exact predictors of an attack?

BRENT: That's right. In the individual. Whole-population-wise, statistically – yes; but not always in individuals, especially not single factors. Look at dietary advice, for instance: if one compares *populations*, coronary heart disease is more common in those populations with high plasma cholesterol levels, and in those – pretty well the same ones – that take the kind of diet that raises the levels. But now, as between *individuals*, while a raised plasma cholesterol increases the risk of coronary heart disease (and we do know the kind of diet that will raise the level) it isn't possible in practice to connect the type of diet an individual is supposedly taking either with his actual cholesterol level or with the likelihood of him actually developing coronary heart disease. Where does that leave one when giving advice to an individual? Maybe one has to be on the right diet for years and years – most or all of one's life – to get an effect: just changing your diet when you're 50 won't do much good.

HUNTER: Any other argument against screening?

BRENT: Yes, people who have no symptoms are pretty unwilling to give up cigarettes or alter their diets just because the doctor says they should, and especially if their families and their next-door neighbors or workmates haven't got to do the same. They don't like to stick out like a sore thumb. Why should anyone act *now* to prevent a disease that the doctor says may occur in him – only *may*, mind you – in 10 or 15 years.

HUNTER: And does the same go for the taking of drugs to lower a raised blood pressure?

BRENT: It does, I'm sorry to say[28] – a raised blood pressure without symptoms. At the moment bringing down a raised blood pressure doesn't seem to affect the risk of developing coronary heart disease very much, though it will reduce the risk of a stroke. Perhaps the coronary damage has already been done by the time the blood pressure is up. Perhaps that applies very largely to various disease-producing factors by the time we screen for them. All of this is why I feel one should start a lot earlier in life, and tackle a whole population in a big way. We're *all* at risk, the way we live nowadays.

HUNTER: And once they have occurred, what about prevention of further attacks of angina – or of coronary thrombosis in the survivors?

BRENT: Yes, that's tertiary prevention. Primary prevention's when you're tackling someone who's perfectly healthy, and in my book that means the young child. Secondary prevention's the sort you practice in screening: when the person hasn't got the disease but has some abnormalities – risk factors – that suggest he might get it. It's odd but, although tertiary prevention's obviously the least hopeful, it's the one that doctors practice most often. They tell the patient about cigarette smoking, diet, slimming, even exercise sometimes, and so on. Now and again, even at that late stage, they get fairly good results.

HUNTER: But now what has actually been done and what has been achieved in the coronary prevention field here in the USA in the last few years?

BRENT: Quite a lot. Not as much as I'd have liked, but still a good deal. Way back in 1965 the American Heart Association suggested[29] a diet for everybody – *everybody*, mind – with less cholesterol in it and more of the right kind of fat than the average American diet has or had, and fewer calories in the case of anyone who was overweight. A lot of people responded. And in 1964 our Surgeon General issued a major warning about cigarette smoking: we now smoke fewer cigarettes than we did. Still too many, but fewer. And then we have jogging, and the other forms of regular exercise that have been promoted. Nothing as radical or as wide-spread as I want to see, but some steady progress.

HUNTER: Are any precise figures available?

BRENT: Indeed. They've been published:[30] between 1963 and 1975 – a decline of 22 percent in consumption of all tobacco products. Per head, that is. Butter down by 32 percent, milk and cream by 19 percent, animal fats and oils by 57 percent; but vegetable fats and oils up by 44 percent.

HUNTER: And has there been any appreciable effect on deaths from heart disease?

BRENT: A slight drop in coronary heart disease deaths between 1963 and 1967 – until 1963 coronary deaths had been going up and up while most other types of death had been coming down. From 1967 there's been a much bigger drop: between about then and 1975 a drop of 20 percent in the coronary death rate among Americans.[31]

HUNTER: A considerable advance?

BRENT: Very considerable; but then coronary heart disease was and still is our biggest killer. I'd like to have seen us do more. Of course, nobody's yet proved the lower death rate *is* due to the changes in our diet, to our smoking fewer cigarettes, and so on; but it seems very likely. Some people say it's just due to differences in diagnosis, or to our having had less influenza – which does often carry off the coronary patient – or simply to better control of high blood pressure.[32] But most of the experts now seem to be thinking along the same lines as myself as regards what the real cause is.

HUNTER: And the position in other western countries?

BRENT: In general, coronary deaths continue to increase: catching up with the American rate. But then, even though I don't think we've done enough in the way of prevention, no other country's done as much.

HUNTER: What about the United Kingdom?

BRENT: There is a suggestion now that your coronary mortality began to drop a few years ago – later than in America. You've been cagier about prevention. In 1974 an expert panel, sponsored by your government, recommended[33] for the prevention of coronary heart disease a reduction of obesity, and diet-wise a drop in consumption of fat and sugar; but its members were definitely against substituting liquid fats for solid animal fats. In 1976 another very important group of doctors *did* recommend[34] the liquid fats, and they were against screening, and they said prevention should really start in childhood. Still that was 11 years after the American Heart Foundation had made more or less the same recommendations.

HUNTER: Were there any unsatisfactory aspects, in your judgment, to that last British report?

BRENT: Yes. They said that diligence and leadership shouldn't, for fear they might induce stress, be discouraged: any stress should be 'managed' by doctors. I'm not sure how you do that in a society that has stress as a built-in factor. I think it should be built out. Also they made no recommendations for government action (they said that wasn't their business), or for special labeling of foods with their content of various types of fat; and they suggested people should get their exercise mainly from leisure pursuits. Mind you, we say that here in the States too; and I think it won't work except for a minority of people. Exercise must be an integral part of life. We must arrange things so that they've just *got* to take some, not to speak of arranging things so that they'll find it darned difficult to find any place to smoke cigarettes in – if they can afford them at the price level I'd like to see.

HUNTER: You are suggesting a more intense, more comprehensive program, backed by government action, though along the same lines as your present American efforts? (*Brent nods*) Tell me, professor: have doctors *en masse* anywhere in the world ever demanded a program anything like that or any other kind of coronary prevention program?

BRENT: Not to my knowledge.

HUNTER: You said an important risk factor for coronary disease is the plasma cholesterol level. Is there any evidence about this level in doctors?

BRENT: I know of only one. Three years after the American Heart Association had made its recommendations on diet 80 percent of American doctors who were tested had a serum cholesterol level above 200 milligrams per 100 millilitres,[35] and anything above that is usually taken to be undesirable. Serum and plasma levels are much the same.

HUNTER: Taken to be undesirable by doctors?

BRENT: By doctors.

HUNTER: No further questions professor. (*Sits*)

JUDGE: You said, professor, that atheroma patches in the lining of the coronary arteries provided the background condition to coronary heart disease. And coronary heart disease has increased greatly in the last 60 or 70 years? – In particular, it presumably became more common in the period between about 1910 and the late 1940s? (*Brent nods*) You are aware there is evidence from post-mortem examinations made in London at those two times that coronary atheroma did *not* increase during those forty years? Indeed, if anything it became less common. [36, 37]

BRENT: I know that work, and I accept its result.

JUDGE: How do you reconcile that drop in coronary atheroma with the increase in coronary heart disease.

BRENT: There is still no completely satisfactory answer, probably because we still do not know the exact cause of either condition. I stick to my point about coronary heart disease being related to coronary atheroma; but atheroma, judge, while nearly always a necessary cause of coronary heart disease, is not a sufficient cause by itself. Many other factors are involved almost certainly: for instance, those factors, especially dietary factors, that lead to thrombosis on an atheromatous patch. And the findings you mention in no way invalidate the list of risk factors for coronary heart disease that I gave, or the corresponding preventive steps that should be taken.

JUDGE: From all you said I gathered that strokes and coronary heart disease have various risk factors in common. Have strokes become much more frequent in the past 60 or 70 years in western countries, like coronary disease?

BRENT: No, judge, they have not; and my last answer partly covers this point too. Atheroma is usually present in people who get coronary heart disease or strokes; but it is not enough by itself to cause either, and the other factors involved are probably not absolutely identical in the two cases. However, some certainly are; and it's interesting that, just as deaths in the USA from coronaries have dropped since 1963, so they have dropped for strokes too.[30] I'd guess this is due mainly to better control of high blood pressure, and to the changes in diet and cigarette smoking in the States that I mentioned earlier.

JUDGE: You said that a raised plasma cholesterol level is a risk factor for coronary heart disease. My understanding is that cholesterol is carried in the blood plasma in a number of different forms, and that a high level of what is known as the high-density type of blood-fat particles actually protects against coronary heart disease while the low-density type has the opposite tendency.

BRENT: You are quite right. I didn't mention this point – it's a recent revival of an old theory – because the story was complicated enough already. But there is now very good published evidence for what you say, especially in the case of people over 50 in whom the *total* cholesterol level is not a very good predictor at all.[38,39] This may be one reason why none of the trials of the effect on the frequency of coronary heart disease of lowering plasma cholesterol levels by changing people's diet has come up with completely convincing evidence of a beneficial effect.

JUDGE: One should perhaps not measure the total cholesterol but the different fractions I mentioned?

BRENT: Right. Of course, another thing is that coronary heart disease takes years and years to develop; so one really needs a dietary trial extending over almost a lifetime to prove what effect, if any, altering the diet may have. Actually, of the three big trials of diet one,[40] in some mental hospitals in Finland, came up with results that a lot of people *did* find convincing, at least for males. But not everybody, I admit.

JUDGE: And it was not just the professional skeptics who were dubious? (*Brent nods*) And the same disappointing results were obtained from trials of drugs that lower the plasma cholesterol level? (*Brent nods*) You said also that modern farming methods result in meat carrying more fat than meat produced by traditional methods. There is published evidence for this?

BRENT: Yes, there is good published evidence.[41] Meat from the free-range animal, the wild animal, has more of the polyunsaturated fats and very much less typical animal storage fat. Monkeys don't get atheroma in the wild state, but they do get it if they're given a typical western diet – plenty of animal fat, butter, eggs, cheese and so on; and if you put them back on to a diet similar to the one recommended to prevent coronaries the atheroma tends to vanish; and it never appears if they're given such a diet all the time.[42]

JUDGE: It has been said[43] that polyunsaturated fats carry certain dangers – for instance, of helping to cause gall stones– and that the polyunsaturates in some of the special margarines have been so treated chemically as to have undesirable effects.

BRENT: To discuss that properly I should have to go into very great technical detail. May I just emphasize that a large number of expert committees has *recommended* the dietary fat changes I put forward?

JUDGE: Professor Brent, I know it may seem inappropriate in a serious forum such as this but, if you were a betting man, on which preventive elements would you put your money as those most likely in, say, 40 or 50 years time to be thought of paramount importance?

BRENT: That's the big question, judge; but I'll give you my answer to it. I think that, if a person were throughout his life to take very regular and very vigorous exercise, he could almost certainly forget about all the other risk factors aside from some rare family disorders of fat metabolism and probably from cigarette smoking; and I'm not sure exercise mightn't even neutralize the effects of cigarettes. However, in second place, a lot further back, I would put abstention from cigarette smoking; and third, though it's a long shot, I'd put plenty of fiber in the diet. In fact, there is already some evidence[44] that these are going to be the first three past the post.

JUDGE: This whole matter of coronary heart disease is complex, professor? There is room for honest differences of opinion? Different doctors have tackled it in different ways, all in good faith?

BRENT: Surely. I do not question the good faith of those who believe strongly in coronary care units or bypass surgery or screening or limited preventive steps. (That's as to the vast majority: there's always a small suspect fringe.) It's their judgment I question, not their good faith.

JUDGE: We could have had doctors here at least as experienced and reputable and honest as yourself who would have spoken up for coronary care ambulances,[45] or would have poured scorn on the diet-coronary-heart disease theory?[43]

BRENT: That is correct.

JUDGE: The lesser mortality in your country in the past 10 years or so might be due to a combination of elements that you criticize – coronary care units, bypass surgery, and so on – and may have had nothing to do with changes in diet, say?

BRENT: It may, as I said.

JUDGE: I wished merely to emphasize the point. And the very radical changes in life-style that you advocate have, in fact, been put forward in the pages of reputable medical journals?[46,47] – There is no conspiracy on the part of a majority of doctors to silence those who hold your beliefs? (*Brent nods*) And, as you have just indicated, the changes in dietary fats that you favor have been recommended by official and mostly medical bodies throughout the world for the general populations of their countries – by 12 such bodies, only two having refused to sanction such changes, and then only in respect of polyunsaturated fats?

BRENT: You are quite right, judge. In fact, forgive me, the number now is 18, not 12. And that to me seems to provide excellent backing for my suggestions as regards diet.

JUDGE: And that is the really contentious issue? No one queries the desirability, in general, of not smoking cigarettes, of taking exercise, and so on?

BRENT: Practically no one, correct. As to the desirability, that is. The method of getting the message acted upon is another thing again. What most of those bodies haven't done is to demand that governments act on their recommendations – take radical comprehensive steps of the kind I outlined. They haven't taken their conclusions the next logical step; and the reason for that, I think, is that such a step means a major attack on our whole western life-style and at the point of recommending that the doctors have chickened out! The medical establishment prefers treatment to prevention, the hospital corridors to the streets. It knows what real prevention would mean. That basically, I think, is why my sort of thinking is not as common as it might be.

JUDGE: We are much obliged to you, professor. And the court is adjourned.

REFERENCES—SESSION THREE

1. *The U.S. Fact Book*, Grosset and Dunlap, p. 65, 1977, New York.
2. Leading Article, *BMJ*, August 27, 1977, p. 537.
3. Leading Article, *BMJ*, May 7, 1977, p. 1176.
4. Trowell, H., *BMJ*, May 14, 1977, p. 1283.
5. Select Committee on Nutrition and Human Needs, United States Senate, *Dietary Goals for the United States*, US Government Printing Printing Office, Washington, 1977.
6. First Report from the Expenditure Committee, *Preventive Medicine*, Vol. I, HMSO, London, 1977.
7. Farquhar, J. W., *et al.*, *Lancet*, June 4, 1977, p. 1192.
8. Edwards, K., *BMJ*, October 16, 1976, p. 938.
9. Astvad, K., *et al.*, March 23, 1974, p. 567.
10. Bloom, B. S., and Peterson, L. L., *NEJM*, May 23, 1974, p. 1171.
11. Baxter, S., *British Journal of Hospital Medicine*, June 1974, p. 875.
12. Mather, H. G., *et al.*, *BMJ*, April 17, 1976, p. 925.
13. Bloom, B. S., and Peterson, O. L., *NEJM*, January 11, 1973, p. 72.
14. Editorial, *NEJM*, January 11, 1973, p. 101.
15. Colling, A., *et al.*, *BMJ*, November 13, 1976, p. 1169.
16. Hill, J. D., Holdstock, G., and Hampton, J. R., *BMJ*, July 9, 1977, p. 81.
17. Hill, J. D., and Hampton, J. R., *BMJ*, October 30, 1976, p. 1035.
18. Hampton, J. R., Dowling, M., and Nicholas, C., *Lancet*, March 5, 1977, p. 526.
19. Liberthson, R. R., *et al.*, *NEJM*, August 15, 1974, p. 317.
20. Hiatt, H. H., *NEJM*, July 31, 1975, p. 235.
21. Panthridge, J. R., and Geddes, J. S., *BMJ*, July 17, 1976, p. 168.
22. Turner, R. W. D., *Lancet*, September 25, 1976, p. 693.
23. Du V. Florey, C., Uppal, S., and Lowy, S., *BMJ*, June 9, 1976, p. 1368.
24. Harnes, J. R., *JAMA*, January 12, 1976, p. 157.
25. Meenan, R. F., *NEJM*, January 1, 1976, p. 45.
26. Editorial, *NEJM*, January 9, 1975, p. 105.
27. Lupien, P-J., Moorjani, S., and Awad, J., *Lancet*, June 12, 1976, p. 1261.
28. Editorial, *NEJM*, December 20, 1973, p. 1369.
29. Bradshaw, J. S., *Lancet*, April 4, 1976, p. 912.
30. Editorial, *NEJM*, July 21, 1977, p. 163.
31. Mulcahy, R., *Lancet*, August 21, 1976, p. 421.
32. Leading Article, *BMJ*, January 10, 1976, p. 58.
33. Department of Health and Social Security, Report on Health and Social Subjects, no. 7, *Diet and Coronary Heart Disease*, HMSO, London, 1974.

34. *Prevention of Coronary Heart Disease*, Report of a Joint Working Party of the Royal College of Physicians and the British Cardiac Society, *Journal of the Royal College of Physicians*, April 1976, p. 213.
35. Warner, W. L., and Shumway, J. E., *JAMA*, November 4, 1968, p. 1307.
36. Morris, J. N., *Lancet*, January 6, 1951, p. 1.
37. Ibid., January 13, 1951, p. 69.
38. Medical News, *JAMA*, March 14, 1977, p. 1066.
39. Miller, N. E., *et al.*, *Lancet*, May 7, 1977, p. 965.
40. Mietinnen, M., *et al.*, *Lancet*, October 21, 1972, p. 835.
41. Crawford, M., *BMJ*, June 19, 1976, p. 1532.
42. Turner, R., *BMJ*, March 20, 1976, p. 710.
43. Mann, G. V., *NEJM*, September 22, 1977, p. 644.
44. Morris, J. N., Marr, J. W., and Clayton, D. G., *BMJ*, November 19, 1977, p. 1307.
45. Briggs, R. S., *et al.*, *BMJ*, November 13, 1976, p. 1161.
46. Bradshaw, S., *BMJ*, February 10, 1973, p. 349.
47. White, L. S., *NEJM*, October 9, 1975, p. 773.

Prevention of Coronary Heart Disease

Editorial, *Lancet*, April 6, 1974, p. 605.
Blackburn, R., Yu, P. N., and Goodwin, J. F. (eds.), in *Progress in Cardiology*, vol. 3, Lea and Febiger, Philadelphia, 1974, p. 1.
Medical News, *JAMA*, February 17, 1975, p. 691.
Tudge, C., *World Medicine*, April 7, 1976, p. 17.
Leading Article, *BMJ*, April 10, 1976, p. 853.
Editorial, *Lancet*, April 10, 1976, p. 783.

Diet and Coronary Heart Disease

Leading Article, *BMJ*, July 6, 1974, p. 4.
Ball, K. P., and Turner, R., *BMJ*, September 21, 1974, p. 740.
Editorial, *Lancet*, August 30, 1975, p. 398.
Shaper, A. G., and Marr, J. W., *BMJ*, April 2, 1977, p. 867.
Select Committee on Nutrition and Human Needs, United States Senate, *Diet Related to Killer Diseases, II*, part 1, Cardiovascular Disease, US Government Printing Office, Washington, 1977.
First Report from the Expenditure Committee, *Preventive Medicine*, volumes II and III, Minutes of Evidence, HMSO, London, 1977.
Mann, G. V., *NEJM*, September 22, 1977, p. 644. (A stimulating and provocative article, highly critical of the notion that there is a relationship between the nature and quantity of dietary fat intake and the prevalence of coronary heart disease.)
Walker, W. J., *NEJM*, January 12, 1978, p. 106. (The first of six letters in a single issue of the journal, all highly critical of the views expressed in the last reference. These letters appeared to have the best of the argument, but the debate will doubtless continue.)

Stress and Psychosocial Factors, and Coronary Heart Disease

Jenkins, C. D., *NEJM*, April 29, 1976, p. 987; and May 6, 1976, p. 1033.

Screening in Coronary Heart Disease

Turner, R., and Ball, K., *Lancet*, November 17, 1973, p. 1137.

Sackett, D. L., *Lancet*, November 16, 1974, p. 1189.

Mulcahy, R. and Hickey, N., *Heart Attack and Life Style*, Irish Heart Foundation, Dublin, 1976.

D'Souza, N. R., Swan, A. V. and Shannon, D. J., *Lancet*, June 5, 1976, p. 1228.

Leading Article, *BMJ*, May 21, 1977, p. 1302.

Exercise and Coronary Heart Disease

Morris, J. N., *et al.*, *Lancet*, February 17, 1973, p. 333.

Paffenbarger, R. S., Jr, and Hale, W. E., *NEJM*, March 13, 1975, p. 545.

Mann, G. V., *NEJM*, April 3, 1975, p. 758.

Treatment of Coronary Heart Disease

Cardiac Rehabilitation 1975, Report of a Joint Working Party of the Royal College of Physicians and the British Cardiac Society, *Journal of the Royal College of Physicians*, July 1975, p. 281.

The Care of the Patient with Coronary Heart Disease, Report of a Joint Working Party of the Royal College of Physicians and the British Cardiac Society, *Journal of the Royal College of Physicians*, October 1975, p. 9.

Short, D., *BMJ*, July 10, 1976, p. 98.

Surgery for Coronary Heart Disease

Leading Article, *BMJ*, August 25, 1973, p. 420.

Corday, E., *JAMA*, March 24, 1975, p. 1245.

Mundth, E. C., and Austen, W. B., *NEJM*, July 3, 1975, p. 13; July 10, 1975, p. 68; and July 17, 1975, p. 124.

Medical News, *JAMA*, March 1, 1976, p. 89.

Editorial, *Lancet*, April 17, 1976, p. 841.

Editorial, *NEJM*, September 22, 1977, p. 661.

Editorial, *NEJM*, December 29, 1977, p. 1462.

DIETARY FIBER

Enter Dr John Hafod

HUNTER (*rising*): You are Dr John Hafod, a consultant physician from South Africa, with a special interest in dietary fiber? Why is it important?

HAFOD: Because there is a group of diseases – diverticular disease of the colon, piles, varicose veins, and appendicitis, and some others – that are common in the affluent countries of the west, but very uncommon in the poorer peoples of Africa and Asia, especially the country dwellers, although these conditions are found to some extent among the better-off Africans and Asians who in general tend to eat a western-style diet. The properties of what is known as dietary fiber provide a reasonable explanation of how those named diseases occur, and perhaps of how others occur too. The diets of people who get all these diseases are known to contain very little fiber while those of the people who do not get them contain a lot. That is the basic story.

HUNTER: And what exactly is dietary fiber?

HAFOD: One kind is what we used to call roughage, the mostly non-digestible material found in unrefined cereals – in the case of wheat it is known as bran. Dietary fiber is also found in fruits, especially as pectin in apples, and in oranges and mangoes; and in many vegetables, such as carrots and cabbage and brussels sprouts. Various gums – guar and sterculia gums – also have certain dietary-fiber-like properties. The dietary fiber in wheat seems to be the most potent, in general. Fruits and vegetables contain a lot of water, of course, and bran contains very little, so that, weight for weight, bran supplies much more fiber. Also the fiber from one of these sources is not always of the same composition as that from another source, though it always has the property of being able to take up a lot of water.

HUNTER: And that accounts for its effects?

HAFOD: To some extent. Partly because of that, and partly because fiber encourages the growth of bowel bacteria, a diet containing a good deal of fiber greatly increases the bulk of the contents of the colon, or large bowel, and so increases the size of the stools that are passed. In westerners it may take three or four days for 'waste' material that is not digested to pass right out through the stomach and intestines in the stools: in African villagers it takes only a day, or a day and a half, and the stools they pass are three or four times as bulky as those of Europeans, and not as dried up.

HUNTER: Most westerners are more or less chronically constipated, the African villagers are not?

HAFOD: Correct. And people taking an in-between diet are in-between as regards the size of stools and the speed with which food residues are passed out.

HUNTER: And black Americans?

HAFOD: They did not become like white Americans in this respect till they gave up eating a lot of maize, and began to take the typical low-fiber western diet: the supermarket diet – refined, packaged, canned. And white South Africans, and the people of France, Sweden, Australia, and so on are like the British and the Americans.

HUNTER: Has the western diet been short of dietary fiber for a long time?

HAFOD: It started to be short of fiber roughly a hundred years ago. In the 1870–80 period a new type of milling of flour – roller-milling – was introduced. It provided a very white flour cheaply for the first time, and people liked it because the flour looked very 'pure', and it made a nice-textured loaf, though some of the proteins and vitamins of the wheat, we now realize, were discarded with the bran that was removed by the new milling process. What's more, the millers liked the white flour because it contained less fat than the previous wholemeal or intermediate flours and so was less likely to go rancid; and it was less attractive to pests like rats and beetles. Also the millers could sell the bran as an animal feeding stuff. All this happened, as I said, in about 1880, and we now realize it takes about 40 years for diverticular disease of the colon to develop.

JUDGE: How do we know that, doctor?

HAFOD: Because in western countries it is not usual in people under the age of 40, but one fifth of people over that age have the condition, and three fifths of those over 80. It was recognizable by doctors, this disease, and recognized, more than a hundred years ago, but it did not start to become at all common until this century; and by 1920 – about 40 years after the very white flour became generally available – it began to be quite common. Another factor, and this has probably been as important for the drop in fiber intake as the introduction of roller-milling, is that at about the same time that white flour was introduced widely the people of western countries also became free, thanks to industrial prosperity and food refining and preservation, to eat a lot more white sugar and fat and meat (none of which contains fiber), and less bread and porridge; and they did so, the total effect being that in the United Kingdom, for example, people are now consuming about one tenth the amount of wheat fiber their great-grandparents took 100 years ago – and the fact that they eat more fruit and vegetables has not compensated for this.

HUNTER: And what about appendicitis, which I think you mentioned?

HAFOD: It first became common towards the end of the last century. In other words, if it is due to a lack of dietary fiber, about 20 years of such a lack is sufficient to produce it; and in fact, appendicitis is now appearing in some African people who have been on a western-style diet for that length of time. We shall have to see whether in due course they also develop diverticular disease of the colon.

HUNTER: Would you describe that condition for us?

HAFOD: It is a disease in which there are little blow-outs, little finger-like cul-de-sacs of the large bowel wall in two rows along the length of it, and these may become inflamed. We know how they are caused because one can take X-ray pictures of the colon when it is active. The muscle of the wall of the colon regularly contracts – squeezes down hard. This is a normal process. But when there is not much bulky material in the colon, this contraction divides it up into a series of self-contained compartments, rather like so many separate balloons. The muscle then contracts further, the pressure in each small compartment rises, and in the end it forces the lining of the colon to 'blow out' as small protrusions – just as one can force out the fingers of a rubber glove by squeezing it when it is full of air and sealed at the wrist.

HUNTER: And how does dietary fiber affect that process?

HAFOD: If there's plenty of bulk in the colon, then those separate compartments are not formed, and any rise of pressure is simply dispersed along the whole length of the colon. It is like a canal with all the sluice gates shut in one case, open in the other. It apparently takes many years of the sort of activity I have described actually to produce the diverticula – the protrusions. But once they are formed one has diverticular disease of the colon: diverticulosis if there are simply protrusions, diverticulitis if they become inflamed.

HUNTER: And the symptoms?

HAFOD: Vague indigestion, colicky pains, bloating, constipation or diarrhea, sometimes a condition very like a left-sided appendicitis (due to a diverticulum becoming badly inflamed), and even peritonitis or abscess formation occasionally.

HUNTER: And how is it treated?

HAFOD: If severe, it may need surgical treatment, or antibiotics and pain relievers. Ordinary diverticular disease is treated nowadays with a high-fiber diet. The patients are advised to eat wholemeal bread, and plenty of fruit and vegetables, and to take half a dozen teaspoons or so of ordinary, preferably coarse-grained bran on their food every day. The optimum amount – to give an easy regular bowel action once or twice a day – varies from person to person.

HUNTER: And the effect on diverticular disease?

HAFOD: Apart from a little flatulence which usually soon passes off, the great majority of patients get marked relief of their symptoms.

HUNTER: And now what *used* to be the treatment? – Say, ten years ago?

HAFOD: The central feature of it was a low-residue diet. And more recently than ten years ago.

JUDGE: Did you say a *low*-residue diet, doctor? You mean one that was *free* of bran, of dietary fiber generally? (*Hafod nods*) But I thought you said, doctor, that a lack of dietary fiber *caused* the disease.

HAFOD: Yes, that is what we now believe; but until this new view of the matter was expounded, it was thought that, as the lining of the colon was inflamed in diverticular disease, any roughage would only irritate it and make things worse.

HUNTER: And why doesn't it, doctor?

HAFOD: Because, as we now realize, when dietary fiber takes up water – for which, as I said, it has a great affinity – it swells into a smooth bulky mass, like a jelly. Someone has suggested it would then be better called smoothage; and certainly, far from irritating the colon, it seems, in a manner of speaking, to soothe it.

HUNTER: For how long was a low-residue diet the usual treatment?

HAFOD: Oh, for half a century or so.

HUNTER: And all the best doctors used it? (*Hafod nods*) The scientifically-minded doctors? The great panjandrums of medicine?

HAFOD: Yes, for what seemed to them to be the best of reasons.

HUNTER: But that were, in fact, the worst of reasons? (*Hafod nods*) And so a lot of people were over a period of decades treated by their doctors in a way that would make their condition worse?

JUDGE: If you hit that nail on the head again, Mr Hunter, it will vanish altogether.

HUNTER (*to Hafod*): Tell me, doctor: will regular use of bran *prevent* diverticular disease?

HAFOD: Well, we do not know yet, of course. It is too early to say. One would guess it would.

HUNTER: But a right diet would be preferable?

HAFOD: Oh yes: a diet naturally rich in fiber – one containing wholemeal bread instead of white bread, little or no sugar, less fat and meat, and plenty of fruit and vegetables; whole fruit and vegetables as far as possible.

HUNTER: And is a high-fiber diet of value in other bowel conditions?

HAFOD: Yes, there are various other disorders of the colon – spastic colon, irritable colon, mucous colitis, and so on – all of which, it seems on the whole, benefit to some extent from such a diet.

HUNTER: And how is appendicitis related to the fiber content of the diet?

HAFOD: The appendix is a short narrow tube closed at one end, a cul-de-sac, leading off the first part of the colon. If it becomes blocked, it gets inflamed. It might become blocked if the muscle at the mouth of it contracted down in the way I described just now for the colonic muscle – and so shut off the rest of the appendix. Or conceivably, if a person is taking a low-fiber diet, a small piece of the resultant hard, dry waste matter in the bowel could become lodged in the appendix and block it. In any case, no sensible person would expect bran to relieve such a blockage once it had occurred, once an acute appendicitis was present, in other words: an operation would normally be required.

HUNTER: And varicose veins and piles, which I think you mentioned?

HAFOD: A person whose stools are small and hard will strain when passing them; and it would come as no great surprise to a doctor, with his knowledge of anatomy, to be told that such straining would after a time dilate the veins of the anus – the back passage – so producing piles, and break down the valves in the leg veins, so dilating them and producing varicose veins. The same explanation might account for the common occurrence of a condition called hiatus hernia, in which a part of the stomach is forced up into the chest through a small gap in the diaphragm, the sheet of muscle between the chest and the abdomen. It too, some people think, may be produced by lack of dietary fiber. It causes heartburn when a sufferer from it bends down or lies on his right side, and it is present in 20 percent of Americans and in only 1 percent of Africans.

HUNTER: And you said there are some other diseases possibly involved in the dietary fiber story.

HAFOD: Yes, although the evidence in their case is not so strong. Two or more of the conditions I have already named commonly occur with one another in the same person, and with one or more other conditions – gall stones, diabetes, obesity, and coronary heart disease. And all these conditions are common in western peoples and rare in rural Africans – with the richer urbanized African and Indian apparently catching up with the western peoples. A diet high in bran causes the bile to contain more of one bile acid that is linked with a lower concentration of bile cholesterol (a substance present in a high proportion of gall stones), and less of another bile acid with the opposite effect on the bile cholesterol. As for coronary heart disease, some of the dietary fibers or similar substances now being investigated do actually lower the plasma level of cholesterol and/or triglycerides, but others do not. This particular part of the picture is rather confused at the moment. However, there is one very reliable recent report[1] that men taking more cereal dietary fiber than their fellows were less liable to get coronary heart disease, though this effect was *not* produced by a lowering of plasma cholesterol levels.

HUNTER: And diabetes and obesity?

HAFOD: A low-fiber diet is almost invariably a diet high in sugar and other substances that make it easy for obesity to develop – and so various other conditions, including coronary heart disease – and possibly diabetes. Also it has been suggested that a high-fiber diet calls for so much more chewing than one rich in refined sugar and refined flour that a person taking such a diet will consume fewer calories, and so be less liable to become obese and perhaps to develop diabetes.

JUDGE: I am right in thinking this is somewhat speculative?

HAFOD: Yes, judge; and so is the theory that a low-fiber diet may be in part responsible for the occurrence of tumors of the colon – though various very plausible mechanisms have been mentioned in that connection. Cancer of the colon, for instance, may well be associated with the breakdown by bacteria in the colon of a particular bile acid – and a high-fiber diet reduces this breakdown – or else with the breakdown of fats. And the types of bacteria in the bowels of people living where colon cancer is common are different from those found where it is not common. Dietary fiber might be responsible for the difference. Certainly any cancer-producing substances in the bowel will be more concentrated and have a longer contact with the bowel wall in people on a fiber-deficient diet – because of their small stools which pass very slowly along the bowel. What is not in doubt is that eating a diet with little or no refined sugar in it will reduce dental decay; and a high-fiber diet is of value here because the chewing of the fiber helps to cleanse the teeth of any food residues, which play a part in causing decay.

HUNTER: To a layman, it seems as though, if only half of this is true, a vast range of common diseases might be preventable.

HAFOD: Oh, yes. A lack of dietary fiber, it has been said, may be causing as much illness as cigarette smoking.

HUNTER: And all these diseases are due or very possibly due to our characteristic western diet with its white bread and other products made from white flour, its sugar, and fat, and meat, its lack of fiber-containing foods in their natural state and in quantity? (*Hafod nods*) And those foods are a product of our western way of life, of its technology and industry? Would you agree too that the complex surgical treatment for some of them (appendicitis, piles, varicose veins, gall stones, diverticular disease of the colon, and perhaps tumors of the colon) is as much peculiar to western civilization as are the causes?

HAFOD: I suppose that is true. I have never considered it in quite that light.

HUNTER: We cause with our right hand and treat with our left? (*Hafod nods*) Do most doctors now accept the dietary fiber theory?

HAFOD: Most of the experts do, along the lines I have indicated.

HUNTER: Has any large-scale action been taken in this field? Have most people started to eat wholemeal bread and so on? (*Hafod shakes his head*) You would agree that would be the right way to proceed? (*He nods*) Have doctors *en masse* made strong representations to government on the topic? Have they in any country, for instance, demanded a high-extraction-rate flour, and perhaps differential taxation to encourage consumption of wholemeal bread or a drop in sugar consumption?

HAFOD: No, but doctors in various countries are themselves eating wholemeal bread, or else bran, in increasing numbers.

HUNTER: To set a good example? Their patients see them . . . ? Tell me, doctor: did this dietary fiber theory emerge from one or more of the western world's great establishments for medical research?

HAFOD: No, in the first place it emerged from the work of a handful of men, mostly operating on their own or with a few colleagues, though at least one worker in Britain was associated with the Medical Research Council there.

HUNTER: And while these men were doing their pioneer studies the brightest stars in the medical firmament were busy advising patients with diverticular disease to take a low-fiber diet – which had caused the disease?

HAFOD: That is not quite how I would phrase it, but – yes, Mr Hunter.

HUNTER: The virtues of a high-fiber diet – in the form of wholemeal bread, etc. – have been extolled for many years? (*Hafod nods*) Mostly by people stigmatized by the orthodox medical profession as unscientific food cranks? Tell me, doctor: would you sooner be alive on unscientific grounds or dead on scientific ones?

HAFOD: We all make mistakes, Mr Hunter. And – well, it was not doctors who invented the roller-milling of wheat in the last century. But now the profession, or at any rate a group of experts from its ranks, is very busy working on dietary fiber, trying to find out what exactly it is that gives it its special qualities. Not a great deal is really known, you understand, about the composition of fiber, and exactly how it works. It is being divided into fractions and sub-fractions, and different kinds of fiber are being studied, and so on. We might be able to make a synthetic fiber; or put an active extract into capsules for people to take. The prospects are endless.

HUNTER: I accept, doctor, that your predecessors did not invent the roller-milling that started a century ago. However, do you know a paper[2,3] that appeared in two parts in the *Lancet*, entitled 'On the Antiseptic Principle in the Practice of Surgery'?

HAFOD: I'm afraid I don't. It sounds rather old.

HUNTER: Or one[4] that appeared in the *British Medical Journal* entitled, 'Description of a New Double Current Inhaler for Administering Ether'? (*Hafod shakes his head*) Forgive me, but the first appeared in 1867 and was by Lord Lister, the father of anti-septic surgery, and the second in 1873 and was by Dr Clover who gave his name to the important anesthetic apparatus described in his paper. Both, you may agree, are crucial papers. And so at the very time the engineers were inventing the roller-milling that would lead to the removal of bran from wheat flour Lister and Clover, using the same type of scientific and technological ap-proach, were making sure it would be possible to treat the ill effects – appendicitis, say – in an operating theater. Would you not say that these doctors and the engineers were brothers under the skin?

HAFOD: It needs a considerable imaginative leap to think so.

HUNTER: You cannot take it? (*Pause*) Then tell me, doctor: what difference will it make to the effectiveness of a high-fiber diet in diverticular disease if every kind of fiber is studied for the next hundred years?

HAFOD: Perhaps none if you put it like that; but one never knows, of course, what might not emerge from the research. And it is always helpful to know just what element in a natural product like dietary fiber is beneficial.

HUNTER: Why is it always helpful?

HAFOD: Well – er – that is the scientific approach.

HUNTER: It is helpful in the way it helps a small child to understand how a clock works if he pulls it all to pieces?

HAFOD: I cannot accept the analogy, Mr Hunter.

HUNTER: Even though doctors were not directly responsible for splitting wheat into white flour and bran, they did not over the decades condemn white flour, did they? (*Hafod nods*) Until recently they rather sneered at the wholemeal-bread fanatics? And they are certainly going to split up dietary fiber into its constituents, and examine each one, and so on?

HAFOD: I'm afraid I do not quite see . . .

HUNTER: That what the doctors are doing now is very like what the millers started to do to the wheat grain a century ago?

HAFOD: I think that is a little far-fetched.

HUNTER: And they are doing it as blithely as the other splitting was done? (*Pause*) Is there more to be learnt from splitting the fiber scientifically, or from the African villagers who have never heard of dietary fiber or of splitting it, but who do not get diverticular disease?

HAFOD: We westerners can learn from both, I believe.

HUNTER: Are you sure, doctor? – You don't think the two are incompatible? You don't think the scientific approach would split the African villagers, their health, their philosophy?

HAFOD: I'm afraid I do not quite follow you.

HUNTER: That is what I have been trying to get you to admit: that you cannot take the high road *and* the low road. Thank you, doctor. (*Sits*)

JUDGE: Two small points, doctor. If diabetes may to some degree be produced by a diet deficient in dietary fiber, has anyone tried the effect of giving such fiber to diabetics in the way in which they have tried that of giving it to people with colonic disease? Or am I being too simple?

HAFOD: Not at all, judge. It has been shown that guar gum,[5] one of the gums I mentioned that behave like dietary fiber, does actually help to control the condition when given to people with diabetes, and even when they are receiving insulin. In the short term, not just in the long term. To a doctor that is a most noteworthy result.

JUDGE: And a query related in a way to what Mr Hunter has just been saying: Has it been shown that broken-down fiber differs in its effects in any way from dietary fiber in its natural state?

HAFOD: Yes, there has been one experiment[6] in which a comparison was made between giving normal people apples and the equivalent in apple purée or the equivalent in apple juice. Apples contain pectin, you may remember, which is a sort of dietary fiber. It was found that the juice – free from fiber, of course – could be consumed eleven times faster than the apples and four times faster than the purée, in which the fiber is disintegrated. Also the juice was less satisfying – that is, as regards reducing hunger – than the purée, which in turn was less satisfying than the apples. And lastly, there were big differences between the three in their effects on blood sugar and blood insulin levels, differences that fit in with the idea that lack of fiber in the diet or broken-down fiber *might* lead to obesity and to diabetes.

JUDGE: So that breakdown or destruction of dietary fiber is undesirable in the kitchen, whatever it may be in the laboratory? (*Hafod nods*) Doctor, you wish to add anything? No? Then thank you; and this court is now adjourned.

REFERENCES—SESSION FOUR
1. Morris, J. N., Marr, J. W., and Clayton, D. G., *BMJ*, November 19, 1977, p. 1307.
2. Lister, J., *Lancet*, September 21, 1867, p. 353.
3. Lister, J., *Lancet*, November 30, 1867, p. 668.
4. Clover, J. T., *BMJ*, 1873, vol. 1, p. 282.
5. Jenkins, D. J. A., *et al.*, *Lancet*, October 15, 1977, p. 779.
6. Haber, G. B., *et al.*, *Lancet*, October 1, 1977, p. 679.

General Reading
Cummings, J. H., *Gut*, January 1973, p. 69.
Burkitt, D. P., *BMJ*, February 3, 1973, p. 274.
Trowell, H., *BMJ*, February 3, 1973, p. 295.
Eastwood, M. A., *et al.*, *Lancet*, May 25, 1974, p. 1029.
Burkitt, D. P., Walker, A. R. P., and Painter, N.S., *JAMA*, August 19, 1974, p. 1068.
Leading Article, *BMJ*, June 14, 1975, p. 580.
Spiro, H. M., *NEJM*, July 10, 1975, p. 83.
Burkitt, D. P., *Royal Society of Health Journal*, August 1975, p. 186.
Eastwood, M. A., *Royal Society of Health Journal*, August 1975, p. 188.
Southgate, D. A. T., *Royal Society of Health Journal*, August 1975, p. 191.
Burkitt, D. P., and Trowell, H. C. (eds.), *Refined Carbohydrate Foods and Disease*, Academic Press, London 1975.
Tudge, C., *World Medicine*, May 19, 1976, p. 47.

Diverticular Disease of the Colon
Painter, N. S., and Burkitt, D. P., *BMJ*, May 22, 1971, p. 450.
Painter, N. S., Almeida, A. Z., and Colebourne, K. W., *BMJ*, April 15, 1972, p. 137.
Painter, N. S., Stahl, W. M., and Almy, T. P., *JAMA*, August 28, 1972, p. 1058. (Three separate answers by two American experts and one British expert to a question about diverticular disease and a low-residue diet; all three favourable to a high-residue diet.)
Painter, N. S., *Diverticular Disease of the Colon: A Deficiency Disease of Western Civilisation*, Heinemann, London, 1975.
Taylor, I., and Duthie, H. L., *BMJ*, April 24, 1976, p. 988.

Brodribb, A. J. M., and Humphreys, D. M., *BMJ*, February 21, 1976, p. 424, 425.

Painter, N. S., *BMJ*, June 5, 1976, p. 1400.

Leading Article, *Lancet*, August 13, 1977, p. 337.

Mendeloff, A. I., *NEJM*, October 13, 1977, p. 811.

Irritable Colon

Smits, B. J., *Practitioner*, July 1974, p. 37.

Leading Article, *BMJ*, June 1, 1974, p. 457.

Dietary Fiber and Bowel Function

Burkitt, D. P., Walker, A. R. P., and Painter, N. S., *Lancet*, December 30, 1972, p. 1408.

Harvey, R. F., Pomare, E. W., and Heaton, K. W., *Lancet*, June 9, 1973, p. 1278.

Eastwood, M. A., *et al.*, *BMJ*, November 17, 1973, p. 392.

Findlay, J. M., *et al.*, *Lancet*, February 2, 1974, p. 146.

Walters, R. L., *et al.*, *BMJ*, June 7, 1975, p. 536.

Cummings, J. H., *et al.*, *Lancet*, January 7, 1978, p. 5.

Varicose Veins, Piles

Burkitt, D. P., *BMJ*, June 3, 1972, p. 556.

Latto, C., Wilkinson, R. W., and Gilmore, O. J. A., *Lancet*, May 19, 1973, p. 1089.

Cancer of the Bowel

Hill, M. J., *et al.*, *Lancet*, January 16, 1971, p. 95.

Malt, R. A., and Ottinger, L. W., *NEJM*, April 12, 1973, p. 772.

Parks, T. G., *Proceedings of the Royal Society of Medicine*, July 1973, p. 681.

Pomare, E. W., and Heaton, K. W., *BMJ*, November 3, 1973, p. 262.

Burkitt, D. P., *JAMA*, February 3, 1975, p. 517.

Dietary Fiber, Cholesterol and Triglycerides in Blood Plasma

Heaton, K. W., and Pomare, E. W., *Lancet*, January 12, 1974, p. 49.

Connell, A. M., Smith, C. L., and Somsel, M., *Lancet*, March 1, 1975, p. 496.

Jenkins, D. J. A., *et al.*, *Lancet*, May 17, 1975, p. 1116.

Durrington, P., Wicks, A. C. B., and Heaton, K. W., *Lancet*, July 19, 1975, p. 133.

Editorial, *Lancet*, August 23, 1975, p. 353.

Heaton, K. W., *Lancet*, November 8, 1975, p. 927.

Brodribb, A. J. M., and Humphreys, D. M., *BMJ*, February 21, 1976, p. 428.

Dietary Fiber and Obesity

Heaton, K. W., *Lancet*, December 22, 1973, p. 1418.

Dietary Fiber and Hiatus Hernia

Burkitt, D. P., and James, P. A., *Lancet*, July 21, 1973, p. 128.

DRUGS

Enter Professor Herbert Hecht

HUNTER: You are Herbert Hecht, a Professor of Clinical Pharmacology here in the United States? (*Hecht nods*) What is clinical pharmacology, professor?

HECHT: It's the study of drugs and the way they act – in the clinical situation as distinct from the laboratory.

HUNTER: I should like, first, to deal with the usage by doctors of some individual groups of drugs – antibiotics, amphetamines, and barbiturates. You know of an antibiotic called chloramphenicol? Will you tell us about it?

HECHT: It is a very effective antibiotic, introduced in the late 1940s. Unfortunately, as was realized after a few years, it has one serious drawback: in about one in every 50,000 people who take a course of it a serious condition, called aplastic anemia, develops, in which the bone marrow stops producing blood cells. Half the people who develop the condition die. Aplastic anemia may develop months after a course of chloramphenicol has ended, and it may develop after quite a short course of the drug; death from it is very distressing for the victim to endure, and for the relatives, the nurses, the doctor, and so on to witness.

HUNTER: When the first of these cases of aplastic anemia was reported, was there a preponderance of them in any particular segment of your population?

HECHT: Yes, among the children of doctors. Apparently doctors who were getting samples of chloramphenicol were handing it to their own children almost like candy: for colds and sore throats and various such minor ailments, for most of which it was probably not of any value anyway.

HUNTER: Because?

HECHT: Because those conditions would often be caused by a virus, which chloramphenicol won't touch, or by a type of bacterium it won't touch; and the patient would get better fairly quickly in any case.

HUNTER: And what happened after the dangers of chloramphenicol were recognized?

HECHT: The American regulatory body, the Food and Drug Administration – the FDA – insisted that warnings be put on the label and the packing leaflet for chloramphenicol, in particular about its being used only for those few serious diseases for which there was pretty well nothing else effective.

HUNTER: And how did the doctors respond?

HECHT: Sales went down at first, but later in the 1950s they picked up again, and by 1960 they were worth 86 million dollars a year. In fact, at one point, years after the dangers became known, chloramphenicol was the biggest-selling single prescription item in the States.

HUNTER: But its use was really essential in only a few conditions? (*Hecht nods*) And it was still causing this very serious disease, aplastic anemia?

HECHT: Correct; and as late as 1967 most people who suffered from an aplastic anemia due to chloramphenicol had been given the drug for some minor or unspecified condition or one for which another, safer antibiotic would have been suitable. I'm talking about the States now.

HUNTER: The drug company concerned was promoting it very heavily?

HECHT: Yes, and very cleverly; but in the end a drug company doesn't sign prescriptions – doctors do. Even as late as 1971 a few doctors were using it as the first-choice drug for most common infections, though in 1968 the FDA had written to all doctors in the States, warning against such usage.

HUNTER: And what was happening in the United Kingdom?

HECHT: Well, in your country too there were warnings in the fifties and sixties about the dangers of chloramphenicol and about it being really needed in only a few conditions; but in 1964, for instance, a million-pounds-sterling worth of chloramphenicol at wholesale prices was prescribed in Great Britain. In 1964 and 1965 family doctors alone had signed a million prescriptions for it. As in the US, it was mostly a minority of doctors who used it. Then in 1967 your Committee on Safety of Drugs issued one of its official warnings.[1] The following year the number of prescriptions had halved, but that was still, by any standard, far too many.

HUNTER: You know the tetracycline group of antibiotics?

HECHT: Do I not? – Oxy-, chlor-, and just plain tetracycline (and one or two newer ones). Broad-spectrum, like chloramphenicol. That means they act against a wide range of bacteria. However, their value for sore throats and so on is very limited indeed; but just like chloramphenicol they've been prescribed pretty freely by doctors for such conditions. In 1972 enough of tetracyclines was manufactured in my country to give a course to half the population – 100,000,000 people.[2]

HUNTER: Does their administration to young children carry any special dangers?

HECHT: If given in the first few years of life, tetracyclines are deposited in the milk teeth; and in some of the permanent teeth when given to children any time up to the age of about eight; they often cause a yellowing of the teeth in which they're deposited, which turns to dark brown or grey. A similar effect on a child's teeth can occur if a tetracycline is given to the mother during pregnancy.

HUNTER: Do you know of any investigation of this effect?

HECHT: Yes, a dentist in Northern Ireland has carried out two investigations.[3] Apart from the discoloration, it is possible to tell if there is a tetracycline deposited in a tooth extracted – for decay or anything else – simply by cutting across the tooth and then examining it under ultraviolet light. If there is a tetracycline deposit, it shows up as a fluorescent band; and in this way one can, in fact, tell the year when a tetracycline has been taken, and on how many occasions a course has been taken – there will be a band for each course. The dentist examined in this way all the second molar milk teeth – the big grinding teeth at the back – extracted for decay from children aged three, four or five, one such tooth for each child being examined; and he did so in 1966–7 and again in 1971–2. The first survey therefore was concerned with tetracyclines prescribed in the early and middle 1960s, and the second with tetracyclines prescribed in the later 1960s and early 1970s. This particular tooth is fully developed by the age of three, so that any tetracycline deposits in it would result from tetracyclines given in the first three years of life (or else given to the mother during pregnancy). The permanent *front* teeth, though, can be stained by tetracyclines given any time in the first five or six years of life. For other permanent teeth it's up to seven or eight years, like I said. In other words, staining of the first milk molars will tend to give an underestimate of likely staining of the front permanent teeth – which are the most important ones for smiling – let alone the other permanent teeth.

HUNTER: And what did this dentist find?

HECHT: There was a slight falling off in the percentage of teeth showing tetracycline deposits and in the number of such deposits per tooth in the very youngest children in the second survey, though the dentist was not sure that this might not have been due to a series of mild winters, which would mean fewer coughs and colds, and so perhaps tetracyclines prescribed less often for the children – mostly unnecessarily anyway – by doctors. However, the broad picture was that about 70 percent of the teeth examined for each age in *both* periods showed some tetracycline deposits, and the number of deposits per 100 teeth was in excess of 200 except for the oldest children in the first survey in whom the number was 141, and the youngest children in the second survey, in whom it was 199.

HUNTER: Two to three hundred deposits per hundred teeth means that on average each child during the first three years of life had received two or three courses of tetracyclines?

HECHT: Right. And the number of courses was rather greater for the children in the second than for those in the first period. If any of the milk teeth contained tetracycline deposits then the permanent teeth certainly would; and it has also been proved quite separately that one in three of the permanent teeth having these tetracycline deposits will show some discoloration, so that at least about 23 percent of all the children involved – one third of 70 percent . . .

JUDGE: I think we understand, professor.

HECHT: Would have visible staining of their permanent teeth. There is no reason at all to suppose that this figure would not be valid throughout the United Kingdom; so, as there were around 1,000,000 births a year in the UK in the 1960s, at least 230,000 children born each year at those times would develop staining of the front permanent teeth due to tetracyclines prescribed for them by doctors.

HUNTER: Mostly unnecessarily prescribed? (*Hecht nods*) So altogether how many children would have permanent tooth staining in the UK?

HECHT: Well, one can only guess. As this dentist showed, the prescribing of tetracyclines for children increased rapidly from the mid-1950s, and was increasing in the early 1960s, and heavy prescribing certainly went on, as he also showed, until the early 1970s – indeed, probably well beyond that, though gradually diminishing. Probably at least something between 2–3,000,000 children in the UK during the 1955–75 period developed staining of the permanent teeth, the result of prescribed tetracyclines. That's a conservative estimate, I'd say.

JUDGE: Any staining of the front permanent teeth is visible when the child – or young person as some of them will now be – when one of them smiles?

HECHT: Yes, judge. That is why I laid emphasis on the permanent front teeth just now, the incisor teeth. (*He smiles*) These front biting teeth, I mean, that always show when one smiles.

JUDGE: How many thalidomide children were there in the UK?

HECHT: About 400, judge.

JUDGE: Why was there much less publicity about this matter of tooth staining?

HECHT: I would guess because it wasn't as dramatic a thing as the thalidomide deformities. The disability per child was much less.

JUDGE: But the numbers involved were enormously greater? (*Hecht nods*) Can the staining, tell me, be removed or disguised?

HECHT: Yes, judge, but only by a dentist putting crowns on the affected teeth; and since the teeth, of course, grow with the child, the crowns have to be renewed every three to five years till the age of 20 or so.[4]

JUDGE: Tell me; tetracyclines are available in the United Kingdom only on a doctor's prescription?

HECHT: A dentist can prescribe them too; but that would represent just a tiny fraction of all the tetracycline prescriptions.

JUDGE: And the staining is absolutely permanent?

HECHT: Yes, judge, it is; and it gets deeper in shade as the teeth are exposed to light.

JUDGE: As, for instance, when a child smiles? (*Hecht nods*) Do go on, Mr Hunter.

HUNTER: It seems, professor, from the figures of this Northern Ireland dentist, that the unnecessary prescribing of tetracyclines by British doctors for young children hardly slackened between the early and the late 1960s. Was there any reason why it should have? Ought doctors to have known of this effect of tetracyclines, or that they were neither needed nor particularly effective for most coughs and colds in children?

HECHT: The answer to both questions is a loud 'Yes'. The undesirability – for a variety of reasons – of prescribing antibiotics for minor nose and throat infections has been preached to doctors for more than 20 years. The effect of tetracyclines on children's teeth was discovered in 1959, and it was publicized again and again in the early and particularly the mid-1960s in British medical journals, standard textbooks and so on,[5, 6, 7, 8, 9, 10] to one or more of which every doctor should have had access. What's more, for those few children with nose and throat and chest infections for whom an antibiotic *was* really needed there were alternatives most of the time that did not affect the teeth.

HUNTER: Could the doctors not have been victims of heavy advertising by the drug industry?

HECHT: Well, sir, leaving aside the question of whether doctors should ever let themselves be victims of industry pressure, the short answer is 'No' – and for the simple reason that in 1966 one of the tetracyclines came off patent, and the others were soon to follow, as the industry well knew; so there was no *heavy* promotion of tetracyclines in the mid-sixties. There had been years previously. There is one other point that I think clinches the argument. When oxytetracycline came off patent a number of firms started to market it, and they went in for a certain amount of advertising for their brands of oxytetracycline – not heavy advertising but noticeable. It so happens that of the three common tetracyclines the one that's least likely to cause the tooth staining is known to be oxytetracycline. In fact, it was recommended for children, when they had to have a tetracycline, for this very reason.[5] Now if doctors were aware of the dangers to children's teeth of tetracyclines, and if drug advertising was influencing the doctors, one would think the combined effect of these two factors would have been to increase, or at the very least to keep steady, the proportion of children receiving oxytetracycline from about 1966 onwards. In fact, the Northern Ireland dentist found, by examining the type of staining, that in his second survey, covering children born in 1966–9, the proportion of teeth containing an *oxy*tetracycline deposit was markedly less in the three-year olds than in the four-year olds, and less in the latter than in the five-year olds, the figures per 100 teeth being 12, 18, and 20 respectively. The corresponding figures for *all* tetracycline deposits were 199, 264, and 258. In other words, as the years went by oxytetracycline – the relatively safe tetracycline – was being used less and less, the drop in usage being more marked than in the case of the other tetracyclines. Perhaps not statistically significant, but . . .

HUNTER: Suggestive that the doctors cannot be exonerated in any way? (*Hecht nods*) Professor Hecht, even though you have taken us into the 1970s, some people might say they would like even more recent evidence on this matter of doctors and antibiotic usage. Is there any?

HECHT: Yes, from the United States this time. First, in January 1975 the Drugs Committee of our American Academy of Pediatrics said there were hardly any reasons at all for using tetracyclines in children aged under eight;[11] but a study[11] in the 1973–5 period showed one in every four doctors surveyed *was* prescribing them for children of that age; and 5 percent of doctors were writing more than half the prescriptions. Second, in the spring of 1974 a study was carried out at the University Health Services Clinic of Duke University, North Carolina, of the value of a protocol – that is, a fixed diagnosis and treatment schedule – for sore throats.[12] The clinic is staffed by doctors, by physician assistants (who are not medically qualified), and by student physician assistants; and the last two groups take some decisions about patients and can prescribe antibiotics. The respective percentages of these three groups using antibiotics for sore throats *before* the protocol was introduced were 56, 39 and 25; and after its introduction they were 18,

17 and 15. In other words, at all times doctors were using antibiotics more than their non-medical assistants.

HUNTER: And should not have been? (*Hecht nods*) And the 'after protocol' figures were more indicative of sound practice?

HECHT: Yes, indeed. The protocol used was agreed by the doctors themselves; and, as you heard, they cut their prescribing of antibiotics from 56 percent to 18 percent. The physician assistants and the student PAs didn't have to make such a big cut because they may have been using antibiotics too often before the protocol was adopted, but they were using them a darned sight less than the physicians. However you look at it, in the mid-seventies some American doctors were treating more than 50 percent of sore throats with antibiotics – nobody could defend a figure like that. Another separate study[13] in 1973 at the same center showed that in two out of every three instances of use of antibiotics either they were not needed or else they were given in the wrong dosage or else the wrong antibiotic was used.

HUNTER: May we turn now to what are called psychoactive drugs – those affecting the mind – in particular, amphetamines and barbiturates. Will you tell us something about the amphetamines, professor?

HECHT: This is a group of drugs of which the first, amphetamine itself, or benzedrine as it was then known, was discovered in the 1930s, although usage of them did not become common until the 1950s and sixties. Dexamphetamine is another, and methylamphetamine – or 'speed' – is a third. ('Purple hearts' contained dexamphetamine plus a barbiturate.) There are various other drugs involved that people, even doctors, do not at first glance realize are amphetamines even though they are, in fact, related to amphetamine chemically or in their action.

HUNTER: Which is?

HECHT: The amphetamines reduce appetite (which is a help in cases of obesity) and they lift depression. In fact, their action in both respects is not very strong or useful. For some years there have been other drugs that reduce appetite, and that do not have the drawbacks of the amphetamines, and for even longer there have been various other, reasonably safe drugs that are of considerable value in cases of depression.

HUNTER: And what are the drawbacks to the amphetamines?

HECHT: They stimulate the brain. They make people feel unrealistically cheerful for a time, and therefore excitable and talkative and full of energy. It's a pleasant feeling, but it wears off after a few hours, there is a let-down. Because of this effect of amphetamines people can become dependent on them, especially people who are unstable or anxious or insecure, and they need gradually to take bigger and bigger doses for the same effect; or most of them do.

HUNTER: Can one classify the sort of people who become dependent on them?

HECHT: Yes, there are two sorts. First, before their dangers were fully realized and in the 1960s *after* they were realized – and even into the 1970s – amphetamines were prescribed by doctors in the UK, USA, and other western countries for obese people trying to stick to a diet, and to people who were a bit unhappy or fatigued or down-in-the-dumps; the over-worked or bored middle-aged housewife was a typical candidate. And she would keep coming back to the doctor again and again for a repeat prescription.

HUNTER: Was there any effect on her obesity or depression?

HECHT: No, very little except in the patient's imagination, or the doctor's.

HUNTER: She had become 'hooked' on whichever amphetamine it was?

HECHT: Right, though she mightn't be increasing the dose very much; and if you'd told her she was a three-quarters drug addict, she'd have been horrified.

HUNTER: But the doctors knew what was happening?

HECHT: After the early 1960s at the latest there was no excuse at all if they didn't, there was so much publicity. You see, the second sort of consumer was a young person who would take amphetamines, usually when with other young people, sometimes by the handful, and even by 'mainlining' them – that is, injecting them into a vein. This sort of consumption can produce serious mental disease.

HUNTER: And where did the young people get their amphetamines?

HECHT: Now and again they'd be prescribed by a doctor – at the request of the young people usually, if it wasn't a threat by them. More usually they'd get them by stealing or purchase from an older person, who had got them on prescription; or else by theft from a pharmacy, forgery of prescriptions, from pushers (who might get them from overseas), and so on.

HUNTER: You are thinking particularly of the United Kingdom in all this?

HECHT: Well, there was a similar situation in various other western countries, including right here in the USA.

HUNTER: How extensive was British doctors' prescribing of amphetamines?

HECHT: In 1960 there were some 6,000,000 prescriptions, in 1966 4,000,000, and in 1969 2,000,000, which was still almost 2,000,000 too many – because by then most experts had for some time been convinced that the usefulness of amphetamines in medical practice was very limited.

HUNTER: How many people were dependent on amphetamines in the UK?

HECHT: In the mid-1960s it was thought there were 80,000 people dependent and getting their supplies legally through medical prescriptions, and 80,000 dependent on illicit supplies.[14]

HUNTER: But doctors continued to prescribe them for years and years?

HECHT: They did; and even in the 1970s doctors were switching their prescribing from 'straight' amphetamines to amphetamine-like drugs, which were just as liable to produce dependence.

HUNTER: And what is the position today?

HECHT: In your country amphetamines and amphetamine-like substances are now relatively little used. This is largely a result of a doctors' voluntary ban on the prescribing of them, which was initiated by one family doctor in Ipswich. Doctors at last woke up to the truth about what they were doing. Also amphetamines are now controlled by the 1973 regulations made under your 1971 Misuse of Drugs Act.

HUNTER: And the position here in America?

HECHT: In the mid-1960s enough amphetamines were produced in the United States to provide 35 doses for every single inhabitant each year.[15] At least half was going into illicit channels.[15] In 1971 tighter legal controls were imposed on amphetamines,[16] but in 1973 it was reported that 78 percent of general-practitioner doctors and 50 percent of internists – specialist physicians – were still prescribing appetite-suppressant drugs of which a substantial number were amphetamines or related substances.[17] When asked to rate the potential for abuse of amphetamines the American doctors polled thought that it wasn't particularly high for prescribed amphetamines, but almost three quarters of them thought it was very high indeed for illicitly obtained amphetamines.

JUDGE: An amphetamine does not alter its character, professor, merely because a medical man has provided it?

HECHT: Not at all, judge. And the dangers of amphetamines are well publicized here in the US.[18]

HUNTER: May we turn now to the barbiturates? For what purposes are they used, and for what purposes are they valuable?

HECHT: Barbiturates were introduced in the early years of this century, and have mainly been used as hypnotics (that is, to induce sleep), or else as daytime sedatives – soothers of the nerves in the anxious or depressed. In fact, we now believe that there are only two main justified uses for them, and one or two very uncommon uses. The two main uses are as an anesthetic, injected into a vein, and for the control of epilepsy. There is practically no need for them to be used as sedatives or to induce sleep.

HUNTER: What is to be used then for these purposes?

HECHT: Well, the best way to tackle insomnia or anxiety, which are commonly treated with drugs, is for the doctor patiently to try and discover the cause and eliminate it. And of course, there are everyday remedies for sleeplessness, which often work. And if a drug is used, then some newer drugs, known as tranquilizers, appear to be safer – just as they are if some daytime quietening of a patient is needed.

HUNTER: In what ways are barbiturates dangerous?

HECHT: The sleep that they induce is not natural, and they leave a hangover. Taken at night or in the daytime they make a patient 'dopey'. One study in your country[19] showed that 93 percent of people over 65 with fracture of the femur (the thigh bone), a serious fracture for an old person – that 93 percent of those who had suffered the fracture between 10 pm and 6 am were taking barbiturates, compared with almost none taking barbiturates among those who had gotten the fracture at some other time in the 24 hours. It was the only way in which the two groups differed. And old people on barbiturates were found to be twice as likely to have frequent falls as those not on them.

HUNTER: What about old people who were taking the newer types of drugs for insomnia?

HECHT: This study suggested they were a little more likely to get a fracture than those not taking any such drug – but only a little more.

HUNTER: And the other drawbacks to barbiturates?

HECHT: They have a complex and undesirable effect on the liver. They are often used for suicidal purposes; and, above all, they often make a patient dependent on them.

HUNTER: They are drugs of addiction?

HECHT: Right. And that doesn't involve only the typical middle-aged or elderly patient taking barbiturates prescribed by the doctor. Since about 1960 they have been used by young people, sometimes injected into a vein, and then they are mostly obtained illicitly (from a pusher, by theft, through forged prescriptions, by paying a middle-aged or old patient for them – 25 pence, or about half a dollar, per capsule is the current going rate in your country),[20] or else by the young person threatening a doctor with a disturbance in his office – surgery, as you would say – if a prescription for a barbiturate is not provided.[20] Barbiturates are powerful agents: they kill more young people than any other drug.

HUNTER: But do their middle-aged and elderly users become dependent on them too?

HECHT: Yes, indeed, the most respectable of people; but they tend not to increase the dose, and of course they don't mainline. It's the amphetamine story all over again. About one in 10 of the ordinary regular users of barbiturates is dependent on them, and quite recently there were about a million regular users in your country.[21]

HUNTER: People can be weaned from barbiturates?

HECHT: Yes, quite often, if a doctor has patience, they can be gradually induced to manage without any drugs at all, or else with one of the tranquilizing drugs I mentioned instead of a barbiturate.

HUNTER: Do these tranquilizers not have any drawbacks?

HECHT: Yes, they have some, and others may emerge with time. They have been available only since the early 1960s. The sleep they provide is not absolutely natural, they cause some hangover, and they can produce dependence; but they are less powerful and less dangerous than the barbiturates.

HUNTER: And have doctors been making a change? In the United Kingdom?

HECHT: They have, but slowly – much too slowly in my judgment. Barbiturate abuse has been well known since the early 1960s; and yet in 1968 there were 25 million barbiturate prescriptions altogether – 17 million for barbiturates as hypnotics, and the rest for barbiturates in smaller doses as daytime sedatives.

HUNTER: The position has improved since then?

HECHT: Well, in England alone in 1967, for example, there were 15 million prescriptions for barbiturates as hypnotics: by 1974 the figure was $7\frac{1}{2}$ million. However, the corresponding figures for tranquilizers in those two years were $14\frac{1}{2}$ million and 20 million; and for other nonbarbiturate hypnotics they were $4\frac{1}{2}$ million and 9 million.

JUDGE: What was gained in one way, professor, was more than lost in another, but the second was considered safer?

HECHT: Right, judge. And as for old people in your country – well, I don't know. The study[19] I quoted just now as regards thigh bone fractures showed that between 1973 and 1976 in the city of Nottingham, in one big group of old people, the percentage being prescribed barbiturates actually *increased* from 41 percent to 51 percent, while the percentage who were getting the newer and safer type of drug had gone down correspondingly.

HUNTER: An unhappy picture?

HECHT: An almost incredible picture. Unhappy for the doctors, and unhappy for the patients.

JUDGE: Does this very wide usage of sedatives or tranquilizers – does it occur in other western countries, professor?

HECHT: It does, especially among women. In 1971, of ten western countries studied, Sweden had the highest consumption of such drugs among women[22]. There was a strikingly low consumption by women in Italy and Spain, almost half that of Sweden.

JUDGE: And what is the position concerning all these drugs in your own country, professor? I mean the hypnotics as well as the others.

HECHT: It is similar to the position in England, judge; though perhaps a shade less depressing. In 1962 we were producing enough barbiturates to supply 24 doses to every man, woman, and child in the USA;[23] but by 1973 the total number of barbiturate prescriptions was down to 20 million;[24] largely replaced, mind you, by the minor tranquilizers – mostly of the newer kind – for which in 1972 there were about 90 million prescriptions.[25] Barbiturates are often abused in my country just as they are in yours; and they're the type of drug most often involved in suicidal attempts and in successful suicides.[24] But again, just as in your country, there's a movement afoot – similar to your successful campaign against the amphetamines – to cut the number of barbiturate prescriptions;[26] so feeling in the United States is certainly moving against them.

JUDGE: Professor Hecht, alcohol and cigarettes are abused, are they not? (*Hecht nods*) Men and women have a tendency to abuse any drug affecting the mind?

HECHT: I agree, sir, but alcohol and cigarettes are on free sale: the drugs I've been talking about are not.

JUDGE: But we have only a very small charge for prescriptions under the British National Health Service. And I believe patients can in any case bring pressure to bear on the doctor to give them what they want.

HECHT: The doctor can resist, judge. And the problem's the same in the States, where we have no free health service.

JUDGE: But then are there not pressures the drug companies can bring to bear on doctors?

HECHT: Oh, yes, they're not angels; you don't have to tell me. But in the end it's the doctor who signs the prescription. I keep coming back to that. And just as I tried to show that the industry couldn't be much involved in the excessive prescribing of tetracyclines in your country in the late 1960s, so I don't think you can involve it in the amphetamine, let alone the barbiturate, position – not to any extent. You see, the patents on barbiturates expired years and years ago, and on amphetamines quite some time back, so it simply wouldn't have paid the drug companies to have spent a lot on promoting them. And doctors are supposed to be informed people, people of good judgment.

JUDGE: And you doubt that they are?

HECHT: Yes, judge, I do – in this respect.

JUDGE: Mr Hunter?

HUNTER: Professor, to summarize the position so far: in the UK, the USA and in other western countries there was, in the 1960s, an epidemic of dependence on amphetamines and barbiturates, and in your view it was in large part the result of careless and ignorant prescribing of them by doctors, and the problem is only now being overcome. Correct? (*Hecht nods*) I came to this hearing forearmed; and I should like, before proceeding to possible remedies for this state of affairs, to strengthen and widen the case against doctors. Will you accept that Sir Derrick Dunlop, first Chairman of the Medicines Commission in the UK, is reported to have said of amphetamines, barbiturates, and other mind-affecting drugs that 'the extent to which such drugs were sought by patients and the extent to which their demands were acceded to by the medical profession was a disturbing feature of modern medicine'?[27]

HECHT: I can believe he said it, and he was fully justified.

HUNTER (*holding up book*): I have here extracts from, and para-phrases of, the official reports of the debates in Parliament on the 1971 Misuse of Drugs Bill.[28] One member of the House of Commons said the main problem, as concerned doctors, was not to control the few black sheep but to control the larger number of gray sheep. The barbiturates that had been used for injection by addicts were prescribed by many doctors. He asked if these doctors knew for whom they were prescribing. If so, awkward questions could be asked. An average of 80 tablets per prescription was a reflection on medical practice and a cause of the tablet overspill that led to abuse. You go along with that, professor, as concerns your own country also?

HECHT: I go along with it, I regret to have to say.

HUNTER: A doctor Member of Parliament said that most cases of overprescribing arose through ignorance. Another MP said that 'the public has been gravely let down by the medical profession' and later a government Minister reported the preliminary views of a subcommittee with a medical chairman: evidence had been given to it that barbiturates were widely and perhaps casually prescribed, and were therefore widely available. It felt strongly that the medical profession should attend urgently to the educa-tion of doctors in the use of barbiturates.

HECHT: I agree. Education is the answer.

HUNTER: And to turn now to doctors prescribing more generally. Will you accept that the Second Chairman of the United Kingdom Medicines Commission is reported as saying[29] that 'doctors of my generation, particularly those in general practice. . . have no idea how to use, I suppose, 90 percent of modern drugs . . . they may very well have acquired some knowledge about drugs, but they were never taught at medical school anything very much' about drugs? (*Hecht nods*) And that a clinical pharmacologist from your country is quoted as saying, 'It is my belief that lack of knowledge and sophistication in the proper therapeutic use of drugs is perhaps the greatest deficiency of the average American physician today'?[30]

HECHT: Yes, like I said, my country's doctors are just as much at fault as yours.

HUNTER: And lastly, in this particular connection, will you accept that the Senior Medical Officer in charge of drug efficiency and safety of the World Health Organization has written, 'The surgeon has to undergo specific postgraduate training for several years, yet a comparable postgraduate training for practising physicians in the rational use of drugs does not exist'?[31]

HECHT: I accept that, and I'd add that sometimes it's worse than just ignorance. I want to mention two recent papers from the UK on prescribing in family practice. The first[32] reported three types of abuse: prescriptions being repeated again and again on the basis of the patients' say-so over the telephone, the message often being taken by the receptionist who then fills in the prescription form for up to half a dozen drugs – for the doctor to sign automatically. Second, diagnosis over the telephone and a corresponding prescription, especially of antibiotics, the patient sometimes telling the receptionist exactly which antibiotic he or she wants. Third, the signing by the doctor of blank prescription forms, the receptionist simply putting in the name of a drug on one of them when some patient comes along later or phones asking for a repeat prescription.

JUDGE: Are these abuses common?

HECHT: It seems so, judge: the second paper[33] reported that of prescriptions for barbiturates 70–80 percent had been written out by a receptionist, over 60 percent of those for drugs for anxiety or depression, and over 20 percent in the case of drugs for heart conditions and so on. The doctor author said his family practice colleagues needed educating on how to wean patients from their tablets.

HUNTER: You know, professor, about a drug called practolol, a beta-blocking drug, introduced in the United Kingdom in 1970?

HECHT: I do. It was withdrawn from general use in your country in 1975 because it was found to be causing serious side-effects –

dryness of the eyes, a form of peritonitis, various skin conditions, and so on.

JUDGE: What, professor, is a beta-blocking drug?

HECHT: The beta-blockers, judge, are a group of drugs, the first of which were discovered in Britain, that are certainly of value in angina, various other heart disorders, high blood pressure, and other conditions. 'Beta-blocking' simply refers to the way they work. Unfortunately, though they have beneficial effects, they can also have undesirable ones: depression, insomnia, stomach upsets – oh, quite a list. On the whole their good effects outweigh the bad ones, but they're still very much at the stage of being tried out.

HUNTER: What I wished to ask you, professor, is whether the carelessness over the prescribing of drugs by family doctors in the UK, which you have described – whether that might not have been responsible for some of the five-year delay in recognizing that practolol had serious side-effects such that its use had to be restricted to hospitals and for just one or two conditions.

HECHT: It's certainly difficult – your Committee on Safety of Medicines has found it difficult – to get the run-of-the-mill doctor to report unusual effects in patients on a new drug. The means for reporting are certainly there but . . .

HUNTER: But the doctors' cooperation is not?

HECHT: I have to admit that is the way it often seems.

HUNTER: So that recognition of the serious side-effects of practolol – which affected hundreds of patients, I think – *may* well have been delayed by the remiss attitude of the doctors?

HECHT: Yes, all right. They need educating as regards drugs.

HUNTER: Then let us look at this matter of curing the doctors of their ignorance and their improper prescribing habits by means of education – in which you believe. First, as to the availability of the education: *The Journal of the American Medical Association* is the official journal of by far the biggest and most important organization of American doctors? (*Hecht nods*) I have here, as an exhibit, a supplement to the journal,[34] published on August 15, 1977 – the year is really immaterial – giving details of continuing educational courses for physicians. (*Hands a journal to Hecht*) How many pages of detail about such courses are there in the supplement?

HECHT: Let me see – yeah, just one hundred and forty pages.

HUNTER: And how many are devoted to courses of postgraduate drug education?

HECHT (*after pause*): Oh, yes, here we are – page 680. Well – er – just over half of a page.

HUNTER: One half page devoted to courses on continuing drug education of American doctors out of 140 pages devoted to continuing education courses generally? Perhaps disproportionately small?

HECHT: Accepted. Mind you, the United States is no worse in this respect than any other country. And we have had for some years now a thing called The Network for Continuing Medical Education, operating on television.

HUNTER: One of its recent broadcasts tested doctors' knowledge of antibiotics, did it not?

HECHT: That's right. You sure get yourself briefed, Mr Hunter.

HUNTER: The report[35] of the test stated that answers to questions in the broadcast 'indicated deficiencies of knowledge and the need for further postgraduate education in the use of antibiotics'. Only 10 percent of surgeons and 15 percent of family practitioners scored 80 percent or better: meaning that, even with the *best* doctors, there would be a one in five chance of them making a mistake with the drugs they were giving a patient? (*Hecht nods*) Drug education might work. That is still your position? (*Hecht nods*) However, there is not much of it; and no evidence of any good effect from the little there is? (*He nods again*) Well now, here is a copy of the *British Medical Journal* for March 18, 1967.[36] (*Hands journal to Hecht*) Will you look at the article beginning on page 671? You are familiar with it? (*Hecht nods*) It came from one of our Medical Research Council workers at a London teaching hospital? Will you tell us what it said?

HECHT: The doctor who wrote it wanted to see if he could link the prescribing of chloramphenicol with – well, with roughly how good a family doctor was. He looked at a group of 200 such doctors, and he gauged how good they were in three ways: first, their degrees and hospital experience; second, how good the local specialists judged them to be on the basis of their knowledge, care and concern for patients, and attendance at special courses.

HUNTER: Their continuing education, in other words?

HECHT: Right. And third, their answers to questions about the organization of their practices, prescribing, and so on. He gauged these 200 doctors, and then compared their ratings with the frequency with which they prescribed chloramphenicol in one month in 1961. By then the dangers of it were known to any conscientious doctor.

HUNTER: And he found? The educated doctors hardly used it at all?

HECHT: No, he didn't. He felt sure, when he started, that the doctors with a high rating *would* prescribe chloramphenicol very little, if at all; and the opposite would be the case for those with a low rating. To his surprise he could not find any link at all between the ratings and the prescribing of chloramphenicol. The good doctors—

HUNTER: The well-educated doctors?

HECHT: Roughly – they were just as likely as the not-so-good to prescribe it. He checked and rechecked his results, and always the conclusion was the same.

HUNTER: It was a reliable paper, one that cannot readily be faulted?

HECHT: Oh, agreed. It's just that it goes plain contrary to all I believe in.

HUNTER: So that, aside from the very small amount of drug education for doctors and their continuing ignorance, even the best-educated, the most knowledgeable do not, in fact, prescribe wisely?

HECHT: That is what this report suggested – for chloramphenicol.

HUNTER: Finally, professor, before we put drug usage into the broader social picture that I am all the time seeking to present I should like to take a panoramic view of the ill effects of drugs. You have heard of the Boston Collaborative Drug Surveillance Program?

HECHT: Surely. Probably the best large-scale investigation of the adverse effects of drugs ever carried out.

HUNTER: I have here a copy of the *New England Journal of Medicine* for October 17, 1974 in which there is a report from the program.[37] I am going to quote, and to calculate, some figures from it. In-patients in the *medical* units of American hospitals comprise one third of all hospital patients, who total 30,000,000 a year. These 10,000,000 *medical*-unit patients receive 90,000,000 courses of drug therapy per year – nine courses per patient on average, that is. A lot of drugs, professor? (*Hecht nods*) 3,000,000 of them, the report said, suffer an adverse drug reaction every year; so, since American hospitals take in 30,000,000 patients a year altogether and drugs are not given only to medical patients, 6,000,000 hospital in-patients suffering an adverse drug reaction is probably a conservative estimate?

HECHT: I'm with you.

HUNTER: The report said that there are about 29,000 deaths attributable to drugs in hospitalized *medical* patients each year – that is, about one in 340 patients – and again one might well double that mortality figure for *all* hospitalized patients, giving a figure round about 60,000. In fact, another 1974 estimate[38] also gave 60,000 as the very minimum likely number of deaths due to drugs in your country each year, so it looks to be about right – if all or most of these patients are admitted to hospital. You know that second report?

HECHT: I know it.

HUNTER: How many motor vehicle deaths are there in the USA each year?

HECHT: Just under 50,000.

HUNTER: So that the doctors in hospitals may be killing more people with their drugs?

HECHT: You can put it like that. Mind you, there was another report[39] from the Boston Study showing that, overall in seven western countries, the proportion of deaths due to drugs was only about one per 1000 medical in-patients. And most of those who died were seriously ill anyway, and in only about a quarter were the deaths possibly preventable.

HUNTER: That would still, in your country's hospitals, represent – let me see – 5000 preventable deaths a year at the least? (*Hecht nods*) Now as to adverse reactions to drugs outside hospital: that first Boston report estimated that there are 75,000,000 adult out-patients in the US taking one or more drugs regularly – that is, at least once a week and usually every day. Getting on for half the adult population? A lot of people? (*Hecht nods*) A lot of drugs? – The report stated that 3 per cent of American hospital admissions are due to drug reactions; and as there are 10,000,000 admissions to their medical units each year, that means some 300,000 patients admitted with drug reactions every year – more if some of the patients, in fact, go to non-medical units. And it leaves aside the obviously very much greater number of patients having minor reactions and not admitted to hospital. Interesting figures, professor?

HECHT: Very striking. Still, you have almost 3000 deaths a year in England and Wales due to drugs – overdosage or adverse effects. And the estimate of the percentage of patients admitted to medical wards who get adverse reactions to drugs varies between 10 and 24 percent.[40]

HUNTER: Your own American figure of 30 percent was bigger, if not better, professor? I am now going to read from the Boston report:[37] 'The benefit-to-risk ratio for the vast majority of commonly used drugs appears to be a reasonable one justifying the proper use of these drugs . . . the large number of hospitalizations resulting from adverse drug reactions is a reflection more of the vast usage of drugs than of their toxicity . . . Thus, if we wish to reduce the amounts of drug toxicity substantially we must reduce the number of drugs that people take.' (*Pause*) 'Reduce the number of drugs that people take'; tell me, professor, how has the total number of prescriptions for drugs altered in your country in the 10 years prior to the appearance of that report?

HECHT: It increased by 50 percent.[41]

HUNTER: And in France, say?

HECHT: By almost 200 percent.[41]

HUNTER: And in the United Kingdom?

HECHT: By 25 percent.[41]

HUNTER: The report spoke of 'proper use' of drugs. If the use of drugs is not proper – which might be thought certainly to be the case by any definition of impropriety – we have established that education of doctors is very likely not going to make it proper? (*Hecht nods*) Now separately, as regards that benefit-to-risk ratio being reasonable for the vast majority of drugs, a value judgment is inevitably involved, is it not? And that judgment would *have* to be linked with the *amount* of prescribing of the drugs, which we've just been discussing? (*Hecht nods*) I mean, some people might say that a chance of one in about 340 – or one in 1000, whichever it is – of dying in a hospital medical unit due to a drug that one had been given there, perhaps unnecessarily, was simply *not* acceptable, might they not?

HECHT: I follow, and I agree a value judgment is involved, and that one can't simply ignore the fact that excessive prescribing does exist today.

HUNTER: You will not dispute either that the report stated 'we have not considered the problems of drug abuse, addiction or overdosage'? (*Hecht shakes his head*) So it would take no account at all of most of the ill effects of the amphetamines and barbiturates discussed by us today?

HECHT: Right.

HUNTER: Will you also accept that it stated 'the study does not provide for the identification of "delayed" adverse drug effects – i.e., those that might develop months or years after a drug is stopped' or of 'the long-term effects of drugs that have recently been marketed'? (*Hecht nods*) So that it might have missed, under that first head, thalidomide, say, or tetracycline tooth staining or even a delayed aplastic anemia due to chloramphenicol; and, under the second head, have failed to prevent a second practolol in the United Kingdom? (*Hecht nods*) And the report could not, of course, deal with what was reported or discussed in five separate papers[42,43,44,45,46] in that same journal within the following two years – that is, that the use of certain estrogens (female hormone substances) for symptoms at the change of life in women, a use that became very prevalent in the 1960s, seems to increase the risk of cancer of the lining of the uterus by five to 14 times?[44] – Making it in white women aged 65 to 74 as common as cancer of the breast, uterine cervix, lung, and stomach combined?[46] There has been an upswing in what is called endometrial cancer in your country since 1960, especially in older women? Yes?

HECHT: Yes, and I admit these were disturbing reports. Of course, one has to balance risks against benefits. And there has been criticism of the reports[47,48] as well as support for them.[49,50,51]

HUNTER: But the consensus is?

HECHT: The consensus is that the reports must be taken seriously. It is in favor of caution in using estrogens for hormonal replacement therapy in post-menopausal women.[52]

HUNTER: Yet these estrogens have been given for menopausal symptoms by all kinds of doctors for some years? – Indeed, some of the very best doctors, the best educated, the most distinguished academically?

HECHT: That is true; but no one could foresee—

HUNTER: One of the papers[43] pointed out that it was cold comfort to say that the increased risk of cancer was no more than one would get from cigarette smoking or over-eating. The comparisons, I suggest, tell us something about our western way of life. (*Pause*) Lastly, I now put it to you, professor, that the real conclusion to be drawn from the figures I quoted from the Boston report, and from all the other evidence we have heard today – on antibiotics, amphetamines, barbiturates, beta-blockers, the carelessness and ignorance of doctors – is that the people of this country and of the United Kingdom and of the western world generally are 'hooked' on drugs, that now to a great extent their lives are managed with drugs; and that doctors, ignorant or knowledgeable about drugs, well-intentioned or indifferent, educated or not educated, are most to blame for this, though they are abetted by the people themselves, by the drug companies, by government, by the media. And that, for as long as people expect a drug for every little ache or pain, every worry, disappointment or frustration, and the doctors continue to encourage and pander to this attitude, for so long one can expect millions of adverse drugs reactions a year, and tens of thousands of deaths. I suggest to you that we are a civilization soaked in our drug technology, and we can see no way whatsoever of getting out of it.

HECHT: I am a doctor, Mr Hunter. I think that one has to go on hoping.

HUNTER: One recent medical paper[53] in your country warned us – or informed us, I'm not quite sure what the right word is – that before too long we may have drugs to alter aggression and sexual desire, to improve memory, make learning faster, and so on. Does that not reinforce what I have just been saying? (*Hecht nods*) I wonder, to fit this matter of drugs on to the larger canvas, if you would now agree that the wide availability of a large range of powerful drugs is a feature peculiar to our modern western civilization? – A characteristic feature?

HECHT: Yes, I go along with that.

HUNTER: And the good effects of drugs, and the bad effects obviously have one and the same source? They are inseparable? (*Hecht nods*) Would you agree also that sometimes the illnesses a drug cures or relieves – the anxieties, the depressions, the indigestion – arise from the nature of work in a multitude of factories broadly similar to the very factories that produce the drug?

HECHT: Yes, I guess that's true.

HUNTER: We cause with our right hand and treat with our left? And we do both faster and ever faster? We are a sick society?

HECHT: I deal with sick people, Mr Hunter. I don't know about a sick society.

HUNTER: You *do* sometimes stop to ask for whom the bell tolls?

HECHT: It's not a bell that tolls, Mr Hunter: it's a bleeper in my pocket that bleeps. And when it bleeps I know it's bleeping for me.

HUNTER: Which is as the bell tolls? No? You cannot admit that? (*Pause*) Thank you, professor.

JUDGE: You wish to add anything, professor? Then the court is adjourned.

REFERENCES—SESSION FIVE

1. Committee on Safety of Drugs, Adverse Reaction Series, No. 4, HMSO, London, 1967.
2. Simmons, H. E., and Stolley, P. D., *JAMA*, March 4, 1974, p. 1023.
3. Stewart, D. J., *BMJ*, August 11, 1973, p. 320.
4. Cooley, R. O., *JAMA*, February 21, 1972, p. 1078.
5. *Drug and Therapeutics Bulletin*, August 4, 1967, p. 61.
6. *British National Formulary*, British Medical Association and Pharmaceutical Society of Great Britain, London, 1966, p. 78.
7. McLeod, J. G., Davidson, S. (eds.), in *The Principles and Practice of Medicine*, 7th ed, Livingstone, Edinburgh and London, 1964, p. 80.
8. Todd, R. G. (ed.), *Extra Pharmacopoeia Martindale*, 25th edn, The Pharmaceutical Press, London, 1967, p. 1024.
9. Leading Article, *Lancet*, April 23, 1966, p. 917.
10. Any Questions, *BMJ*, November 12, 1966, p. 1185.
11. Ray, W. A., Federspiel, C. F., and Schaffner, W., *JAMA*, May 9, 1977, p. 2069.
12. Grimm, R. H., Jr, *et al.*, *NEJM*, March 6, 1975, p. 507.
13. Castle, M., *et al.*, *JAMA*, June 27, 1977, p. 2819.
14. *Drug Addiction*, Office of Health Economics, London, 1967, p. 15.
15. Sadusk, J. F., *JAMA*, May 23, 1966, p. 707.
16. Anderson, B. J., *JAMA*, November 11, 1974, p. 900.
17. Lasagna, L., *JAMA*, July 2, 1973, p. 44.
18. Cohen, S., *JAMA*, January 27, 1975, p. 414.

19. Macdonald, J. B., and Macdonald, E. T., *BMJ*, August 20, 1977, p. 483.
20. Leading Article, *BMJ*, September 27, 1975, p. 725.
21. Bewley, T. H., *Proceedings of the Royal Society of Medicine*, February 1968, p. 175.
22. Balter, M. B., Levine, J., and Manheimer, D. T., *NEJM*, April 4, 1974, p. 769.
23. AMA Committee on Alcoholism and Addiction, *JAMA*, August 23, 1966, p. 107.
24. Editorial, *NEJM*, October 10, 1974, p. 790.
25. Blackwell, B., *JAMA*, September 24, 1973, p. 1637.
26. Editorial, *Lancet*, September 6, 1975, p. 441.
27. Drugs in Use, *Pharmaceutical Journal*, London, November 22, 1969, p. 623.
28. Bradshaw, S., *Drug Misuse and The Law*, Macmillan, Basingstoke, 1972, quoting from *House of Commons Parliamentary Debates, Weekly Hansard*, vol. 803, col. 1749 *et seq.*, and vol. 808, col. 549 *et seq.*, HMSO, London, 1970.
29. Gould, D., *New Scientist*, May 23, 1974, p. 462.
30. Koch-Weser, J., quoted in Friebel, H., *WHO Chronicle*, February 1973, p. 59.
31. Friebel, H., *WHO Chronicle*, February 1973, p. 59.
32. Bliss, M. R., *Lancet*, July 31, 1976, p. 248.
33. Freed, A., *BMJ*, November 20, 1976, p. 1232.
34. 'Continuing Education Courses for Physicians', Supplement to *JAMA*, August 15, 1977, p. 680.
35. Neu, H. W., and Howrey, S. P., *NEJM*, December 18, 1975, p. 1291.
36. Meade, T. W., *BMJ*, March 18, 1967, p. 671.
37. Jick, H., *NEJM*, October 17, 1974, p. 824.
38. Talley, R. B., and Laventurier, M. F., *JAMA*, August 19, 1974, p. 1043.
39. Porter, J., and Jick, H., *JAMA*, February 28, 1977, p. 879.
40. Leading Article, *BMJ*, February 21, 1976, p. 413.
41. Gould, D., *New Scientist*, May 23, 1974, p. 465.
42. Smith, D. C., *et al.*, *NEJM*, December 4, 1975, p. 1164.
43. Ziel, H. K., and Finkle, W. D., *NEJM*, December 4, 1975, p. 1167.
44. Editorial, *NEJM*, December 4, 1975, p. 1200.
45. Weiss, N. S., Zzekely, D. R., and Austin, D. F., *NEJM*, June 3, 1976, p. 1259.
46. Mack, T. M., *et al.*, *NEJM*, 3 June, 1976, p. 1262.
47. Baggs, W. J., *NEJM*, October 14, 1976, p. 897.
48. Editorial, *Lancet*, March 12, 1977, p. 577.
49. Doll, R., *et al.*, *Lancet*, April 2, 1977, p. 745.
50. Leading Article, *BMJ*, July 23, 1977, p. 209.
51. Gordon, J., *et al.*, *NEJM*, September 15, 1977, p. 570.
52. Proudfit, C. M., *JAMA*, August 23, 1976, p. 939.
53. Editorial, *NEJM*, April 4, 1974, p. 800.

Chloramphenicol and Tetracyclines

Wilson, C., *Prescribers' Journal*, 1961, vol. 1, p. 60.
Wintrobe, M. M., *Prescribers' Journal*, 1964, vol. 4, p. 2.
Ory, E. M., and Yow, E. M., *JAMA*, July 27, 1963, p. 273.
Inglis, B., *Drugs, Doctors, and Disease*, André Deutsch, London, 1965, p. 121.
Huguley, C. M., Jr, *JAMA*, May 2, 1966, p. 408.

Leading Article, *BMJ*, March 18, 1967, p. 649.

Mintz, M., *By Prescription Only*, 2nd edn, Beacon Press, Boston, 1967.

Today's Drugs, *BMJ*, June 8, 1968, p. 607.

Manten, A., Meyler, L., and Herxheimer, A. (eds.), in *Side Effects of Drugs*, vol. VII, Excerpta Medica, Amsterdam, 1972, p. 362.

Editorial, *Lancet*, February 16, 1974, p. 251.

Amphetamines and Barbiturates

Connell, P. H., *JAMA*, May 23, 1966, p. 718.

Today's Drugs, *BMJ*, March 23, 1968, p. 753.

Drug and Therapeutics Bulletin, 26 April 1968, p. 33.

Working Party's Report, Control of Amphetamine Preparations, *BMJ*, November 30, 1968, p. 572.

Report by the Advisory Committee on Drug Dependence, *The Amphetamines and Lysergic Acid Diethylamide (LSD)*, HMSO, London, 1970.

Department of Health and Social Security, Reports on Public Health and Medical Subjects, No. 124, *Amphetamines, Barbiturates, LSD, and Cannabis, their Use and Misuse*, HMSO, London, 1970.

Leading Article, *BMJ*, December 7, 1974, p. 552.

Over-Prescribing in the USA

Dunea, G., *BMJ*, July 23, 1977, p. 240.

Beta-Blocker Drugs

Prichard, B. N. C., *Practitioner*, October 1977, p. 501.

Leading Article, *BMJ*, June 14, 1975, p. 577.

Commentary from Westminster, *Lancet*, February 12, 1977, p. 377.

STRESS

Enter Mr Harold Buck

HUNTER: Mr Buck, you are an English general surgeon? Perhaps, as most of those in the courthouse are American, I should explain that in the United Kingdom surgeons, however well qualified, are invariably addressed as 'Mister', not 'Doctor'. An old tradition. I want to deal first, Mr Buck, with the different types of modern stress, and with their psychosomatic and psychoneurotic consequences. Do you think stress important in the production of disease?

BUCK: Of some importance. I see the end result of it fairly often in my practice.

HUNTER: Is there more stress today than in the past?

BUCK: No, that is in my view a fallacy. Famine, plague, war – man has always had stresses to cope with. In many ways twentieth-century man is much *less* subject to stress than his forbears. He leads a relatively easy, protected life.

HUNTER: Stress is not particularly oppressive today? And it isn't of overwhelming importance in causing disease?

BUCK: That is my position.

HUNTER: But there are types of stress peculiar to our time? (*Buck nods*) Such as?

BUCK: Oh, the general rush and bustle of life.

HUNTER: More specifically, mechanical sources of stress, say? – The motor car, the plane, the bulldozer, the road drill, the big factory machine?

BUCK: Well, yes – though I don't see the motor car as such a big source of stress.

HUNTER: Accidents are the most common cause of death of people under the age of 40 in all western countries, and car accidents are the most common kind of accident? (*Buck nods*) Awareness of the possibility of sustaining or causing death might be construed as a source of stress?

BUCK: Obviously.

HUNTER: And are you aware that car driving can raise the pulse rate to as high as 200 beats per minute in the case of racing-car drivers, and 140 in the case of ordinary drivers?[1] And that in the case of the racing drivers there are also marked increases in the levels in the blood of adrenalins – to as much as 20 times the normal value[1] – and of certain fatty substances,[1,2] which, it is suggested,[2] might be involved in the development of the atheroma present in coronary heart disease? And that speaking in public has a similar effect and also produces clear abnormal changes in the electrical activity of the heart as well as a pulse rate up to 180?[3]

BUCK: Public speaking is not a common activity, Mr Hunter, or peculiar to our time.

HUNTER: But car driving is? And a rapid pulse rate is the same, and probably has the same effects in a person who is immobile, however it is caused?

BUCK: Possibly.

HUNTER: The normal pulse rate is 72 beats a minute, give or take 10 beats or so? (*Buck nods*) Therefore it is doubled or trebled in car driving or in public speaking?

BUCK: So it is if one takes very vigorous exercise.

HUNTER: But do you see no difference between the heart pounding away very fast if a man is running – say, from a wolf or a tiger, as he once commonly did – and when a man is sitting in a comfortable seat in a car or standing, addressing an audience.

BUCK: Obviously there is some difference.

HUNTER: I am relieved to hear it – because the *absence*, as a result of exercise, of the abnormal changes in the heart's electrical activity that *do* occur in public speaking, has been demonstrated.[4] One might reasonably expect the *presence* of those changes to be associated with deleterious effects on a person's body if the changes were often repeated?

BUCK: Yes, quite probably.

HUNTER: Did you know that aeroplane pilots have during a flight a marked increase in the amount of one kind of adrenalin in their blood,[5] and that the pulse rate of pilots may rise to double its normal value at take-off and landing?[6] And that certain changes in the blood and urine are detectable for as long as two days after a flight?[5] And something similar happens to plane passengers?[5]

BUCK: I have read all this. Myself, I sit back and look at the newspaper.

HUNTER: You are not suggesting the pilot should do the same? (*Pause*) It has been said that man has a stone-age body with all its stone-age responses in modern stressful circumstances where those responses can find no outlet.[7] You would not dissent? Today the responses are often quite inappropriate and are internalized? In other words, the bracing of the whole body that was needed to run away from the wolf or the murderous neighbor, or to turn and fight them – this occurs today but finds no outlet.

BUCK: Every age has its stresses, Mr Hunter. We have to live with the motor car and the plane.

HUNTER: Would you agree that today, as well as 'mechanical' forms of stress, we have what might be called 'alienating' forms of stress that are peculiar to our time? – The dehumanization, the sense of strangeness implicit in our wealth of gadgets, in computers or atomic power stations or motorways, or in large impersonal corporations or huge public utility companies, or in, say, the underground systems or the airports at large cities?

BUCK: I think that's a bit far-fetched myself.

HUNTER: Have you ever done battle with a computer, Mr Buck? You did not find it frustrating, a source of resentment and even anger?

BUCK: Oh, one has to learn to live with these things.

HUNTER: Have you ever learned to live with a nuclear power station down the road? Or with Concorde going over your head twice a day?

BUCK: No, neither have most people.

HUNTER: Do you know the subway stations at Times Square in New York, or at Oxford Circus in London? – They are not sources of stress at rush-hour periods for those tens of thousands who use them?

BUCK: Yes, but there are troubles in everyone's life.

HUNTER: Do you use any London underground station regularly in the rush hours?

BUCK: No.

HUNTER: It is easy – is it not? – to be philosophical about other people's stress, and distress?

BUCK: A doctor cannot afford to take all his patients' troubles to heart, Mr Hunter. I imagine the same applies to lawyers. You asked a straight question, and I gave you a straight answer.

HUNTER: Medicine itself causes stress, does it not? – For instance, your operating theater, Mr Buck – or operating room as they say here in the States – is, I imagine, full of instruments and machines and gadgets; all, I'm sure, very necessary. But do you not think that some of the patients who enter the theater conscious must be frightened, distressed, even terrified, however mistakenly, by what they see and hear?

BUCK: My team of nurses and doctors and I myself do everything we can to reassure any conscious patients. No, I do not think any substantial proportion is made afraid in the theater.

HUNTER: Do you think most people would be made afraid by waking, fully conscious but paralyzed, during an operation?

BUCK: Yes, but that is an extremely rare phenomenon.

HUNTER: I have here the issue of the *Journal of the American Medical Association* for March 22, 1976, in which, following the appearance in that journal of an earlier paper[8] reporting on six such patients, there were letters[9, 10, 11] from three readers reporting the same experience of being awake and paralyzed in the operating theater, two of the three being doctors; and in only one case was there any kind of medical 'excuse' for what had happened. The paralysis is commonly due, of course, to the curare-like muscle relaxants often used in anesthesia today. Well, Mr Buck?

BUCK: I have already said it is extremely rare. The tens of thousands who do not have such an experience do *not* write to any journal to say so.

HUNTER: As compared with an operating theater, there is an equal or greater plethora of gadgetry in an intensive care unit or a coronary care unit? (*Buck nods*) Do you accept that some doctors believe patients in such units *are* often afraid, that some of them may even be literally frightened to death? (*Pause*) Do you wish me to quote the doctors who have expressed that view? – I have some relevant papers[12, 13] here, in particular one[13] entitled 'Emotional Stresses of Patient-Physician Encounters'.

BUCK: I accept what you say, but it is like news – only bad news gets reported.

HUNTER: For every patient who dies of fright there may be ten – twenty – who suffer agonies of mind without dying? I have said all that about medicine, Mr Buck, to show that doctors themselves – I am sure unwittingly – sometimes inflict stress, and so are perhaps inured to its presence in their patients' lives.

BUCK: We are not all as indifferent to suffering as you imply, Mr Hunter. I will say no more.

HUNTER: There is something of a social element to the second kind of stress I mentioned, the alienating kind? (*Buck nods*) But will you accept that there is a more narrowly defined kind of social stress? – As from, say, unemployment or fear of it, bad housing, unsatisfying work, marital trouble, and so on? – Psychosocial factors, as they are called.

BUCK: Such things have existed in every country in every age.

HUNTER: Would you say then, for instance, that what is called the rat race and all that goes with it – the lust for status, power, and money, the jealousy and scheming and trickery – would you say *that* has always existed?

BUCK: In one form or another, yes.

HUNTER: As intensely, to fill the whole of life? (*Pause*) And has any age but ours lacked the support, the easement that can be provided by religion, by neighbors, by the extended family? Has any age been quite so nakedly ruthless in its lust for material possessions?

BUCK: I am sorry to disappoint you; I think probably other ages have been as bad, at least in that last respect.

HUNTER: Well, let us move on now to the effects of stress. You will accept that it may have a directly adverse effect? – For instance, physical stress (excessive heat, say, or prolonged loud noise) may directly produce physical disease or damage in the body? Or social stress – due to poverty, for instance – may have a readily comprehensible effect via malnourishment or exposure to cold? (*Buck nods*) But stress most commonly acts by arousing emotions of anger, fear, resentment, apprehension, and so on, which, if prolonged, may result in physical disease? The changes in various bodily mechanisms produced by the emotions I mention and that might be expected to result in physical disease are known and have been carefully investigated? Or stress may produce mental disease on occasion – chronic states of depression, anxiety, and so on? Or perhaps both? (*Buck nods*) And would you agree that sometimes the main factor in setting off such changes is not so much stress of an overwhelming immediate kind as the mental make-up of the recipient of the stress which may have been inherited or have had its origin in some earlier stress, perhaps in childhood?

BUCK: You mean over-emotional people, neurotics?

HUNTER: There is a note of disdain in your voice.

BUCK: I am sorry you should think so.

HUNTER: Is it because you do not understand such people, and so are afraid of them? Or because you fear that inside every surgeon there is a neurotic trying to get out?

BUCK: If so, you will not induce one to come out of me.

HUNTER: Do most doctors share your view of neurotic or over-emotional patients, or of those with social problems?

BUCK: Most doctors get on with their job of helping individual people, Mr Hunter, as best they can.

HUNTER: There is some evidence on this matter. Do you know what self poisoning is? Would you care to define it briefly for the court?

BUCK: It describes the act of someone, usually a young person who, because he or she, though most of them are female, has some kind of personal emotional problem – a psychosocial stress factor, you would call it – takes a dose of tablets, often aspirin or sleeping tablets, and usually short of a lethal dose in the hope that a hospital will see to it that death does not result but that the shock involved will induce repentance in the boy friend, or the parents, or whomever it is, and ensure that in future they will do whatever it may be the young lady concerned wants them to do. It is a form of emotional blackmail. It has become very common in this country in the last 10 or 15 years.

HUNTER: Will you accept that one recent study showed that 44 percent of junior doctors and 25 percent of senior doctors in a hospital felt hostility towards such patients whereas there were none who felt hostility towards patients admitted with coronary heart disease?[14]

BUCK: I understand their attitude even though I do not share it.

HUNTER: You are aware that doctors and many lay people know that two of the three main risk factors for coronary heart disease are indulgence in cigarettes and indulgence in certain types of food?

BUCK: Yes, but it is a very long-term process.

HUNTER: Long-lived self-indulgence is less culpable than the short-lived kind? (*Pause*) And do you know that self-poisoning patients are discharged as soon as possible, and that it has been suggested that a failure by a doctor to deal properly with such patients may result in them having a second try and killing themselves?[15,16]

BUCK: That is to be deeply regretted, of course; but if people are determined to tread an emotional tightrope. . . .

HUNTER: Would it disturb you at all, Mr Buck, to know that two thirds of suicides have visited their general practitioners during the month before death, and that the drugs used by 80 percent of persons attempting suicide with drugs have been prescribed by doctors?[17]

BUCK: It is not always easy to tell when a person is suicidal. And a person who is determined to end his life will always find some way. And as doctors are almost the only source of powerful drugs it is inevitable that those who take their lives with drugs will nearly always have got them from doctors. It does not mean that doctors are negligent.

HUNTER: The court may or may not be convinced of that, Mr Buck. However, perhaps I can now revert to the main theme. There is a range of psychosocial stress factors, perhaps present in a neurotic personality, sometimes even overshadowed altogether by it, that can in the long term produce bodily diseases, and these are known as psychosomatic disorders. For instance, coronary heart disease, a raised blood pressure, asthma, migraine, ulcerative colitis, duodenal ulceration, some skin conditions, some women's complaints, obesity, many types of headache – all of these are psychosomatic?

BUCK: True, though some of them are only partly psychosomatic; and that element is not usually of great relevance by the time the patient gets into the hands of a doctor, especially a surgeon like myself. By then the disease is established – a physical disease needing physical treatment very often, perhaps an operation.

HUNTER: Is that not a strong argument for doctors to pay more attention to any psychosocial factors at an earlier stage?

BUCK: Many family doctors do so; but the patient often does not visit the doctor in the early stages. And it might not be very healthy if it were the normal thing for a person to run to a doctor with every little trouble. Most troubles don't end in disease. And some doctors – community physicians, health educators, and so on – do give a lot of attention to psychosocial factors on a broader front, to the extent that they can, and mostly behind the scenes, not face-to-face with individual patients.

HUNTER: And not in any radical way? And there are not many of them? And they are rather looked down on by their fellow doctors? (*Pause*) The real business of doctors is the diseased body? – Or for a few the diseased mind? Never the diseased society that makes people ill?

BUCK: Society isn't responsible for all illnesses. There are such things as bacteria, Mr Hunter.

HUNTER: But it is society that may allow sewage to seep into a drinking water supply and so enable some bacteria to cause disease? Or that may let people go hungry with the result that their bodies cannot resist bacteria? (*Pause*) I take it you would not agree with the Edinburgh professor who wrote, 'It is encumbent on every doctor to take some account of every variable which might influence his patient's distress and then to respond to his real needs. Sadly, so often the psychosocial ones are neglected. . . .'[18]

BUCK: I agree with him, but I have only so much time. I can operate fairly quickly on a duodenal ulcer, Mr Hunter. I cannot operate at all on stress or psychosocial factors. I am not a sociologist or a politician.

HUNTER: Though some surgeons do *operate* for anxiety and tension – distress, in other words – in psychiatric patients, do they not? They destroy a small part of the brain by inserting a fine electrode, and coagulating the brain tissue?[19]

BUCK: And it is sometimes an effective procedure. That is within my province. To alter people's whole lives is not. Doctors are devoted to the relief of individual suffering; they are not revolutionaries.

JUDGE: Apart, of course, from Dr Ché Guevara, Dr Allende of Chile, and so on. The late Dr Guevara, the late Dr Allende . . . Are you saying, Mr Buck, that doctors do not have time to attend to psychosocial factors or that to do so is not really their concern?

BUCK: It is their concern only in part, judge. Certainly we do not now have the time; and I am doubtful, if we did have it, just how successful we should be.

HUNTER: Will you accept, Mr Buck, that an illness, as well as being caused or worsened by psychosocial factors, may have psychosocial consequences – loss of a job and so on, which may maintain the illness, as may the original factors if they persist; and that all of these need attention too?

BUCK: Yes, and again we do what we can, but we cannot perform miracles.

HUNTER: And that psychosocial factors play *some* part in causing and maintaining *most* diseases?

BUCK: Many diseases, yes – lung cancer, for instance, or a cancer of the cervix, which is more common in women who start sexual activity early. But they still need a physical treatment by the time they reach doctors like myself.

HUNTER: But there is, in other words, a huge field that doctors, for whatever reason, have tended to neglect? (*Pause*) Is the treatment doctors actually give to psychosomatic or psychoneurotic complaints very successful?

BUCK: Sometimes. We can nearly always provide relief of symptoms.

HUNTER: Does it commonly include the use of tranquilizers to relieve the tension and anxiety – hyperarousal, I think, is the medical term – associated with these conditions, and sleeping tablets to relieve insomnia? And antidepressive drugs?

BUCK: Yes, not infrequently.

HUNTER: Do you know how many prescriptions for such drugs were issued in England alone in 1973? – I can tell you: it was 45,000,000.[20] In the United States in 1972 it was 144,000,000.[21] And some were doubtless for people with psychosocial problems, the earliest stages of what may in time become psychosomatic disorders or psychoneuroses? (*Pause*) And are these very drugs, when they fail to provide any real relief, not used in the self-poisoning that many doctors find so distasteful?

BUCK: Yes, I see your point; but the vast majority of those receiving these drugs do not use them for self-poisoning. They get relief from them, some kind of relief.

HUNTER: But are doctors not saying to patients, when they prescribe in that way, that they have to put up with the stress and the bad social conditions that often produce it – unemployment, bad housing, poor education – instead of perhaps fighting to change them? Are the doctors not acting as agents of the established order?

BUCK: We do what we think best for our individual patients. You will be suggesting next that we are government agents.

HUNTER: That, Mr Buck, is what I am suggesting.

BUCK: I must look more closely at my next pay check.

HUNTER: Mr Buck, in your view which are the most widely-read, general medical journals in the English-speaking world?

BUCK: The *Lancet,* the *British Medical Journal,* the *Journal of the American Medical Association,* and the *New England Journal of Medicine.* Two of them are probably also the best general medical journals in the world.

HUNTER: Will you accept that in the year 1975 these four journals published between them about 1500 original articles and 1000 leading articles? (*Buck nods*) Will you also accept that with the solitary exception of the *Lancet* not one of them, according to their indices, had a single item of any kind on the subject of psychosomatic disorders in that year? – Not that the *Lancet* was anything to write home about in this regard: it had one letter on the topic and one review of a book on it. I have the 1975 journal indices here if you wish to check my statement.

BUCK: I accept it.

HUNTER: So that your lack of any deep interest in the causes of psychosomatic disorders seems to be common in the profession? (*Pause*) I now want to move on to some related topics. As well as with disease, physical or mental, people can react to stress by taking cigarettes, alcohol, or drugs? Though there are often, of course, other elements than stress involved.

BUCK: I know some doctors say one common reason for cigarette smoking is to relieve anxiety and tension, and another is to 'pep' oneself up so that one is better able to deal with stress.[22] But there are always plenty of theories on why people smoke.

HUNTER: There is also a large number of deaths due to cigarette smoking? It causes or helps to cause coronary heart disease, lung cancer, chronic bronchitis, emphysema, and so on, does it not? Do you know how many deaths cigarettes cause? Will you accept about 100,000 a year in the United Kingdom, of which 25,000 are premature deaths[23] – that is, deaths of people in the prime of life – and a total of well over 300,000 deaths a year in the United States?

BUCK: Yes, but this is one field in which you can't criticize doctors. In both those countries more than half the doctors who used to smoke cigarettes have given them up.

HUNTER: To set a good example to other people?

BUCK: I've no doubt their motives were mixed, as people's motives usually are.

HUNTER: There has been a substantial drop in cigarette smoking among other men in social class I? And it has been shown at one British university that the proportion of medical students who smoke cigarettes is no smaller than the proportion of other science students who don't?[24]

BUCK: Correct; and I am much more pleased by the fact that many other people are giving up cigarettes than put out by the fact that doctors are not as unusual in this respect as we used to think.

HUNTER: There is evidence that less than half the students at one medical school could remember being warned against cigarette smoking by the staff.[23] And how many anti-smoking clinics are doctors running in the United Kingdom now? Will you accept that there are hardly any?

BUCK: Because the results from them were very poor.

HUNTER: But how much research have doctors put into methods of helping people to stop smoking? As much as into proving beyond a doubt that smoking did cause certain diseases? Is not the reason that the latter was an interesting prestigious topic for research whereas the other is not?

BUCK: That is an unworthy suggestion, Mr Hunter.

HUNTER: I have here a copy of the *Lancet* for April 17, 1976, containing an article[25] dealing with Specialized Centers of Research – or SCORs – here in the United States, and the large sums of government money they attract. It describes how 'millions of dollars are being spent by SCORs in the name of early diagnosis, especially in regard to those diseases characterized by airways obstruction': that is, I think – but correct me if I am wrong – diseases often caused by cigarette smoking. The article says that 'Such expenditures take place despite all the currently available evidence suggesting that early diagnosis makes not one scrap of difference to survival-time. . . . The ingenuity that goes into constructing the gadgets used for early detection is awesome. . . . Were all the ingenuity and money that are being invested in SCORs dedicated to finding out why people start smoking, and how to persuade them to stop, then something tangible and worthwhile might result.' Do you still think my suggestion was unworthy? (*Pause*) And is it not a fact that for some years the British Medical Research Council received practically no applications at all for grants in connection with research into the cigarette habit? (*Pause*) Tell me, Mr Buck, is it more impressive that thousands of doctors in this country and in Britain have given up cigarettes or that thousands of them are still smoking?

BUCK: Oh, you get black sheep in every profession. Doctors have been in the forefront of all anti-cigarette propaganda.

HUNTER: Have they ever marched in white coats through the streets of New York or London to demand an end to all cigarette advertising?

BUCK: That is not the kind of thing . . .

HUNTER: Yes, do go on. (*Pause*) Were you not going to say that it is not the kind of thing respectable doctors could be expected to do? But they have done it, have they not, Mr Buck, in the United

Kingdom? – To demand better pay for themselves? And they have gone on strike or partial strike – have they not – for the same purpose? And they have acted similarly here in the United States for more money for themselves and in West Germany, and in Italy, and ... need I continue? (*Pause*) As to the effectiveness of doctors' propaganda against cigarettes, I have some figures here for total tobacco consumption per adult: for this country they are 11 pounds in 1963 and 9.2 pounds in 1973; and for the United Kingdom in those years 6.6 pounds and 6.2 pounds respectively.[26] An improvement, but hardly a dramatic one in the UK?

BUCK: An improvement.

HUNTER: But one that the doctors of Switzerland, West Germany, France, Italy, the Netherlands, Belgium, and Norway – to mention a few countries – have not been able to achieve for *their* populations. You will accept that in each of those countries between 1963 and 1973 consumption of tobacco per adult – on average, that is – went up, as did the number of cigarettes consumed per adult?[26] (*Buck nods*) So any success western doctors have had one might describe as patchy? (*Pause*) Now alcohol, Mr Buck, another response to stress: it has been said that to a doctor an alcoholic is someone who drinks more than himself.

BUCK: Nobody likes to label a person an alcoholic.

HUNTER: I thought doctors were agreed that alcoholism was a disease, not a moral fault. An official family doctor estimate of the number of alcoholics in England and Wales some years ago was 10,000,[27] whereas other estimates suggested the real figure at that time was at least 200,000.[27] What other common chronic disease is there the diagnosis of which is missed 19 times out of 20 by family doctors?

BUCK: None, but most people want to have their illnesses diagnosed. The alcoholic doesn't – he's expert at keeping away from doctors, and, if he does come up against one, at concealing his weakness. And then alcoholism still carries a stigma in the eyes of lay people.

HUNTER: You don't think the real reason is that to drink alcohol is a socially accepted custom, and that doctors are great social conformers?

BUCK: Another way of putting it would be to say they are good citizens.

HUNTER: The management of alcoholism involves dealing with a number of social and psychological factors, does it not? And until recently doctors had not been trained to do that – had they? And they have no natural gift for it, or interest in it? They tend to shy away from it.[28] Alcoholics Anonymous, a lay organization, is much better at it than doctors, would you not agree?[29]

BUCK: One of the two founders of Alcoholics Anonymous was a doctor.

HUNTER: Why not both? Are you aware that 39 percent of senior *psychiatrists* and 44 percent of junior psychiatrists were reported in one British study[30] to take an unfavorable attitude towards alcoholism? A higher proportion than for any other condition surveyed except drug dependence. And that they believe the proportion of general practitioners who take an unfavorable attitude is much the same, and of general physicians and surgeons is very much higher – around 80 percent of general surgeons, they were reported to believe, take an unfavorable attitude to alcoholism.

BUCK: Alcoholics can be infuriating people to deal with. That is probably the main reason why doctors feel about them as they do. You are not a doctor, Mr Hunter. It is easy to moralize about something you have not experienced.

HUNTER: But doctors are supposed to be above that sort of thing? No? There has been an increase of alcoholism and offences associated with alcohol in various western countries during the last 25 years? The alcoholism of affluence, to which I am suggesting doctors have shown an inadequate response. Perhaps you will accept that there are now some millions of alcoholics here in the United States, and about 500,000 in Britain, where consumption of alcohol per head is now higher than it has been for 60 years.

BUCK: Yes, but that is not a purely medical problem. It is a malaise of society. Doctors cannot be expected to provide a complete answer.

HUNTER: Cirrhosis of the liver is due to alcohol? (*Buck nods*) How many deaths does it cause each year in the United Kingdom?

BUCK: Around 2,000, I think.

HUNTER: And alcohol causes many thousands more deaths, directly or indirectly, including road-accident deaths? (*Buck nods*) Tell me: how many thousand deaths does cannabis cause each year?

BUCK: Hardly any, but it causes harm in other ways.

HUNTER: How many people use cannabis regularly? Certainly far fewer than the number who take alcoholic drinks regularly? (*Buck nods*) Why then are doctors so ready to condemn cannabis? Why have they put such great efforts into trying to find out what harm it may do to people?

BUCK: The fact that one drug that can do harm – alcohol – is freely available does not mean we should let another drug become freely available even though it may do less harm. In regard to cannabis doctors are simply showing their traditional attitude of caution towards drugs.

HUNTER: Such as they showed towards thalidomide? Or chloramphenicol or tetracyclines? Or amphetamines and barbiturates? – Which we heard about yesterday. A few years ago there were some 80,000 people in the United Kingdom alone dependent on prescribed amphetamines, and more recently some 100,000 dependent on prescribed barbiturates.

BUCK: Lamentable figures, I agree; but doctors in the United Kingdom have reacted to them so that the prescribing of amphetamines and barbiturates is now very much less.

HUNTER: After some years of inactivity?

BUCK: I regret to have to say 'Yes'.

HUNTER: In fact, doctors are not very concerned about drug dependence – are they? – so long as *they* have prescribed the drug or when the drug, as in the case of alcohol, is widely used legally and by themselves; but they are strongly opposed to lay people, especially the younger ones, having access to other drugs affecting the mind, no matter how harmless. Is that not the position?

BUCK: Cannabis is not a harmless substance.

HUNTER: But it is not as harmful as alcohol or barbiturates, and probably not as harmful as amphetamines? (*Buck nods*) Is not all this yet another example of the doctors' inability to face up to psychosocial problems? Are they not schizophrenic about cannabis *vis-à-vis* other drugs affecting the mind? (*Pause*) I have here the *Lancet* of August 4, 1974, and I am going to read an extract from an article[28] on page 453: 'There is unfortunately a certain amount of evidence that many doctors simply do not want to know about the patient as a person: they would on the whole prefer it if they could study and treat the pathological process in, say, the heart or the liver without having to have those organs lodged in a human frame. As the Army has technical exercises without troops, so we might have clinical medicine without patients.' Well, Mr Buck?

BUCK: That is not the sort of clinical medicine I practice, Mr Hunter; and I am not unique in my profession.

HUNTER: Well, finally, even though you do not think stress any more common today than in previous times, you would at least agree that the use of sedatives and tranquilizers for stress disorders is peculiar to our time?

BUCK: Obviously. They're a typical product of our western industrial society.

HUNTER: And the same could be said about cigarettes.

BUCK: Yes.

HUNTER: One has to see all things in their context?

BUCK: Yes, including doctors, Mr Hunter. And the context is not a black-and-white one.

HUNTER: Thank you, Mr Buck. (*Sits*)

JUDGE: Mr Buck, I wonder if there is anything you might like to add? No? Then I have something to say to you from which I think Mr Hunter, your – er – brother under the skin, would not dissent. You have undergone a long and difficult, though I think always fair, cross-examination. I should like to say that everyone in this court must be aware that there are many occasions in life when we are only too happy to put ourselves in the hands of doctors: for instance, if we sustain a fracture or a wound; or if we – our wives or daughters – are going to have a baby; or if we have a fever or a sudden severe pain or some condition obviously calling for surgical skill. I am not prejudging the issue; but the fact that the profession might be found to have made mistakes on occasion does not mean that it stands totally condemned. Its members are human beings. There is certainly a good deal to be set in the balance in the profession's favor; and tomorrow we shall resume our consideration of any counterbalancing arguments. This court is now adjourned.

REFERENCES—SESSION SIX
1. Taggart, P., Gibbons, D., and Somerville, W., *BMJ*, October 18, 1969, p. 130.
2. Taggart, P., and Carruthers, M., *Lancet*, February 20, 1971, p. 363.
3. Taggart, P., Carruthers, M., and Somerville, W., *Lancet*, August 18, 1973, p. 34.
4. Taggart, P., Parkinson, P., and Carruthers, M., *BMJ*, July 8, 1972, p. 71.
5. Carruthers, M., Arguelles, A. E., and Mosovich, A., *Lancet*, May 8, 1976, p. 977.
6. Carruthers, M., *Lancet*, May 12, 1973, p. 1048.
7. Carruthers, M., *Proceedings of the Royal Society of Medicine*, July 1973, p. 429.
8. Blacher, R. S., *JAMA*, October 6, 1975, p. 67.
9. Silbergleit, I.-L., *JAMA*, March 22, 1976, p. 1209.
10. Michael, R., *JAMA*, March 22, 1976, p. 1210.
11. Archer, J., *JAMA*, March 22, 1976, p. 1211.
12. Baxter, S., *British Journal of Hospital Medicine*, June 1974, p. 875.
13. Editorial, *JAMA*, February 26, 1973, p. 1037.
14. Patel, A. R., *BMJ*, May 24, 1975, p. 426.
15. Leading Article, *BMJ*, September 13, 1969, p. 610.
16. Leading Article, *BMJ*, February 20, 1971, p. 419.
17. Birtchnell, J., *BMJ*, July 26, 1975, p. 230.
18. Aitken, R. C. H., *BMJ*, March 15, 1975, p. 611.
19. Laitinen, L. V., *Lancet*, February 26, 1972, p. 472.
20. *Medicines Which Affect the Mind*, Office of Health Economics, London, 1975, p. 19.
21. Blackwell, B., *JAMA*, September 24, 1973, p. 1637.
22. Russell, M. A. H., *Practitioner*, June 1974, p. 791.
23. *Smoking or Health*, Royal College of Physicians, London, 1977.

24. Brunskill, A. J., *BMJ*, January 15, 1977, p. 165.
25. Round the World, *Lancet*, April 17, 1976, p. 852.
26. Lee, P. N. (ed.), *Tobacco Consumption in Various Countries*, 4th edn, Tobacco Research Council, London, 1975.
27. *Alcohol Abuse*, Office of Health Economics, London, 1970.
28. Bennet, G., *Lancet*, August 24, 1974, p. 453.
29. Glatt, M. M., *Lancet*, February 22, 1975, p. 447.
30. Macdonald, E. B., and Patel, A. R., *BMJ*, May 24, 1975, p. 430.

Self-Poisoning
Leading Article, *Lancet*, March 8, 1969, p. 598.
Patel, A. R., Roy, M., and Wilson, G. M., *Lancet*, November 25, 1972, p. 1099.
Smith, A. J., *BMJ*, October 21, 1972, p. 157.
Alderson, M. R., *Lancet*, May 25, 1974, p. 1040.
Rosen, D. H., *JAMA*, May 10, 1976, p. 2105.

Alcoholism
Committee on Alcoholism and Drug Dependence, *JAMA*, May 10, 1971, p. 1011.
Evans, M., *Practitioner*, June 1974, p. 801.
Ritson, E. B., *BMJ*, April 19, 1975, p. 124.
Editorial, *NEJM*, October 2, 1975, p. 719.

Psychosocial Factors in Disease, etc., and Doctors' Attitudes
Morris, J. N., *Proceedings of the Royal Society of Medicine*, March 1973, p. 225.
Boyd, P., *Proceedings of the Royal Society of Medicine*, September 1975, p. 566.
Leading Article, *BMJ*, September 29, 1973, p. 653.

Psychosomatic Disorders
Munro, A., *Practitioner*, January 1972, p. 162.
MacCulloch, M. J., *Practitioner*, May 1972, p. 704.
Morgan, D., *Practitioner*, July 1972, p. 114.
(These last three papers figured in a 1972 *Practitioner* series of papers on psychosomatic medicine.)
Brown, J. J., *et al.*, *Lancet*, June 5, 1976, p. 1217.
Editorial, *Lancet*, May 21, 1977, p. 1089.

PATTERNS OF ILLNESS AND OF REMEDIES

JUDGE: This is the last of the seven sessions that constitute the first of the three parts of our enquiry. In the first session we heard of mistakes that doctors had made in the past. In the next five sessions we heard, among much else, of mistakes that they are allegedly making today in relation to a variety of modern diseases and treatments. The present session is important because in it we are to take a wider view of the health scene, and of the position of doctors in it; and I shall myself begin the questioning of today's witness.

Enter Professor James Larkin

You are James Larkin, a Canadian Professor of Social Medicine? What is social medicine, professor?

LARKIN: It is the branch of medicine that deals, not with individual patients and their individual aches and pains, but with populations, with the broad picture of disease in them, with what causes the diseases, what prevents them, and so on. With health and disease in the community.

JUDGE: And where have these topics been most carefully studied?

LARKIN: England and Wales, undoubtedly.

JUDGE: And are England and Wales fairly representative in health matters of the western world generally? (*Larkin nods*) Well then, would you say their population is a healthy one? Healthier than other populations?

LARKIN: If you mean physically healthier, judge, than the population of, say, a medieval European country, then the answer is certainly 'Yes' in most respects. If you mean physically healthier than the English and Welsh population a century ago, then again the answer is certainly 'Yes'. If you mean physically heathier than the people of other western countries today, then the answer is 'No' in some cases, 'Yes' in others – though the differences are not great. If you mean mentally healthier than those in underdeveloped countries, then my personal answer is 'No'. But physically healthier? Oh, yes.

JUDGE: Which western countries are healthier than England and Wales?

LARKIN: If one uses what one might call, after their compiler, the Maxwell figures[1] – published by McKinsey and Co., Inc., the American management consultant firm, in 1975 – if one uses the Maxwell amalgam of mortality rates at various periods of life (that is, the death rates of infants, of mothers in connection with child-

birth, of middle-aged men, and so on), then Sweden, the Netherlands, Norway, and Switzerland are clearly ahead of England and
Wales; while in turn England and Wales are just about level with
Denmark, and Japan, and Finland; ahead of France, Spain, Italy,
and West Germany; and well ahead of the United States.

JUDGE: But does the United States not spend relatively more on
health than any other country?

LARKIN: It does, judge: since 1971 it has been spending more on
health than on defense,[2] and in the 1966–76 decade it spent as
much on health as in the previous 35 years.[2] But health does not
always go hand in hand with expenditure on health. By these
widely accepted Maxwell criteria of health the United States is
next to last in the western league: below, not merely England and
Wales, but below Austria, Luxembourg, Ireland, and Belgium –
to mention just a few. Only Portugal, of 22 western nations, is
below the USA. And yet American health expenditure per head
is about three times that of Italy or of Ireland, and about twice that
of Germany or France.[1] And even as a proportion of the gross
national product American expenditure on health is the highest.

JUDGE: But the United States – all western countries – are healthier
than underdeveloped countries?

LARKIN: Physically healthier – yes, in a majority of respects.

JUDGE: If the health of western countries does not vary with their
health expenditures, does it vary with their relative numbers of
doctors?

LARKIN: No, judge, it isn't really possible, as between one western
country and another, to link the health of the people with the concentration of doctors.[1] The two just do not go together. There is
an apparent connection when the density of doctors is low, as in
underdeveloped countries; but even there the link is probably not
a direct one. It's just that, if a country is not materially prosperous,
its people are usually, for various reasons, not physically very
healthy either, and, again for various though different reasons, it
doesn't produce or attract many doctors. But one shouldn't jump
to the conclusion that doctors lead to health, or a lack of doctors
leads to ill-health.

JUDGE: If England and Wales are fairly healthy and are fairly
typical of the western world, when did they start to acquire this
health they have?

LARKIN: Roughly in the 1850–60 period. Physical health we are
talking about. There was a steady improvement between then and
the mid-1930s, and an accelerated rate of improvement between
the mid-1930s and the mid- or late 1950s. Since then there hasn't
been much change.

JUDGE: By 'improvement' meaning?

LARKIN: First, that the expectation of life increased. In 1870 the average expectation of life of a boy baby in your country was only about 40 years; by 1910 it was about 50; and by 1950 it was about 66 years. A baby girl had a greater expectation of life throughout this period: in 1950, for instance, *her* expectation of life was 72 years.

JUDGE: And secondly?

LARKIN: Deaths from certain diseases have become less common – which, of course, accounts for the increased expectation of life at birth – particularly deaths from infectious diseases like typhoid and cholera and, above all, tuberculosis. In general, it was infants, children, and younger people who died from these more than older people, and so it was they who mostly showed the benefits; infants later than children and young people. Life expectancy for the middle-aged westerner, in fact, especially for the middle-aged man, hasn't improved all that much in the last 100 years. If you got through to middle age a century ago your chance of living to be 70 or 80 wasn't so much worse than today. This was partly because older people did not benefit greatly from the drop in infectious-disease deaths, partly because some relatively new diseases have appeared in the last fifty years, especially coronary heart disease and lung and other cancers.

JUDGE: And also the other twentieth-century diseases we have been hearing about all this week? (*Larkin nods*) You said there was a slow, steady improvement in health until the mid-1930s?

LARKIN: Yes but, although it was relatively *slow*, much more of the actual improvement in health and in life expectancy of the last hundred years or so had been secured by then than has been secured since. There was a greatly accelerated *rate* of improvement between the mid-1930s and the late 1950s, but the actual improvement secured was not so great in quantity during that later period.

JUDGE: And why should there have been an accelerating rate since the mid-1930s?

LARKIN: Because it was roughly from then on that many life-saving drugs were quickly discovered, and various vaccines began to be used.

JUDGE: Prescribed by doctors?

LARKIN: Yes, but nearly all discovered or developed by the drug industry. It doesn't call for any great expertise to give a vaccine, or to know when an antibiotic really *is* needed – even though, as Professor Hecht said, antibiotics are often prescribed for people who don't need them.

JUDGE: The doctors deserve little credit?

LARKIN: They deserve some – but certainly not the biggest part – of the credit. And in any case, as I said, most of the improvement in health had been secured previously.

JUDGE: Well, and to what extent had doctors played a key role in that earlier phase?

LARKIN: To only a limited extent. The improvement in health secured between about 1860 and the mid-1930s, and to some extent beyond, was due mainly to improvements in nutrition, sanitation – pure water supplies, for instance – hygiene, housing, and so on, and also to a smaller family size. Food and sanitation were probably the main factors.

JUDGE: And, if not due to the doctors, these improvements were mostly due to?

LARKIN: To the increasing material wealth of our industrial society; and to all kinds of people, engineers, scientists, teachers, central and local government personnel, as well as public-health doctors, farmers, builders, and politicians – who helped to shape a gradual social improvement based on prosperity, and with a corresponding gradual improvement in health. The doctors advised on the medical aspects, of course, and they staffed and were important in the setting up of special clinics, school health services, and so on; but these latter played only a minor part in the total process.

JUDGE: Can you quote any supporting evidence for this?

LARKIN: Yes – a study[3] of the life span of Italian Renaissance artists. They were chosen for study simply because there were good records of their life spans. It was found that their usual age at death was over 60 – pretty well the expectation of life for the average baby in this country in about 1930. Why? – Because the artists lived with wealthy patrons who, in Renaissance Italy, had good hygiene, good sanitation, good food, and so on. What they didn't have was modern medicine of any kind.

JUDGE: Is the view you have propounded now the orthodox medical view?

LARKIN: It is the orthodox view among various experts in social medicine – or public health, as it used to be known. Lay people and even many doctors don't appreciate it. For instance, you will find some otherwise very well-informed doctors – pure clinicians – saying that tuberculosis was conquered by the introduction in the late 1940s of the anti-tuberculous drugs. Now this is just not true. By the late 1940s the death rate from tuberculosis among young people (aged between 15 and 45, that is) was about a tenth of what it had been in 1870. It is certainly true that the remaining deaths were very quickly eliminated with the help of the new drugs; but *most* of the improvement had been secured by social changes long before those drugs became available. Not that the doctors invented the drugs anyway. The drug companies did – as well as some dud items, and some me-too products. And yes, their selling methods have sometimes been dubious; but in the forties and fifties it was they who made most of the big modern therapeutic discoveries.

JUDGE: You have a paper there, professor. Is it relevant to what you are saying?

LARKIN: Yes, as I thought I might be asked about all this I brought with me a paper[4] printed in the *British Medical Journal* some years ago, which was the text of the Harveian Oration delivered by Lord Platt to the Royal College of Physicians of London – of which he was for some time the President. He had also been for some years a professor of medicine, and is a medical man of very great distinction. May I read from it?

JUDGE: Certainly, so long as you are prepared to leave it as an exhibit.

LARKIN: Lord Platt said, 'The adoption of the scientific method in the Harveian tradition by clinical medicine has been recognised by the appointment of about 43 wholetime professors of medicine or of therapeutics in the United Kingdom alone. The growth of departments of academic medicine in the United States has taken place at the same time on an even larger scale. Their contributions to the understanding of disease are established, real, and secure, and they have helped to make possible the deployment of the discoveries of modern medical science, both in relation to treatment and in diagnosis. Yet we must face the fact that these departments have not been responsible for, nor even seriously involved in, any of the discoveries in therapeutics or preventive medicine which I have just enumerated.'

JUDGE: Which were?

LARKIN: He had been referring to diseases like tuberculosis, poliomyelitis, pernicious anemia, diabetes, plague, and malaria. He then pointed out that the sulphonamides and all the antibiotics except penicillin came from industrial laboratories, and penicillin was developed in such a laboratory. Much the same could be said, he went on, of the antituberculous drugs, polio vaccine, the new penicillins, and vitaminB_{12}. Liver for pernicious anemia, insulin, and stilboestrol – a female hormone substitute – are the only three substances he mentioned as having come from an academic unit (and only liver had come from an academic *medical* unit), though the credit for cortisone should go partly to an academic non-clinical scientist, partly to a clinician, and partly to a drug firm. He concluded: 'To continue the recital would be tedious, but the findings are essentially the same when we look into the origins of anaesthetics, tranquillizers, vitamins, anti-malarials, antihistamines, hypotensives, sex hormones, and oral contraceptives. Not one originated in a department of academic medicine or therapeutics.'

JUDGE: And would you also deny, professor, that the great improvements during the last 50 or 100 years in surgery and anesthetic practice and midwifery and in our hospital specialties generally have made a big difference to the health of the people?

LARKIN: If you are asking, judge, whether they have made a *big* difference to the death rates or life expectancy, then the answer is 'No' in general – though, of course, they have made some difference, they have saved some lives. If you mean, 'Have they relieved a great deal of pain and suffering, made life easier for a lot of people, and cured many non-fatal diseases as well as some that would previously have been fatal?' then the answer is certainly 'Yes'. However, I am bound to add that some of the work done by hospitals could have been done – and most certainly could now be done – as effectively or almost as effectively outside hospital, and certainly more cheaply; and that some of what is done in hospitals today is of little or no *proven* benefit. I am thinking of the developments of the last 20 years particularly. I am not criticizing the doctors and nurses who are doubtless very dedicated and hard-working. I am merely saying that in the last two or three decades the health expenditure pendulum has swung unjustifiably far – and on the whole unfruitfully – in the hospital direction and away from the community.

JUDGE: You sound very sure of all that you have been saying, professor.

LARKIN: We are 95 percent sure, judge. There are some uncertainties: for instance, rheumatic fever has become very much less common than it was 30 or 40 years ago, and deaths from measles or whooping cough started to fall long before there were any suitable drugs or vaccines for doctors to use; and we just don't yet know why these things happened. It may have been the general social improvement I mentioned earlier. It certainly wasn't the doctors. One thing, however, I am absolutely sure of is that doctors are simply not credible when they say – as some of them do, more or less – 'We conquered the old diseases; so just leave the new ones to us, and we'll conquer them too in the same way.' They didn't conquer the old diseases: they played some part in society's conquest of them, and in any case many of their old methods of approach to disease are probably quite inappropriate today.

JUDGE: You numbered food among the factors that started to improve about a hundred years ago; and yet we have been told in this court in the last few days by your colleagues that food is responsible today for obesity, for the diseases due to a lack of dietary fiber, and in part for coronary heart disease. So how can it have improved? Would your view and theirs not seem to be irreconcilable?

LARKIN: No, judge, it's like this: a hundred years ago the food of the ordinary people in your country and other western countries was sometimes inadequate in quantity and often in quality – it might be adulterated or pest-ridden, or be deficient in certain vitamins. Rickets or scurvy, for instance, due to a lack of vitamin D and vitamin C respectively, were common and continued to be common until well into this century. Now in all these respects – quantity, and the quality aspects I mentioned – it has improved in the last hundred years. (Indeed, in some ways food began to improve in the eighteenth century.) Scurvy and rickets are almost unknown in your country today except for some rickets among immigrants. Food is not adulterated, or is certainly not adulterated in the same crude way. Pests rarely get at it. However, we have now come to realize that some of the *other* changes that have occurred in the last hundred years have not been improvements, though they were commonly thought to be so at the time of their introduction. The provision of plenty of cheap white sugar and of cheap white flour, and the provision of large amounts of relatively cheap animal fats, and of a very large variety of foodstuffs fairly cheaply – so that almost anyone could afford to eat more food than he or she needed – all this, we now realize, was undesirable, and indeed has helped to cause new diseases. The pendulum has swung too far from a lack of food, and that not particularly good food, to an excess that is sometimes defective in quite different ways; in a sense from dangerous nutritional poverty to an almost equally dangerous nutritional affluence – in over-processed foods.

JUDGE: Thank you, professor. Mr Hunter?

HUNTER (*rising*): Professor Larkin, you said that the increase in life expectancy in the mid-1930s to mid-1950s period was to a great extent due to the large number of new and effective drugs and vaccines, mostly produced by the drug industry. (*Larkin nods*) Has the flow of these items now ceased?

LARKIN: No, but it has become much less.

HUNTER: And at the same time has an almost correspondingly *increased* amount of time and expertise been devoted to licensing and controlling and testing and discussing at length any new drugs and vaccines that do come along?

LARKIN: That is certainly true. We have various regulatory agencies, and a new medical discipline, called clinical pharmacology.

HUNTER: And the only thing it lacks is enough important new drugs on which to exercise itself? (*Larkin nods*) The two go together? The whole operation has become counter-productive?. The stable door's been bolted after the horse has gone?

LARKIN: I should hesitate to say categorically what the relationship was, but yes, it certainly looks as though there is one.

HUNTER: I should like to take you up now on the failure of western countries in general to secure any great increase in life expectancy in the past 20 years or so. Why was that? – Presumably not just the absence of new drugs and vaccines.

LARKIN: No, that was merely one element. But before I start my answer I should say that not only has life expectancy either failed to increase or else increased only a little in the last 20 years, but for certain sections of the people in certain countries it actually fell between the mid-to-late fifties and the mid-to-late sixties – especially among males, older males particularly.

HUNTER: In one or two countries?

LARKIN: No, some World Health Organization figures[5] showed it to have dropped in 10 out of 25 countries studied for males aged 15; and for males aged 65 in 15 out of 25 countries studied. In other words, if you reached either of those ages in the countries concerned during the 1965–9 period your remaining span of life was on average going to be shorter than it would have been if you had reached either of those ages 10 years earlier. What's more, there is some indication that a similar trend may be starting for females in some countries.

JUDGE: Might not a levelling-off, professor, of the gradient of increasing life expectancy simply indicate that on average people are now achieving their three-score years and ten; and that it is unrealistic to expect a further massive improvement?

LARKIN: That is certainly a big factor, judge; though there is nothing sacrosanct about the biblical figure. A very distinguished and more recent authority[6] says we should be able to look forward to most children living to be active octogenarians. And levelling-off aside, a *drop* in life expectancy must always be taken seriously, especially if it is not just a small, temporary drop affecting merely one or two countries.

HUNTER: And this drop is a result of? What is it that is killing people?

LARKIN: Well, in young people in Britain[7] and other western countries – from age 15 up to, say, 45 – the main causes of death now are accidents, especially road accidents, and suicide (England and Wales, and Switzerland being the only western countries to show a drop in deaths from these causes, at any rate for the population as a whole, in the 1960s[1]); and also certain cancers, and coronary heart disease – the last especially among the older males in this group.

HUNTER: And the middle-aged?

LARKIN: In your country[7] the main causes of death for them are coronary heart disease (especially in men), cancer (especially lung cancer in men and breast cancer in women), strokes in the older members of this group, and bronchitis, asthma, pneumonia, and influenza; and much the same pattern is prevalent in other western countries. For many of these conditions that are killing the young and middle-aged – killing people prematurely, that is – there isn't a great deal one can do in the way of curing, in hospital or anywhere else, once they have developed. And of course, they often put people off work and sometimes into hospital, quite apart from in the end killing them. They exact a high cost in every way, in other words.

HUNTER: And we mostly know what causes these conditions?

LARKIN: Yes, we know or else strongly suspect what factors are mostly involved: cigarettes, air pollution; too much food, especially saturated fat, and fiber-deficient sugar and white flour; possibly cancer-producing foods besides fats, or even food additives (modern adulterants, you could say), and cancer-producing chemicals and so on at the place of work; lack of exercise – the result of sitting watching the television, for instance; the automobile; and stress with no natural outlet, and with drugs and alcohol as the only answer.

HUNTER: And these causative factors are characteristic, central features of the western way of life – absolutely peculiar to our time?

LARKIN: Nearly all of them are, yes; and as possible everyday features of life for almost an entire population every single one of them is.

HUNTER: And the conditions they cause are, by and large, also peculiar to our modern western society? Characteristic of it?

LARKIN: Yes, by and large. Bronchitis and pneumonia have always occurred, of course, to quite some extent; and suicide and accidents – though not road accidents in such numbers. If one looks at the USA for one moment: more than 100,000 deaths due to accidents a year – almost half of them automobile accidents – and more than 10,500,000 people injured in accidents generally.[8] Terrifying figures.

HUNTER: They could come only from a technology-ridden society?
LARKIN: Yes. And then suicide occurred before but it has never previously been the most common cause of death among a group of young people, as it is now among young people between the ages of 17 and 20 in France. And most of the big killing diseases – heart disease, lung cancer, and so on – are special to our time.

HUNTER: Would you also describe as characteristic diseases of our civilization those that were earlier described as being due to a lack of dietary fiber, but that do not normally kill? Diverticular disease of the colon, and so on.

LARKIN: Yes, and dental decay due to the excess of sugar in our diet, and, of course, the side-effects of drugs; and obesity, and diabetes, and some mental illnesses; and to some extent cirrhosis of the liver due to alcohol, though, like diabetes, it *can* often kill, and, though common in the west in our time, is not peculiar to us in time or place. And then there's the whole spate of modern psychosomatic disorders, which often don't kill people but can disable them – those you discussed with Mr Buck – due to unsatisfying work, or unemployment, or unhappy personal and social relationships, and so on.

JUDGE: Professor Larkin, most of the causative factors you mention are characteristic of affluence, or produced by it? (*Larkin nods*) So you are saying that affluence is now productive of disease? (*He nods again*) And yet an earlier affluence, manifesting in better housing and nutrition and so on, was responsible for a steady improvement in health in the western world from about 1860 to the 1950s; so somewhere in between affluence presumably began to be productive of more ill-health than health, to be counter-productive of the latter?

LARKIN: Correct.

HUNTER: And by and large this affluent way of life is the one favored by doctors?

LARKIN: Yes, very much so, aside from cigarette smoking.

HUNTER: And it is spreading to the richer strata of society in under-developed countries (*Larkin nods*) And now the treatments these diseases of affluence receive – the operations, the maneuvers of the coronary care unit, the antibiotics, and the various other drugs: are they also as characteristic of our time as the diseases and their causes? (*Larkin nods again*) They are all engineering or chemical or mechanical approaches? Rather similar to the factors – the automobile, the cigarette-making machinery, the white bread and sugar factories, the television set, the elements producing stress in the cities and in industry – that cause the diseases in the first place, or that produce their causes?

LARKIN: Yes, I agree that is true.

HUNTER: And on the whole the treatments, you say, are not particularly effective?

LARKIN: Correct. Almost certainly we would not produce results any worse than we're getting at the moment if a lot of money was switched from the hospital-centered approach at a late stage to a community-centered preventive approach before ever the conditions had developed.

JUDGE: Professor Larkin, you seem to be saying that hospital medicine – the predominant type – if it has not quite reached the same counter-productive stage as affluence, is none the less relatively powerless to deal with this flood of new conditions. As the expectation of life is at best fairly static, any good that hospital-style medicine is doing is presumably being matched by the evil done by the excess of affluence? (*Larkin nods*) And, as Mr Hunter suggested, the affluence and the hospital medicine of today are branches of the same tree? (*He nods again*)

HUNTER: Are you optimistic, professor, about the results of a community-centered approach to these modern conditions?

LARKIN: I am personally, but even those who doubt we can achieve much with prevention have to admit that something ought to be done when life expectancy for some people in the west is going down at the same time as health expenditure is going up – on hospitals mainly.

HUNTER: Could the one be leading to the other: the increased hospital expenditure to the decreased life expectancy?

LARKIN: Yes, in a way: if you build more and more hospitals, and fill them with more and more expensive machines, and their car parks with automobiles, the lesson you teach lay people is that they needn't bother too much about taking responsibility themselves for *preserving* their health. They can carry on as they are doing, as the doctors are doing; and then, when something goes wrong, the brilliant hospital doctors will put it right – with tablets or injections or an operation. And of course, the hospital doctors, no matter how brilliant, very often can't.

HUNTER: The emphasis should be much more on individual responsibility and prevention?

LARKIN: And on the family doctor. He is needed for some of the preventive work, and to encourage the individual in the rest; and he can treat a lot of patients at home – they needn't go into hospital.[9] There needs to be a better distribution of family doctors too, and very often they can delegate work to other members of the health team – and so save more money again.

HUNTER: When, for instance?

LARKIN: Well, we mentioned some common diseases that disable people but don't kill them, or don't usually kill them — thanks often to the great ability of modern medicine simply to keep people alive. And there are others. I'm thinking particularly of mental illness and mental defect, and of some of the degenerative diseases of old age — arthritis, deafness, perhaps bronchitis, and so on. They're undramatic, but they cause a lot of suffering and inconvenience, and yet they are relatively neglected medically. The skills of a nurse or social worker or even a home help are as likely to be as useful in these cases as the skills of a doctor.

HUNTER: Is it not proposed, however, in the UK[10] and in the USA[2] to shift health service money into the areas you mention during the next few years, and away from acute hospital care?

LARKIN: That is true, but man proposes and God disposes.

HUNTER: And in the present context God wears a white coat, you mean? (*Larkin nods*) And what you are suggesting goes against all the medical trends of many years past?

LARKIN: Correct. The medical system ought to be judged as much by the quality of the *care* it provides as by the number of *cures*; and yet more and more money has been spent on hospitals, especially acute, purportedly 'curing' hospitals. In the UK the proportion of National Health Service money going to hospitals increased from 56.5 percent to 67 percent between 1954 and 1974, and in the same period the proportion going to family doctors dropped from 10.5 percent to 6.5 percent.[11] Each technological advance costs more to introduce into a hospital than the last one, and the returns are much less, if indeed the value has been properly assessed at all. The number of doctors and nurses and other staff for every hundred beds goes on increasing: a new medical sub-specialty is invented every couple of years; often, especially here in the United States, some very expensive apparatus will be purchased by more than one hospital in one quite small area. And so on. Sooner or later the process has got to stop, if only because the supply of money isn't inexhaustible.

HUNTER: But why are doctors so keen on hospitals if their value is limited?

LARKIN: The public is keen on them too. Partly because for some conditions their value is very real, and has been for decades: for nearly all routine operations (assuming the patient does really need the operation), for the proper diagnosis and treatment of fractures, the treatment of major wounds, and of certain special infections, the management of difficult childbirth, the diagnosis of any kind of difficult condition – for these and many other purposes a hospital is certainly the best place to be, and so doctors tend to think it should be best for *all* purposes.

HUNTER: Anything else?

LARKIN: Yes, many of the big advances in medicine – in medicine, not in health – in this century and the last occurred in hospitals or else depended on hospitals for clinical testing, even when the actual discoveries were not made there. So the idea got fixed in the minds of doctors and of lay people that hospital medicine must be superior to medicine practiced elsewhere. There is a superior status attached to being a doctor in a hospital. Life and death are clearly involved. And there's more money involved too. And the work is more interesting, anyway more interesting on a scientific and intellectual level. (*Pause*)

HUNTER: Yes?

LARKIN: Yes, I'll stick my neck out and say it. I agree with a quotation you read to Mr Buck yesterday. I think the biggest single reason in a curious way why hospitals get all the limelight is that doctors want, not so much to get away from patients, as to get away from the rawness of life. In a hospital the doctor's a god, he can keep the patient at a distance, take X-ray pictures of him, stick needles into him, operate on him – but he doesn't need ever to get involved with the patient as a human being in a human situation, perhaps a tricky situation. I'm not saying all doctors are like this, but some are; and it's largely, I think, an unconscious motive. To go out into the community, to get mud on your shoes, dirt on your nice clean white coat – this doesn't appeal to most doctors, no matter what it might achieve for their patients. Being a doctor in a hospital all the time's like – oh, like being a landscape artist who never, but never, leaves the studio.

HUNTER: And yet we are now faced with a completely new pattern of disease, which calls for a new type of approach? The days of the sudden dramatic illness and the quick dramatic hospital cure are gone?

LARKIN: Correct, for what they were ever really worth. We now know nearly all the scenarios for dramas of that kind, and we can guess the very few that are going to be written in the next few decades. A preventive, grass-roots approach is needed, just as it produced most of the real improvements in health in the past. The present Director General of the World Health Organization is on record[12] as being for devolution of health care – right down to the man-in-the-street – and of prevention, and of what he calls a demystification of medical technology; but he thinks doctors are a long way from ceasing to confuse health with the conventional medical wisdom.

HUNTER: That might be thought to be directed more at the underdeveloped world. As we are in the United States and speaking mainly of western countries, do you have anything that is obviously relevant to them?

LARKIN: Yes, our Canadian Minister of Health and Welfare – you can't get any closer to the States than that – has come out[13] in favor of Canadians themselves being made more responsible for maintenance of their health, and for alterations to the environment and to their life-style that will make for health; and has suggested a shift of emphasis away from expensive hospital-centered medicine and towards prevention, and towards more care for the old and the mentally ill.

HUNTER: I now want to ask you one final question, about which I should like you to think very carefully before answering. Are doctors and lay people not so used to the hospital-style approach to health and illness, so convinced of its value, so carried along by its momentum, that nothing short of a revolutionary change of attitude – politically or ecologically induced – will make them willing to take part in the kind of prevention that is clearly needed, which is a radical change in life-style?

LARKIN (*after a pause*): No, I do not agree with that.

HUNTER: You think it can be achieved without a new type of doctor, without a new type of motivation, without a total change in our society having to occur first? (*Larkin nods*) Thank you, professor. (*Sits*)

JUDGE: Professor, you wish to add anything?

LARKIN: Just that, if I did not believe that it *is* possible to achieve the kind of preventive action I have been suggesting without some kind of major upheaval, then I should be a very unhappy man – I should be in some different occupation. Preventive medicine, I am sure, can be effectively practiced in every part of the health field; and it is the medicine of the future.

JUDGE: Thank you kindly, professor; and that seems an appropriate note on which this court might adjourn for the present.

REFERENCES—SESSION SEVEN

1. Maxwell, R., *Health Care: The Growing Dilemma*, 2nd. edn, McKinsey and Co., Inc., New York, 1975.
2. Rogers, D. E., and Blendon, R. J., *JAMA*, April 18, 1977, p. 1710.
3. McManus, T. C., *Lancet*, February 1, 1975, p. 266.
4. Platt, Lord, *BMJ*, November 25, 1967, p. 439.
5. *World Health Statistics Report*, No. 10, World Health Organization, Geneva, 1974, p. 677.
6. Doll, R., *Royal Society of Health Journal*, August 1977, p. 167.
7. *World Health Statistics Report*, No. 9, World Health Organization, Geneva, 1974, p. 622, 636.

8. Medical News, *JAMA*, April 19, 1976, p. 1662.
9. Editorial, *Lancet*, November 12, 1977, p. 1016.
10. Department of Health and Social Security, *Priorities for Health and Personal Social Services in England*, HMSO, London, 1976.
11. *The Cost of the NHS*, Information Sheet No. 29, Office of Health Economics, London, July 1976.
12. Mahler, H., *Lancet*, November 1, 1975, p. 829.
13. Lalonde, M., *A New Perspective on the Health of Canadians*, Gouvernement du Canada, Ottawa, 1974.

General Reading

Cochrane, A. L., *Effectiveness and Efficiency: Random Reflections on Health Services*, The Rock Carling Fellowship, 1971; Nuffield Provincial Hospitals Trust, London, 1971.

Davies, B. M., *Community Health and Social Services*, 2nd. edn, English Universities Press, London, 1972.

Hobson, W. (ed.), *The Theory and Practice of Public Health*, 4th edn, Oxford University Press, London, 1975.

McKeown, T., and Lowe, C. R., *An Introduction to Social Medicine*, 2nd edn, Blackwell Scientific Publications, Oxford, 1974.

McKeown, T., *The Role of Medicine: Dream, Mirage, or Nemesis?* The Rock Carling Fellowship, 1976; Nuffield Provincial Hospitals Trust, London, 1976.

Prospects in Health, Office of Health Economics, London, 1971.

Disorders Which Shorten Life, Office of Health Economics, 1966.

The Age of Maturity, Office of Health Economics, 1969.

Medicine and Society, Office of Health Economics, 1972.

The Health Care Dilemma, Office of Health Economics, 1975.

NHS: How Well Does It Work?, Which, London, August 1975, p. 232.

PART II
What Doctors Are

THE DOCTORS

Enter Dr Harry Jaeger

HUNTER: You are Dr Harry Jaeger, an American internist – what in the United Kingdom call a consultant physician? And you have held various positions in the medico-political life of your country? (*Jaeger nods*) Dr Jaeger, will you listen to this quotation? – 'What motivates the good doctor' is 'the chance to help a faltering person and the professional motive of winning the esteem of his fellows ... the ordinary physician is not moved by the dubious chance at wealth but would rather have regular and adequate income, the feeling of security and freedom to devote himself in an uncompromising way to his calling.' You agree with what it says?

JAEGER: Without reservation.

HUNTER: It comes from an article[1] written by a member of the editorial board of the *Journal of the American Medical Association*. It suggests three elements in the good doctor: help to others, desire for peer esteem, and a wish for only a fairly modest income. You agree? (*Jaeger nods*) No qualifications, no provisos? (*Jaeger shakes his head slowly and repeatedly*) Well now, in 1975 did not large numbers of doctors in California and New York refuse for a time to treat any but emergency patients? And was not this because they had been asked to pay very high premiums for insurance against malpraxis suits (malpractice, as we say in England): that is, where a patient takes a doctor to court or threatens to do so on account of some alleged negligence?[2] And in 1976 did doctors in California not have another 'strike' for the same reason?[3]

JAEGER: That is true, Mr Hunter, but insurance premiums sometimes carrying *increases* of $20,000 a year[2] – or up in 1976 300 percent on the 1975 figure[3] – left them no option. What do you do if your insurance premium is $60,000 or more?[3, 4] Here in the States, Mr Hunter, your legal colleagues operate on a contingency basis in malpraxis cases – that is, the amount they receive depends on the amount of money they manage to get for the person who comes to them and is thinking of suing. Win nothing, get nothing. So do they advise going ahead or do they not? Even if a lawyer advises an out-of-court settlement he stands to get some thousands of dollars. And sometimes, if a case is won, the patient gets only 16 or 17 cents out of each dollar awarded – the rest goes to the lawyers and the hangers-on.[3, 5] And hundreds of thousands of dollars have been awarded in some cases.[3, 5] Why, you even have lawyers ringing up people who've been in accidents and offering their services.[3] Professional men! Some states took legislative action to curb them. Still the doctors are beginning to hit back: they're suing lawyers and patients who bring a suit and lose it, and they're getting damages.[5]

HUNTER: The relevant upshot of all you have said is that doctors *will* occasionally renege on their obligations to 'help a faltering person', but they will do so only under the most extreme provocation. That is your position? The premiums were absurd? And few, if any, of these malpraxis suits were justified.

JAEGER: Very, very few. Correct.

HUNTER: But in 1975 did hospital house staff in New York, Chicago, and Washington[5,6] not walk out on their patients in support of a claim for shorter working hours?

JAEGER: The public was with them. They had been under great, acknowledged provocation for a very long time in the matter of hours of work. They did it for the ultimate good of their patients.[7]

HUNTER: Almost selflessly? (*Pause*) You may be aware, Dr Jaeger, that in the United Kingdom, also in 1975, the junior hospital staff took industrial action lasting some weeks to obtain more money for themselves, and that they did it again in 1976; and that senior hospital staff for a time in 1975 and 1976 treated emergency cases only – because they objected to a decision by the elected government to remove private beds from National Health Service hospitals.[8,9] And in Ireland junior doctors went on strike in 1973 for more money.

JAEGER: Yes, I heard about all of that.

HUNTER: Extreme provocation, would you say? Money in one form or another seems to be enough to make doctors forget about that first obligation of theirs, does it not? And yet did you not agree that doctors wish for only a fairly modest income?

JAEGER: They do. Money is not the main motivation of doctors.

HUNTER: Well, let us turn for a moment to that second element in their motivation – the esteem of their fellows. PSROs is short for Professional Standards Review Organizations, is it not? (*Jaeger nods*) Now correct me if I am wrong about their genesis, will you? The US government through its Medicare and Medicaid and Maternal-and-Child-Health program provides payments for doctors who attend the old, the poor, and certain maternity cases respectively? The cost of these grew from some $11,000,000,000 in 1969 to some $15,000,000,000 in 1972.[10] The government was concerned about the increasing cost.

JAEGER: Good medicine costs money.

HUNTER: Well, shall we just say that doctors do? You are aware that your government has revealed that in 1974 no fewer than 207 doctors in the USA earned more than $100,000 each from Medicaid work, one doctor even earning over $450,000?[11]

JAEGER: Yes, and it later admitted the list was full of mistakes. It included a doctor who'd died in '74, and others who'd actually retired.[3]

HUNTER: But, as to any who hadn't retired or died, was it not calculated that they would have had to work a 72-hour day right through the year to make these amounts?[11] And has a later report not got doctors earning – I mean 'making' – more than $500,000 a year out of Medicaid?[12] (*Pause*) But now to revert to PSROs: in order to ensure that doctors providing medical care under Medicaid and the other government schemes were not admitting patients to hospital unnecessarily or keeping them there too long or being otherwise over-assiduous in performing duties that would determine their level of remuneration the government arranged that these bodies, the PSROs, should be set up all over the country – sponsored by doctors and controlled by doctors who would lay down what were reasonable standards for hospital admissions, for management of various conditions, and so on; and see to it that those doctors who diverged very markedly from the standard were informed of the fact – in the first place so that they might mend their ways, though penalties might be involved.[10,13] The ultimate result may be that an American doctor will have to be recertified as competent every few years.[14] Is that an accurate summary of the position, Dr Jaeger?

JAEGER: It is – for an English attorney.

HUNTER: Well then, will you tell an English attorney why it is that the establishment of PSROs has met with such vehement opposition from many American doctors?[15,16,17,18,19]

JAEGER: Because we don't like government interference in medical practice.

HUNTER: But the PSRO system was partly established in response to the avarice shown by doctors in relation to government health money; and the surveillance is to be conducted, at any rate for the present, by the doctor's own peers – his fellow doctors.

JAEGER: We Americans don't like snooping from anyone.

HUNTER: And do your fellow Americans like paying taxes to give doctors incomes of over $500,000 a year? (*Pause*) You agreed earlier that a main motivation of doctors was the desire for the esteem of their fellow doctors. Does this not necessarily imply that some doctors will get something less than esteem under any dispensation? They cannot all score 100 percent. Why then should it be wrong for such disesteem to be given under the aegis of PSROs

– so long as they are set up and controlled by doctors? Is it because there would be a lot of disesteem?

JAEGER: Frankly, I think you're trying to trap me with words.

HUNTER: Well then, here are some figures in relation to the need for the establishment of PSROs. I have here an article[20] from the *Journal of the American Medical Association*, reporting a survey of the use made by 33 doctors of laboratory services for patients they were attending in one particular hospital. The laboratory cost per patient for the heaviest doctor user was no less than 17 times as high as that for the lightest user. A seventeen-fold difference; and it was about two and a half times the average of the cost for all the doctors. (Incidentally, the corresponding figures for drugs was a four-fold difference between the heaviest and the lightest doctor users.) And a lot of that testing would be purely defensive? Just in case of a malpraxis suit?

JAEGER: Yes, but you can't be too careful with lawyers on your tail.

HUNTER: We have now disposed of two of the factors that you felt unreservedly, Dr Jaeger, characterized the good doctor: helping people, and desire for peer esteem. The third was his being 'not moved by the dubious chance at wealth'. Well now, those American doctors who were earning tens of thousands of dollars a year from Medicaid – sometimes somewhat dubious dollars – are not at all exceptional in their incomes, are they? – United States doctors commonly have earnings in the $60,000–100,000 range, do they not?[21]

JAEGER: And think of the education and training and hard work and responsibilities they have.

HUNTER: But you said that a wish for only a fairly modest income was a characteristic of doctors. Is $100,000 fairly modest? (*Pause*) Is their work not interesting? Are they ever in danger of unemployment? (*Pause*) Well now, will you accept that most people in the States – who do not have interesting work very often, or any job security – have an income in the $10,000 to $15,000 range?[21]

JAEGER: I don't know what the figure is.

HUNTER: Is it not an item of knowledge that any doctor who is looking at his patients as persons should have?

JAEGER: Plenty of businessmen and lawyers earn more than doctors.

HUNTER: And you are not the only American doctor who thinks that perhaps they shouldn't.[22,23] (*Pause*) Is medicine a business? Of course, even in Hungary, a communist country, despite its national health service, doctors make charges and patients get priority according to what they pay. The cost of delivering a baby is the average monthly wage of a worker, and for removal of an appendix twice that.[24] The ethics of doctors seem to transcend national and even ideological frontiers, do they not?

JAEGER: Yes, freedom will out, even under communism – with doctors in the lead.

HUNTER: I agree they're in the lead: the Canadian federal revenue department's green book on taxation for 1973 gave average rounded-off incomes (in Canadian dollars) as follows:[25] doctors, 43,000; lawyers, 37,000; engineers, 34,000; accountants, 27,000; farmers, 9,500; fishermen, 9,000.

JAEGER: The laborer is worthy of his hire.

HUNTER: I'm sure Canadian farmers and fishermen would agree. (*Pause*) In Australia there was in 1976 a government-backed scheme for payment of medical expenses, called Medibank. I now quote from what was said in the *Lancet*[26] about it: 'Misuse by doctors is regularly in the headlines. . . . Private pathology laboratories are common in the cities; and automated analyses are believed to be yielding huge takings for these "medical factories". "We'll have to do something to curb the pathology bonanza" was a comment heard in Canberra. The open checks for doctors may now be too open for the good of Medibank and the nation – and, in the final analysis, for the doctors themselves.'

JAEGER: Do I have to answer for the southern hemisphere too?

HUNTER: Well, let us stick to the northern. You may find the figures for the UK easier to defend, though even there the incomes of most doctors are way ahead of those of most people and yet, as in your country, they have interesting work and are immune to unemployment. I have here the issue[27] of the *British Medical Journal* for June 4, 1977, giving salary scales for doctors. Again I've rounded off the figures. That for junior doctors training in hospital ranged from £4,500 a year to £8,500, though with various extra payments for overtime and so on it was said that some junior doctors, even in 1976, were earning as much as £15,000 a year. The net average annual income for a family doctor was £9,000. The range for consultants – that is, specialists – was from just over £8,000 to just under £11,000 (their income goes up automatically with length of service); but in addition for the 12,000 or so medical and dental consultants there were over 5,000 special 'merit' awards in addition to their salaries, and these awards ranged from £2,000 a year to £8,000 a year (and some part-time consultants can make a great deal more extra income than that from private practice). You may agree that a total income of approximately £20,000 a year, if it does not make a man rich beyond the dreams of avarice, is substantial when compared with, say, a British old-age pension.

JAEGER: You should compare like with like, Mr Hunter.

HUNTER: The court has noted your sentiment, I am sure, doctor.

(*Pause*) The British Medical Association, mind you, has protested because the incomes of British doctors are the lowest of the doctors in any Common Market country. In 1974 a doctor could earn two or three times as much in Denmark or Belgium or West Germany, and even in Luxembourg. The Association said in 1976 that British doctors would start emigrating to Europe,[28] though the next year the Association's journal was saying they wouldn't, after all, because Europe already had too many doctors.[29] All drawn into the profession by a desire to help suffering humanity?

JAEGER: You can't expect highly trained men to work for peanuts.

HUNTER: But is there nothing, doctor, between the peanuts and the caviar? Especially as they say they don't *want* to make a lot of money. *You* said it. (*Pause*) Well, having established that they do reluctantly make a lot, and so disposed of all three of your alleged medical motives, I should like to move on to the question of how some doctors – some North American doctors, at any rate – make it. And the answer is, in a nutshell, unnecessary surgery.

JAEGER: I will not accept that for a moment. It's been debated over and over again, and no-one's certain of the truth.

HUNTER: There are twice as many specialist surgeons for every 100,000 people in the USA as in the United Kingdom?[30]

JAEGER: I believe so. You'll catch up one day.

HUNTER: And there are also, oddly enough, twice as many operations for every 100,000 people.[30] You do not deny it? (*Pause*) Do you really think there is *twice* as much sickness calling for surgery among the Americans as among the British?

JAEGER: No, I'd guess the truth is you haven't enough surgeons to do all the work that's needing to be done; but, as I said, you'll catch up one day maybe.

HUNTER: You are aware of a study of the actual total charges made in 1973 by American doctors for various operations and so on, performed under the Medicare scheme? It appeared in the *New England Journal of Medicine*.[31]

JAEGER: I believe I glanced at it.

HUNTER: I have done more than that. The charges made by family doctors – I stress, family doctors – for removal of an appendix averaged 280 dollars, the extremes of charges being 100 and 500 dollars; for removal of the gall bladder they averaged 431 dollars, the extremes being 275 and 750 dollars; and for removal of the uterus they averaged 481 dollars, the extremes this time being 150 and 765 dollars. These were 1973 figures. Specialists on the whole charged a little more.

JAEGER: So? These are major operations. And think of those

HUNTER: Removal of an appendix from start to finish often takes half an hour or less? (*Jaeger nods*) 560 dollars an hour is a satisfactory rate of remuneration, no? (*Pause*) Anyway, I just wanted to set the scene, the very relevant monetary scene, for what is to follow. If, as you suggested, there are some diseases in British people calling for surgery but not receiving it because of a shortage of surgeons, one would expect – would one not – that deaths or disability from those diseases would be a lot more common in the UK than here in the USA? Do you know of any reports to that effect?

JAEGER: I can't recall any off-hand.

HUNTER: And yet one would expect some if half the operations that need to be performed in the UK are not, in fact, performed? And one would expect a knowledgeable doctor like yourself to have read some of them? So the *simple* explanation of Americans having double the number of operations that the British undergo per unit of population is that the Americans have twice the number of surgeons. And what is the simple explanation for your having twice the number? That surgery, as the figures I have just quoted strongly suggest, is a very lucrative branch of American medicine.

JAEGER: What you certainly do have in your country is waiting lists for surgery.

HUNTER: Which would you prefer, Dr Jaeger? A line of people waiting for operations, or surgeons waiting to operate on people?

JAEGER: There are no medical queues of any kind in my country.

HUNTER: Oh? Not even of doctors in the richer parts and of patients in the poorer parts: in Appalachia, say, where it is difficult to get doctors to settle? Though it's been suggested[32] by one American doctor, who was angry about conditions there, that, what with all the Medicare-Medicaid money there is in Appalachia, and the large numbers of docile sick people, and low malpractice rates, and cheap land, and *some* beautiful scenery – that it's really an ideal spot for an American doctor on the make.

JAEGER: I regard that as offensive; and there are parts of your country that are under-doctored, as you well know, both in respect of family medicine and hospital medicine. Some areas are much better off for medical and financial resources than others. A doctor can expect reasonable social and educational facilities where he lives. Anyway in the States he can and he does.

HUNTER: And other people? And how many more materialistic motivations are you going to give us for doctors? As to under- and over-doctoring, it is a fact, coming from your own Rand Corporation and appearing in the *Journal* of your own American Medical Association,[33] that the number of active non-government physicians per 100,000 people in your country varies from 195 in some of the big cities to 42 in some of the rural areas; and that in 1971 there were 133 counties in America with no active doctor in them at all – representing almost half a million doctorless people. (*Pause*) Come, Dr Jaeger, your profession can't really expect to have haloes *and* golden tie clips to match, can it? Shall we discard the haloes? (*Pause*) You are acquainted with another study[34,35,36,37] – of those doctors who performed surgery in four areas of the USA, covering the 1970–72 period, and published in 1976? (*Jaeger nods*) It showed that 30 percent of the doctors said they specialized to some extent in surgery, and 25 percent of doctors starting their hospital residency periods (their senior training periods, that is) enter surgical units. Of all those performing operations in these four areas rather less than half were actually surgical specialists – the remainder being general practitioners doing some surgery on the side, or medical specialists doing even less. Of the surgical specialists rather less than two thirds were board-certified: that is, had the appropriate specialist qualifications. You accept that these were the findings?

JAEGER: I can't recall exact figures after all this time.

HUNTER: I have the original reports here if you wish to refresh your memory. (*Pause*) The conclusion of the study was that there are too many doctors doing surgery in the States; that, as a result, at least some of them are not getting enough actual surgical practice to keep their hands and minds as active as one would like in someone performing operations; and that in one way or another their number should be reduced, and the doctors eliminated should go into family practice. Now why do so many American doctors perform surgery? Well, I've given you the fees charged for some individual operations; but this study reported[36] on the annual amounts earned by the 'surgeons' in the study. It was well over $40,000 a year (in some places it was almost $60,000 a year), and 20 percent above the income of other doctors. And that was in 1971, Dr Jaeger. (*Pause*) I won't ask you if two and two make four; but I want now to move across the border into Canada. You are aware of a study appearing in the *New England Journal of Medicine*[38] that compared surgical rates in Canada and Britain? (*Jaeger nods*) Will you tell us about it?

JAEGER: It showed that surgery was more common in Canada than in England and Wales.

HUNTER: Overall some one and a half times to twice as common? For 10 out of 12 operations that are what is called elective and discretionary – that is, the surgeon and patient can choose to have them performed or not – the Canadian rate was higher than the

England and Wales rate. Removal of the tonsils five to six times more common, removal of the uterus twice as common, of the breast three times as common, and of the gall bladder five times as common for men and seven times as common for women.

JAEGER: And inflammation of the gall bladder is also more common in Canada.

HUNTER: I think, doctor, the true position is that it has been claimed to be more common, and this has been disputed by the author of the study with which we are dealing.[39] And no such explanation has been put forward to explain why the Canadian operation rate *overall* is higher than the rate in England and Wales. What is not in dispute is that deaths from gall bladder disease in people over 65 in Canada are about twice as high as in England and Wales, and the author of the study thought this or some part of it might be due to the extra gall bladder operations.

JAEGER: It *could* be, as I said before, that there's a need for surgery in your country that is simply unmet. I mean not just for gall bladder disease.

HUNTER: Except that, as the author of the paper pointed out – and as you may recall I mentioned more generally in relation to diseases in your and my country – if that *were* the case then one would expect to find a higher death rate in England and Wales from, say, cancer of the uterus and cancer of the breast (you'll remember both were removed much more often in Canada), but in fact the rates from those cancers are *not* higher. In other words, there are not a lot of patients with those conditions in England and Wales who should be operated on but who die because they are not. There *does* seem to be unnecessary surgery of the uterus and the breast in Canada – or there was. And so it seems that the extra Canadian deaths in older people from gall bladder disease may *well* have been due in part to the unnecessarily high operation rate for removal of the gall bladder.

JAEGER: That was the author's conclusion. It isn't mine.

HUNTER: And do you agree with the author's suggestion as to why surgical rates are higher in Canada? Let me refresh your memory again: he said, first, that there were one and a half times the number of surgeons per 100,000 people in Canada than there are in England and Wales, and more 'acute' beds. (And overall, you will remember, surgery was about one and a half to twice as common – exactly the same picture as in the US except that here you have *twice* the British concentration of surgeons and *twice* as much surgery.) Second, he said that nearly all operations in England and Wales are performed by specialists whereas in Canada a lot of general practitioners still do surgery. And third and perhaps most important, in England and Wales nearly all surgeons are paid a fixed salary whereas in Canada a surgeon's income depends on how many operations he performs – at any rate, to a very great extent.

JUDGE: No comment, Dr Jaeger? (*Pause*) Your charge is a serious one, Mr Hunter.

HUNTER: I am mérely, judge, retailing what was said in the paper reporting this study; and Dr Jaeger has not disputed that it was said. The paper gave two extra arguments, which may be regarded as clinching the matter. In Portland, Oregon, under a pre-payment scheme known as the Kaiser-Permanente program surgeons are paid a fixed salary, and the surgical rate there is almost the same as in England and Wales, and a lot less than in Canada, though the population of Canada resembles the Kaiser-Permanente membership as to age and sex. Second, the surgical rate in two Canadian groups, in the same city and alike except in one single respect, have been compared. They differed only in that one group was in a pre-paid medical program whereas the other group had the usual fee-for-item-of-service system. The first group had lower rates for all operations studied. Any comment, Dr Jaeger?

JAEGER: Freedom always carries a price tag.

HUNTER: And the one carried by a freedom to operate for cash is sometimes death?

JUDGE: I think you go too far, Mr Hunter, as regards this witness. The facts you have presented may warrant what you have just said, but not in relation to Dr Jaeger.

HUNTER: I withdraw the remark, judge.

JAEGER: And you didn't mention the way operation rates for the same condition vary a great deal between one region or hospital in your country and another. They do; and so do hospital death rates for the same condition, and so does the length of time people are kept in hospital – or even in bed – after an operation, even after a simple hernia or appendicitis operation. There are all kinds of inequalities in your own National Health Service.

HUNTER: Are you suggesting that has some sinister significance? Or that it is due to the same kind of factors as we have just been discussing in relation to American and Canadian surgical rates?

JAEGER: I didn't say sinister, and I don't say sinister for the US or Canada. I say one man does this and another man does that, and they're both honest.

HUNTER: But in the United Kingdom there is almost no financial inducement, in the case of surgeons or indeed any other doctors, for them to be otherwise? (*Pause*) Shall we get back to the United States? – In the same issue of the journal that carried the report of the study we've just considered was a leading article,[40] which indicated it is four times more risky for an American over 65 to have cold surgery (you know what that means, of course: 'Come in and have the operation when it's convenient for you') – to have such surgery for a hernia, a rupture, than it is to have no surgery at all, and simply to run the risk of it strangulating and having *then* to submit to an emergency operation. It said too that, in Vermont as operation rates go up, so do overall death rates. It went further: it said the higher death rates up to age 65 in your country, as compared with Britain and Sweden, for example, may in part be due to too much surgery. (*Pause*) No comment, doctor, on what an American medical journal says about America? It is a commonplace among doctors that at least 90 percent of the operations in your country for removal of the tonsils are quite unnecessary – except presumably to the surgeon's bank balance? (*Pause*) Still no comment? Is it not a fact that the American Board of Surgery – that is, the United States specialist certifying body, judge – has now introduced a scheme whereby every surgeon certified by the board will have to be regularly re-examined?[41]

JAEGER: That is so; and a fine tribute to the high standards demanded for American surgeons.

HUNTER: Unless it could be evidence for the previously existing low standards.

JUDGE: Yes, Dr Jaeger? – You have been anxious to say something?

JAEGER: I've been wanting to say, judge, in reply to Mr Hunter's monologue that, on May 9, 1974, the same *New England Journal of Medicine* he's been quoting at me had an article[41] showing that the operation rates in California for a group of doctors, male and female, and their spouses were as high as or even higher than the corresponding rates for their socio-economic equivalents – ministers, lawyers, or businessmen. A variety of operations was involved. Now did they have themselves or their spouses operated on for the sake of the money they'd make out of it? No, sir. They had the surgery because they thought it necessary.

HUNTER: I too have studied that paper, doctor. Now please correct me if you think any of the statments I make are wrong. The study showed that at age 30 no less than 20 percent of male doctors had had their appendixes out, compared with only 7 percent of the general US male population at that age and 7 percent of the male population of the Oxford area in my country at that age. Do you *really* think American doctors are almost three times more likely to have diseased appendixes than their brother Americans or their English cousins? Is it a contagious disease, peculiar to hospitals? Or do the figures not suggest the doctors to be hypochondriacs? You are aware it has been shown in the German Federal Republic, where removal of the appendix is two-three times more common than in other countries, that three quarters of the appendixes removed are quite normal,[40] but deaths from appendicitis are three times as common too – because of this unnecessary surgery?[40]

JAEGER: I haven't yet heard of Californian doctors dying off like flies.

HUNTER: Or–er–drones? Second, it was shown in the study you quote that at age 60 more than 50 percent of the wives of the male American doctors involved had had a hysterectomy – removal of the womb, judge – whereas for the general American population the figure was only 30 percent, and for the women of the Oxford area of England it was only 15 percent. Third, the authors of the paper stated that their results certainly showed the likely trend in future *demand* for surgery by lay people, but not that of the *need* for it.

JAEGER: That was their opinion.

HUNTER: Do you really think that the wives of American doctors *need* a hysterectomy more than three times as often as the women in the Oxford area of England, and nearly twice as often as other American women? Or is it just a method of birth control, or of getting rid of what they consider a superfluous organ?[42] Are you aware too that in an editorial the *Journal of the American Medical Association*,[43] referring to this study, indicated its limitations but implied that the American lay public, as they became more knowledgeable, would demand and *need* as many operations as those American doctors and their spouses are having already – which was quite the opposite of the conclusion implied in the original report of the study? (*Pause*) The Association has always been devoted to the interests of the American doctor, has it not? Especially his financial interests? It has for decades resisted any suggestion of a Health Service like the British National Health Service.

JAEGER: Yes, sir, and a very good thing too.

HUNTER: Because that would mean an end to the system of more operations equals more money for the doctors? (*Pause*) Does the study in question not suggest the very sinister and disturbing truth that many American doctors have brain-washed themselves and their spouses even more than they have yet succeeded in brain-washing the public on the need for meddlesome, interfering, and even dangerous surgery? And that, when they do succeed in brain-washing the ordinary people to the same extent, they'll be pocketing even more in the way of fees than at present? And perhaps America will be even further down the western health league than she is now?

JAEGER: I resent that. I deeply resent that.

HUNTER: And do you resent the fact that between 1968 and 1973 the annual rate of hysterectomy among American women aged 15 and over increased from 6.8 per thousand to 8.6 per thousand?[42] – So that it does seem as though the American general public is catching up with the doctors' wives – helped by the doctors. Perhaps you could learn a lesson from Canada.

JAEGER: Meaning what?

HUNTER: Meaning, doctor, that between 1964 and 1971 the number of hysterectomies in the Canadian province of Saskatchewan increased by 72.1 percent whereas the number of women over 15 increased by only 7.6 percent;[44] so a committee of the College of Physicians and Surgeons of Saskatchewan, having some lay members on it, was formed in 1972, and it drew up a list of acceptable reasons for the operation – those performed for other reasons being regarded as unjustified. Also it looked at what the position had been in certain hospitals in 1970, and what it was in others in 1973. Well now: between 1970 for the first hospital group (1973 for the second group) and the year 1974 the percentage of unjustified hysterectomies in the hospitals as a whole dropped from 23.7 percent to 7.8 percent; and between 1970 and 1974 the total number of hysterectomies in Saskatchewan dropped by 32.8 percent. The doctors in the province knew about the committee and its list, of course. In other words, once they knew the operation was under scrutiny they became more careful about performing it. Now – will your country be taking a cue from Canada, doctor?

JAEGER: Not if those operation rates on doctors and their spouses are any guide.

HUNTER: Well then, let us look more closely at the health of doctors themselves. We established the other day, with the help of Professor Brent, also an American, that serum cholesterol levels were not lower in American doctors than in other Americans. You may also accept that doctors are admittedly slow in seeking treatment for themselves when they have cancer[45] or a psychiatric illness.[46] It has been said that they pay more attention to the health of their patients than to their own.

JAEGER: That's right: they're too busy with other people to be bothered about themselves.

HUNTER: I said nothing about them being busy, doctor, or not busy; though I shall say something in a moment. 70 percent of doctors also omit, for themselves, the regular check-ups that 90 percent of them recommend to their patients.[45] That was found in a study of some American doctors. It also showed that about 46 percent of the doctors had *significant* unknown diseases (there was an average of almost five new, unknown diseases per doctor). These figures were very similar to those in a group of business executives; and in fact, 38 percent of all the diseases found in the doctors needed treatment compared with only 24 percent of the executives' diseases. And 87 percent of the doctors who were found to have significant unknown diseases needed treatment, compared with only 57 percent of the executives with such diseases. 'Significant', judge, meaning 'worth paying attention to' – conditions such as tumors, heart disease, hernia, or diabetes.

JAEGER: That's right, Mr Hunter. I remember this little study. The doctors had more heart disease and peptic ulceration than the executives, which probably meant they were under more stress; and someone else showed coronary heart disease was the commonest killing disease among doctors, even in the 1940s and fifties,[45] and someone else said doctors were too busy to lead a healthy life;[45] and someone else found a majority of doctors didn't have a doctor of their own,[45] *et cetera, et cetera.* So?

JUDGE: You do not feel, doctor, that you and your colleagues should practice what you preach?

JAEGER: Yes, judge, but we're a very busy profession. We don't *make* diseases for ourselves.

HUNTER: Or even imagine them, doctor? Now: you are perhaps acquainted with a 30-year study[46] of a group of United States doctors – they were medical students at the start – as compared with a group of non-medical graduates.

JAEGER: I know it. The doctors were a lot more likely to have had a poor marriage or a divorce, and to have misused drugs or alcohol, and more likely to have had psychiatric treatment.

HUNTER: In fact, nearly half the doctors had had marriage difficulties, and a third had had trouble with drugs and alcohol; and indeed, in all respects they had experienced more difficulties than the non-medical people, although this was a sample of doctors supposedly healthier than most of their colleagues. Do you remember what this poor showing on the part of the doctors was put down to?

JAEGER: Yes, it was their childhoods – things like their relationships with their mothers and fathers, their health as children, the general atmosphere at home, and so on.

HUNTER: Yes, and it was *not* overwork that got the doctors into difficulties – it was the demands of dependent patients when the doctors themselves had their own barren childhood backgrounds to cope with. You are aware also that doctors under 40 are at least four times as likely as other people to commit suicide – American doctors anyway?[47] That a conservative estimate has it that 17,000 doctors in this country – 5-6 percent of all the doctors – are now adversely affected by alcoholism, drug abuse, or mental illness?[47] And that the wives of doctors often complain of marital difficulties, have trouble with drug or alcohol misuse, and suffer from depression or bodily symptoms; and that this seems to arise because they find their husbands undemonstrative, cold, rigid, and uncommunicative?[48] And the doctors tend to meet all their difficulties by working harder, by turning their aggression on themselves, by denying to themselves what they would certainly recommend to their patients, even when they realize they are not well?[46,47,48]

JAEGER: They channel all their energies into helping their patients. What's so wrong with that?

HUNTER: And away from their wives and families when they should be turning to them to give and receive support?

JAEGER: We're talking about a minority of doctors.

JUDGE: But, doctor, a very substantial minority. Almost a half of the doctors in the 30-year study Mr Hunter mentioned had had a poor marriage. If a substantial proportion of doctors behave like this to themselves, and to their families, what hope is there of them understanding the psychosocial problems we were hearing the other day affect a lot of their patients?

JAEGER: That study,[46] judge, said they might make excellent clinicians even though their rearing and childhood had been mixed-up – in fact, because of that.

HUNTER: But would you not draw the conclusion, doctor, that perhaps there should be a different selection procedure for medical students? At the moment it is those students who do well in examinations, who are already striving too hard and are imbued with guilt, that get into medical school.[49] And trainee family doctors, it has been shown,[50] are rigid, unimaginative, lacking in humor and culture and interest in social matters and indeed in any minority-type interest. They show conventional responses, they respect authority, they conform, they believe in dominance, they have narrow technical interests. In other words, they are the sort of people who will keep their hand to the plow, but will never wonder about a better plow or whether their kind of plowing is necessary at all.

JAEGER: Well, Mr Hunter, *you* have a lonely furrow to plow if you intend to alter the medical profession.

HUNTER: Hard perhaps, but I'm not so sure about its being lonely. My next topic is medical migration world-wide. About 100,000 doctors are now migrating across the world in one direction or another each year.[51] Let us look first at the position as it affected the United States up to 1977 – when the position changed greatly, though we'll deal with that later. You have a large number of foreign medical graduates – FMGs as they are known – in your country?

JAEGER: Of our more than 300,000 American doctors[51] about 20 percent were trained in foreign medical schools.[52] Something in many ways to be proud of.

HUNTER: About 10,000-12,000 FMGs were known to enter the USA each year in the early-to-mid-1970s, mainly from Asia, Europe, and South America?[53]

JAEGER: Correct, although about 5,000 or so annually were what we call exchange visitors[53] – that is, they came for specialized training with a view to returning to their own countries after a few years. Mind you, a lot of them either stayed, or else returned home with the intention of coming back here, or else came back because they became disillusioned at home. They didn't always find back home the intellectual satisfaction that they expected.[51]

HUNTER: That they had been led in the United States to expect? (*Pause*) Or else they didn't find the money they had been led to expect. (*Jaeger nods*) There was an examination that foreign medical graduates were advised to take before coming to the United States, set by the Educational Commission for Foreign Medical Graduates, and commonly known as the ECFMG? And only those foreign medical graduates who had passed it could enter approved training programs in what are called accredited hospitals – as interns or residents (junior medical staff, that is). And most of the 10,000 or 12,000 annual medical entrants we just mentioned did eventually pass the ECFMG?[54] Once a foreign doctor had passed it he was at least eligible eventually for full licensure, which would enable him to practice quite freely? He got it by taking an exam called FLEX – the Federal Licensing Examination. But there was also the restricted licensure that some States in your country issued to foreign doctors who had not passed the ECFMG, and even to some who had?[54,55]

JAEGER: That is correct. Many of the doctors who received such provisional licensure worked – and still work – in non-accredited hospitals: not running approved training programs, that is; often mental hospitals,[51,54,55] and sometimes only under supervision. We appreciated what they did.

HUNTER: They received little or no proper training? (*Jaeger nods*) And some worked under supervision in hospitals without having any licence, or even as technicians and so on? Some even worked outside the health field, perhaps trying to pass the ECFMG or get a license? All these doctors were and are sometimes known as the medical underground?[51,54,55]

JAEGER: Yes, but the number of such FMGs is really unknown.

HUNTER: Well – do correct me if I am wrong – one estimate had it that between 1961 and 1971 some 9,000 foreign doctors entered the USA completely unknown to the authorities: unknown as physicians, that is. [54] Another had it that there were recently well over 10,000 foreign doctors actually working in the health field not fully licensed and not in approved training programs. [55] And even of those FMGs who *were* in such programs there was a much smaller proportion in hospitals affiliated to medical schools (that is, in general, the better hospitals for training purposes) than was the case for American medical graduates. [54,55] (*Jaeger nods*) In 1973 how many foreign medical graduates received a full licence?

JAEGER: About 7500, as I recall. [56]

HUNTER: And how many extra licentiates were there in all in that year?

JAEGER: Nearly 17,000. [56]

HUNTER: And you would accept that in 1972 the corresponding figures were almost 7,000 [53] and 14,000 [56]?(*Jaeger nods*) So that in those two years, despite the factors operating against the FMGs, nearly a half of the new fully licensed doctors in the USA came from foreign countries? (*Jaeger nods*) Also, what is apparently not in any doubt is that in 1971 some 10,500 medical graduates entered your country while your own medical schools turned out only 9,500 graduates. [51] (*Pause*) You are aware it has been suggested that, at least in part, the lower rate of licensure among foreign as compared with United States domestic medical graduates was not necessarily due to any lack of competence in the former, [57] but due to a form of discrimination, the methods of licensing being different for the two types of graduate? – American graduates didn't usually take FLEX, they took Part III of the American Boards exam? Also that the state licensing boards, in using the power they had to give limited licenses to FMGs – to practice only in certain areas or even in certain institutions – were steering them to where there was a marked doctor shortage thanks to the unwillingness of American doctors to practice there? And that FMGs with an American immigrant visa or who had become American citizens were much more likely to be given a full license than those who were in your country only as visitors, competence aside? [57] So that the latter constituted a reservoir of doctors to be tapped as and when it suited your country's convenience? [57]

JAEGER: You shouldn't believe everything just anyone tells you, Mr Hunter.

HUNTER: I don't. I believe in fact, doctor, and facts are what I am giving you. And you must not jib at them if they are unpleasant.

In 1974 18,000[58] of the interns and residents in *approved* hospital training programs in the USA were FMGs; and 41,000 were non-FMGs – that is, mainly graduates of United States medical schools.[59] So that, if as a conservative estimate we allow for the fact that two thirds of the junior staff in the *non*-approved programs consisted of foreign medical graduates, it would be true to say that, until very recently, one third at the very least of all United States interns and residents – junior hospital doctors – were foreign medical graduates?[60]

JAEGER: That is true. We were very conscious of the problem.

HUNTER: Their salaries were often lower than those of other doctors, were they not?[54] Sweated labor, as you might say? The medical slave trade? It was calculated that, if the 12,000 or so foreign medical graduates the United States imported in 1973 were to be replaced by US graduates, the educational cost would be around 600 million dollars.[55] Now, the rate of importation of FMGs increased greatly in the late 1960s and early 1970s, doctor. Why was that?

JAEGER: In 1965 my country enacted that priority should be given, for immigration purposes, to people with special professional or technical skills.[51]

HUNTER: Because it was felt the USA needed such people, never mind their own countries? Your Department of Labor said you were 50,000 doctors short, did it not?[53] And would you dissent from the following rounded-off figures for inflow of FMGs for the years 1966 to 1973 in sequence: 7,000, 8,500, 9,000, 7,000, 8,000, 10,500, 11,500 and 12,500?[53] There were also, of course, the extra numbers of immigrants unknown as physicians whom I mentioned just now? (*Pause*) And would you dissent from the statement that the increase in numbers mostly represented doctors from Asian countries?

JAEGER: No, I would not. The numbers of Asian doctor immigrants increased sevenfold between 1965 and 1970. By then they represented more than half of all the new immigrant doctors.[51]

HUNTER: I put it to you that the first eight countries of origin of foreign medical graduates in United States graduate programs in 1974 were in the following rank order by numbers involved: India, the Phillipines, Korea, Formosa, Iran, Thailand, Mexico, and Pakistan.[58]

JAEGER: I don't dispute that. As I said, we were very conscious—

HUNTER: New York State is, for a lot of Americans, the epitome of the United States, is it not? Will you accept that about two out of every five doctors in New York State are from foreign medical schools?[60] (*Jaeger nods*) What was the concentration of doctors in the US in, say, 1970? Perhaps you will accept that it was 15.4 per 10,000.[51] And that for some of the leading donor countries the figures were: India, two per 10,000 people; Iran, 2.6; Korea, 3.7; and the Philippines, 7.5.[51] These countries – some of them certainly – could ill afford to lose any doctors – if, that is, doctors serve a useful purpose?

JAEGER: No question.

HUNTER: In some of them babies and young children were dying and are still dying for want of the most elementary medical care? (*Jaeger nods*) And yet doctors from those countries helped to staff the intensive care units in your country that were keeping alive – if that is the right word – septuagenarians or octogenarians for a few more months, and at enormous cost? (*Pause*) Tell me, Dr Jaeger, what is the current and projected annual output of your own American medical schools.

JAEGER: That I can tell you because I'm involved in this one. For 1975–6 it was around 13,500, and the projections for the succeeding five years are 14,000, 14,500, 15,000, 15,000, and 15,500 – these last two figures being for 1979–80 and 1980–81.[61] They're round figures, of course. Between 1966 and 1976 we increased our number of American medical schools from 88 to 114,[61] I'm proud to say.

HUNTER: And yet in 1970, when all this must have been at least mooted, if not already planned, had not your Congress – in response to your Department of Labor's repeated assertion that doctors were still in short supply in the USA – had it not very largely waived the previous requirement that exchange visitors coming to your country for post-graduate training had to leave it for at least two years after the training was finished?[51, 53] (*Jaeger nods*) In effect, giving *carte blanche* to any foreign medical graduates to enter your country and stay here?

JAEGER: I guess so. We were very—

HUNTER: Well now, let us look at the consequences. In a report mentioned yesterday, prepared by the American management consultant firm of McKinsey and Co., Inc.,[62] it was shown that, if one graded 22 western countries according to seven different criteria of health in 1971–72 – infant mortality, maternal mortality, mortality in the middle-aged, and so on – then the first seven countries were, in this order, Sweden, the Netherlands, Norway, Switzerland, Denmark, Japan, and England and Wales; the 21st and next-to-last country being the USA. Will you accept that each of those seven countries had a lower concentration of doctors in 1970 than the USA?[62] And that during the 1960s the percentage change in that concentration had been lower in every one of them except Sweden – which started from much the lowest base of all seven – than it was in the USA?[62] (*Jaeger nods*) So where was the sense in importing all those foreign medical graduates? And where was the sense in planning to increase the output of your own medical schools? Where is the sense now in increasing it?

JAEGER: You can't have too many doctors.

HUNTER: And yet increasing their total numbers didn't seem to bring any increase in health at all commensurate with the doctor increase. It could even be argued that after a certain point it brought less health.

JAEGER: What you're saying undermines the whole American concept of life.

HUNTER: Dr Jaeger, you said that money and intellectual satisfaction attract foreign medical graduates to the USA. And yet they are very often needed much more in their own countries.

JAEGER: Yes, but a lot of the work is in country areas, understand, and is pretty elementary stuff, so they just don't want to know about it.

HUNTER: Although it might improve the health of the people as a whole much more than the American – the western – style of medicine that they practice for a minority of people, for the richer people, in their own cities, where the doctors tend to congregate? – Those who do stay in their own countries, I mean. Why do they *want* that intellectual satisfaction? What is it makes them think along the lines of western scientific hospital medicine all the time?

JAEGER: Because that's the way they're brought up as medical students.

HUNTER: By Americans sometimes? Is it not a fact that quite a number of the medical schools in the underdeveloped countries are largely staffed by doctors from America and other western countries?

JAEGER: Yes, sir. The brain drain in reverse. It's give as well as take.

HUNTER: But if it encourages a hundred times as many brains to emigrate to America . . .? Are you aware that the Pahlavi medical school in Iran is a carbon copy of an American school, that all teaching is done in English, and that nearly all the teachers are British or American?[63] And do you know also that just a few years ago nearly 90 percent of the doctors graduating from Pahlavi University emigrated to your country? Nearly 90 percent, doctor. Suppose the training of these people had been more appropriate to the health needs of their own country? Less highbrow, less scientific, less geared to the intensive care unit and more to the ordinary people of the villages and their ordinary health problems? Whether or not you called the end product 'doctor' wouldn't matter. You know this has been suggested?[64, 65] It might have stopped the emigration, might it not? You don't defend that massive emigration, do you? You don't defend a position in which, as once happened, a whole year's output of doctors in Thailand chartered a plane as soon as they had qualified and flew off immediately to the United States?

JAEGER: No, but there's a thing called the liberty of the subject. You can't, Mr Hunter, just keep people out because you think they . . .

HUNTER: Yes, doctor? – Were you not going to say 'because you think they shouldn't come'? But is that not exactly what your country is *now* planning to do to nearly all foreign medical graduates who might wish to settle here? – Except that you want to keep them out, not for the good of their countries, but for that of yours. The Health Professions Educational Assistance Act of 1976 (PL 94-484), signed into law by President Ford, was designed for that purpose, was it not? The Carnegie Council on Policy Studies in Higher Education had reported[66] that, what with the USA's increasing output of doctors and those Americans who had qualified in foreign medical schools returning to their home country, there was no longer a doctor shortage. What's more, quite a few FMGs had begun to take their specialty examinations and were competing for the top medical jobs in the US with American citizens, were they not?[67] And so it was decided that medical immigration should be pretty well ended by 1980:[68] the FMGs had been fine for the menial jobs, but they mustn't start getting uppity; and anyway, some people thought there'd soon be so many American-born doctors that *they* could fill *all* the country's medical posts. Why, if the FMGs weren't kept out, there might even be unemployed doctors.[66] American doctors.

JAEGER: You make it sound decidedly nasty, Mr Hunter, and it wasn't like that.

HUNTER: If facts sound nasty, so be it, doctor. Now – correct me if I'm wrong – the new law laid down that any FMG wanting to get into the States to work would, as from January 1977, first have to pass what is known as the National Boards Examination, Parts I and II (or some equivalent) plus an English test. The catch was that, while you could sit the old ECFMG exam *outside* the US, you can't take the National Boards exam except *inside* the US; so the law meant, in effect, 'No more foreign medical graduates unless they're prepared to come here at the fairly high risk of not being accepted as doctors – or unless specially invited because possessing a very special skill wanted by the US.'[66] Some people here thought this was a bit precipitate. They weren't all against the thing in principle, but some of them felt there might be snags if it was done in a rush. And the State of Illinois very obligingly provided some supporting evidence.[68] It had 127 FMGs without a federal license practicing in its mental hospitals; and in January 1977 it compelled them all to take the FLEX exam, and every single one failed – not surprisingly, as most of them had qualified years before – and they were all forthwith suspended from duty. Virtue was triumphant. Right, doctor?

JAEGER: Right on facts, not on the gloss you're putting on them.

HUNTER: Well, that left the American doctors working in Illinois mental hospitals with quite a lot of extra work to do; and they protested loud and long, and so did a lot of other people, who'd seen the FMGs doing a good job year after year for which there were no American takers.[68] So after a time the Governor of Illinois said yes, *he*'d find it difficult, he thought, to pass a law exam after his 18 years in practice; and special legislation was passed, graciously permitting the FMGs to go back to work till March 1978 – when they had to sit the exam again. Washington had been getting the message too. First, the Secretary for Health, Education, and Welfare gave a one-year waiver for the National Board exam requirement;[68] and then in September 1977 a new exam the Visa Qualifying Exam or VQE – was introduced. If you were an FMG, you had to pass this, and pass an English test, and so get your visa; and then take FLEX for full licensure[69] – though you *could* still get in if you were persistent enough. But all jobs for FMGs must be training jobs, not just service jobs;[70] and FMGs will normally be restricted to a two-year stay; which, as nearly all residency programs – leading to a specialist qualification – last for three years, means no or very few FMGs will be qualifying as specialists here in future.[68, 70] Now all this is an excellent way – is it not? – of making sure there'll be jobs for all the American medical boys, even if it does put some FMGs who've been working hard in the United States for years into a difficult position.[71] A turnabout from 1973? You'd have them when it suited you but not when it didn't.

JAEGER: I'll say one thing for you, Mr Hunter: apart from those last remarks I'd guess you could pick your way through a minefield blindfolded. But we're not the only country to play at this game. Canada, just a few years back, was getting even more doctors from overseas, mostly from Asia, than from its own medical schools,[72] and in November 1976 it said 'No more'. And there's always your own country.

HUNTER: Oh yes, we have a net loss of about 500 of our own medical graduates each year[72, 73] – until recently to the USA and Canada,

Australia, and so on – and we have a net annual gain of 700 foreign medical graduates, mostly from Asia. Actually about 3000 doctors come every year, but most of them go home eventually. [72]

JAEGER: And *your* hospital service would collapse without them.

HUNTER: Oh yes, doctor. I was not suggesting the United States had a monopoly in this respect. About one in four of all doctors in the United Kingdom is from a foreign medical school, mainly Asian; [72] well over 50 percent of the junior staff in hospitals, and about one in eight of all consultants [74] plus about one in six of all family doctors [74] are the same. And like yourselves, we do not train all the immigrant doctors properly; we use them to a great extent as cheap labor in hospitals and in specialties that our own junior doctors will not usually favor. Each of our consultants – as we call most of our specialists – must have his retinue of junior staff, most of whom therefore cannot hope ever to be specialists themselves. With about 12,000 specialists and 19,000 junior staff, the former holding their posts for 30 years or so, it is quite obvious that most of the juniors, even the British juniors, must either stay as juniors or become family doctors or emigrate; the foreign medical graduates have the extra option of returning home.

JAEGER: I'm relieved that you admit the British have faults too.

HUNTER: We have at least one fault that even you Americans cannot boast: we have now begun to 'export' some of our own highly-trained specialists to oil-rich countries in the Middle East, where they are very well paid. At Heathrow Airport our own doctors get on Concorde for the Middle East, and on the next runway doctors from India are getting off a plane from that country – to settle with us. Actually they're now settling in somewhat smaller numbers than they were a few years ago: in June 1975 we introduced a special clinical and language test for certain overseas doctors – the TRAB test, so called because it is set by the Temporary Registration Assessment Board of the General Medical Council – and about two thirds of the would-be immigrants who take it fail. [75] The Board was set up in response to doubts about the ability of some immigrant doctors, especially their ability in English; but it did more or less coincide with an appreciation, similar to what you have had in the States, of the fact that the increased output of our own medical schools might lead to unemployment among British doctors. But now, in view of this picture of migration – and we have, of course, left out the relatively small movement of doctors from Australasia, and from Canada to the United States, and so on – what conclusions about doctors can one draw?

JAEGER: That they respond to the forces that motivate most people.

HUNTER: But they're not like most people, doctor; or so they pretend. Do you not remember the quoted words with which I began my questioning of you: 'The ordinary physician is not moved by the dubious chance at wealth but would rather have regular and adequate income, the feeling of security and freedom to devote himself in an uncompromising way to his calling'? Is he not called to serve his fellow citizens within the borders of his own country, which has educated him? Or *must* he go to Manhattan or London to follow his calling in an uncompromising way? Would the doctors even in an underdeveloped country have a grossly inadequate income? Would it not be far in excess of that of most of their patients? Just as that of American doctors or of British doctors is far in excess of the incomes of most of *their* patients. Would you not say these doctors from underdeveloped countries have been seized by two virulent infections? That of desire for money, and that of intellectual pride? And that they have caught both infections from the doctors of the west?

JAEGER: I find you melodramatic again. Once these countries are developed countries then they'll all be able to afford the hospitals and laboratories and clinics and so on that are essential to the practice of good medicine.

HUNTER: Such as has secured an almost static life expectancy for middle-aged American males? Are you aware that the United States sucks in, not only doctors, but all kinds of scientists and technologists from other countries? That this inflow was valued in 1970 at no less than $3,700,000,000, which was above the entire United States non-military foreign aid for that year?[76] How could an underdeveloped country become like the USA – even if one assumes that to be desirable – if the USA is importing most of the country's best brains, fully trained, year in, year out?

JAEGER: Life is not quite so simple as you make out, Mr Hunter.

HUNTER: No? I want now to show what doctors *could* do. You have heard of the Lincoln Pediatric Collective, doctor?

JAEGER: Have I not? A bunch of long-haired young medics operating from Lincoln Hospital in the Bronx. Community-conscious they called themselves. As though I'm not community-conscious.

HUNTER: The Bronx is a poor district of New York City, has a lot of unemployment and crime, a large black population, and few doctors? The Lincoln Hospital serves around half a million people? In 1970 a group of about 30 pediatric house staff and students formed the Lincoln Collective? (*Jaeger nods*) A doctor, who was clearly being quite objective about it, wrote an article[77] on the topic. At the suggestion of the judge, and as the quotation is not a short one, and as my reading of it could be construed as emphasizing what was not emphasized in the original, or as playing down what was not played down, we shall have it projected on to the screen against the back wall of the court, where everyone may read it as it originally appeared in cold print. There are one or two paraphrases or linking or explanatory passages (to which I do not think anyone would take exception) written by myself. (*The quotation is projected.*)

From the collective's recruitment brochure: 'There is an increasing number of medical students and house officers who have a socially and politically conscious orientation toward their role in medicine, who are concerned with practicing medicine in such a way as to effect social change . . . in an environment which now generates disease. . . .' In the hospital itself they carried on with their pediatric clinical work; and their main work in the community was to arouse people's consciousness of the need for the approach they were advocating. As an allied group in the Bronx put it: 'We want free health care for all people. . . . We want community-run health clinics on every block to deal with minor health problems. . . . We want door-to-door preventive care to deal with sanitation control, nutrition, drug addiction, child day care, and senior citizen services. . . . We want educational programs that expose the leading health problems, such as unemployment, poor housing, racism, malnutrition, police brutality, and all forms of exploitation.'

The author of the article wrote that the type of revolutionary physician involved in the collective attacked 'the traditional approaches to medical training as rigidly authoritarian, extremely demanding personally, and initially involving some subjugation to an élitist structure . . . It is obvious that the revolutionary physician is deeply occupied with life style. He resists the depersonalization of technological society, which is considered by him to be "the central malaise in American life today".'

The revolutionary physician believes 'that the medical establishment, especially medical schools, but also governmental agencies such as comprehensive health-planning agencies, have acted in a pseudo-conspiratorial manner to secure control over resources intended for health and used them in a way that has resulted in personal aggrandisement rather than improved health status. The solution proposed is community control of health services.' (This is the author of the article, of course, speaking.) The revolutionary physician usually put all social and economic problems under the heading of 'health problems', and usually felt that for a few physicians and some middle-aged do-gooders merely to plod on as best they could – that this would make little impact on the immense health needs that exist, and might simply blunt 'the edge of confrontation.'

The author continued: 'I have found the collectivists . . . have not succumbed to viewing the individual as an organ or a pathologic entity. They are concerned about all the factors that influence and usually impair the patient's ability to achieve health . . . and are interested in seeking the advice and opinions of many others at the professional and the nonprofessional level. Within the hospital itself, they have tried to introduce many of the cherished values long associated with the traditional family doctor. In place of a succession of nameless white-garbed house staff, they have tried to introduce a person who has as his major personal goal, continuity of care for his patients. This is viewed as an end in itself. . . . They see the solution of the health-care crisis only in terms of change in the total fabric of society. They wish to escape being dehumanised. They challenge the more materialistic values of society, and they believe the prevailing order to be discredited. . . . In many ways this' – that is, the approach of the collective – 'seems to represent a direct reaction against the traditional competitive, egocentric, isolated, social structure so common in medical-school education and residency training.' And lastly: 'The tradition of the absolute worth of the individual and its elaboration in the Hippocratic Code must be carefully distinguished from a more recent tradition of largely economic individualism.'

HUNTER: In other words, Dr Jaeger, in that last part of the quotation this author is saying that the worth of the individual, as traditionally seen by doctors, is not to be confused with the value of the individual as a money-grubbing entrepreneur.

JUDGE: You wish to comment, doctor?

JAEGER: The Lincoln Collective was a bunch of way-out commies, doubtless smoking marijuana on the side.

JUDGE: You have evidence on that score?

JAEGER: You don't need evidence, judge, for that kind of thing. You just know.

JUDGE: I fear that, in my perhaps old-fashioned judicial way, I do like evidence, doctor.

JAEGER: Well, anyway, where did they get to? A bunch of long-haired kids taking on the American nation?

JUDGE: Well, their – and your – ancestors 200 years ago did take on the British nation with a measure of success – or what some would call success.

JAEGER: There'll be no Boston tea party in the Bronx, judge.

JUDGE: A pot party perhaps? Mr Hunter?

HUNTER: I should like finally to turn back to some eminently non-revolutionary physicians. First, doctor, as it seems to summarize all I have said about American doctors, I want to quote from an article by a doctor writing from Chicago – the very heart of America – for the *British Medical Journal*[78] not long ago: 'In the last year, health insurance premiums have gone up by as much as 30%, and General Motors . . . recently announced it was spending more money on health than on steel . . . it is reported that Medicaid patients have twice as much surgery as the rest of the population. . . .' He wrote too of 'investigations and newspaper exposés of fraud and unlawful practices. These include unnecessary operations, gross overprescribing, inflating costs, "kickbacks" from laboratories to physicians ordering tests, double billing, and billing for services that were not rendered . . . it has long been the theme of government officials that this is the medical profession's last chance to put its house in order – or someone else will have to do it for them – meaning the government.'

JAEGER: We've heard all this stuff already, Mr Hunter; and why do you keep going for the USA?

HUNTER: I'm now going to look at my own country for you, doctor. In 1972 the British Medical Association held its Annual Clinical Meeting in Cyprus. Four hundred British doctors attended.[79]

JAEGER: And why not? Doctors have got to go places, see the world.

HUNTER: Cyprus is a center of scientific medical excellence?

JAEGER: Well no, I guess, but still—

HUNTER: Do you think it appropriate that the opening address was on moral problems facing the medical profession at the present time? (*Pause*) In 1973 the British Medical Association held its annual meeting jointly with the Canadian Medical Association in Vancouver on the west coast of Canada.[80] Three hundred British doctors and their wives attended.

JAEGER: Why not? – A beautiful city, Vancouver.

HUNTER: Pleasant to have a break in, thousands of miles from home? (*Jaeger nods*) Then in 1974 the Association held its Annual Clinical Meeting in conjunction with the Medical Association of Jamaica – in Kingston and Montego Bay, Jamaica.[81, 82] Five hundred and seventy-five people from Britain attended, including presumably more doctors than constitute the entire medical population of Jamaica, especially if one allows for the brain drain. Jamaica is, of course, like Cyprus, a center of scientific medical excellence? A medical Mecca?

JAEGER: Well no, it's not exactly Baltimore or London. . . .

HUNTER: It perhaps has a lot of disease problems relevant to the interests of British doctors? Diseases the British doctors none the less cannot see in Britain? (*Jaeger shakes his head*) It does, however, have sunshine and a lot of nice beaches and nice hotels, does it not? Rather like Cyprus and Vancouver. Well away from the poorer parts.

JAEGER: But what's so wrong with combining a little pleasure with one's business?

HUNTER: You mean one's profession, do you not? It was perhaps appropriate that the opening address was on coronary artery disease, to which, as we heard from Professor Brent, good living, and also stress and lack of exercise – as from overmuch air travel – may contribute. This meeting was held in April 1974, doctor, just six months after the Middle East oil crisis had sent oil prices rocketing upwards.

JAEGER: Well, doctors can't be at the beck and call of a couple of oil sheikhs.

HUNTER: Unless the sheikhs are ill perhaps? (*Pause*) The following year British doctors, doubtless including some of those who went to Jamaica, started an 'emergencies only' campaign against the British government's plan to phase private beds out of the National Health Service. It could not have been because they feared they might not, if the plan succeeded, have the money to go to Jamaica next time? In June 1976 some 1200 Canadian doctors[83] flew to Dublin for a joint annual general and scientific meeting of the Irish, British, and Canadian Medical Associations. At the meeting one Canadian doctor complained that Canadian doctors weren't getting paid enough.[84]

JAEGER: And what's wrong with them going to Dublin to meet up with old friends?

HUNTER: The cost of registering at the meeting to a British Medical Association member was £40, and to him the basic cost of the visit to Dublin ranged from £65 to £155.50 – no meals or drinks included, of course.[85] You may recall that at the time Britain had about a million and a quarter unemployed. Some of the doctors at these meetings will doubtless have claimed tax rebates in respect of their expenses.

JAEGER: And wouldn't you?

HUNTER: What was the British old-age pension in June 1976? Will you accept that it was £13.50 for a single person per week?

JAEGER: All right, all right.

HUNTER: So that even a very restrained doctor, going to that Dublin conference might confidently be expected to spend far more in its five days than the total income of an old-age pensioner for 10 weeks? – That is, assuming he did not go to any of the optional events organized in connection with this scientific meeting, such as a visit to an Irish tavern, a cabaret show, and a horse-race meeting. (*Pause*) In February 1974, only three months after the Middle East oil crisis, the British Medical Association was advertising a golf competition between British and American doctors, to be held in Ayrshire, Scotland.[86] There was to be no medical meeting, no clinical or scientific aspect – simply a golfing competition. In other words, some hundreds of American doctors, many doubtless with their wives and children, were to come to Britain just to play golf – and they'd usually come by jet plane – at a time when there was a grave shortage of oil. Within the two months previous to the appearance of that golfing advertisement in the *British Medical Journal* there had been two letters[87, 88] in that same journal about a shortage of plastic syringes – and, of course, the raw material for plastics is oil. 'Whom God would destroy, He first sends mad'?

JAEGER: You've sure got your head in the clouds, Mr Hunter, haven't you?

HUNTER: Well, a lot of doctors seem literally to have theirs in the same place, don't they? Lastly, did you know that the choice for the 1979 British Medical Association's Annual Clinical Meeting was between Hong Kong and Gibraltar,[89] the former being chosen? And Gibraltar for '78? Centers of medical excellence?

JAEGER: Well no; but interesting places, both.

HUNTER: But these are purportedly scientific meetings; and the medical population of Hong Kong and of Gibraltar is tiny. And journeys to them from Britain are not cheap.

JAEGER: Oh well, your British doctors don't get such a lot out of life anyway.

HUNTER: You wouldn't think they should go to the Bronx? (*Pause*) One brief final glimpse of medico-scientific America, doctor: in the issue[90] of the *Journal of the American Medical Association* for September 26, 1977 there was an announcement of the Association's 1977 31st Winter Scientific Meeting, to be held at Miami Beach, Florida. A single room in a hotel would cost a doctor between $22 and $44 per day; and a suite up to $110 a day. The course fee was up to $70 per half day. The front page of the program carried six pictures: one of the beach and adjacent hotels, etc., at Miami; one of some flamingoes; two of a yacht, anchored in one, speeding through the water in the other; one of Miami lit up at night; and one of a nubile, scantily-clad young lady surfing.

JAEGER: Oh, just the human kind of bait to get doctors hooked on the scientific line.

HUNTER: Yes, Dr Jaeger. (*Pause*) One final question, doctor. Would you not agree that western doctors are in the mainstream of modern western society, both as individuals in the ordinary conduct of their lives, and as practitioners of scientific medicine? (*Jaeger nods*) Their science is the science of the west, their life-style is the life-style of the west, their ambitions and expectations are those of the west?

JAEGER: And why not?

HUNTER: They are siblings to the engineers, the chemists, the businessmen, the physicists, the airline pilots, the molecular biologists, the oil explorers, the computer technologists of the western world?

JAEGER: They're at home among such people, they use their inventions and methodology, yes. They're among the scientific élite. But doctors have their own ethos, of course.

HUNTER: Of course, as we have seen at today's session. The radioactive know-how they utilize in hospitals is utilized also to make the warheads of the American and Russian ICBMs? (*Pause*) At least, doctor, the cloud in which I have my head is not mushroom-shaped. No further questions.

JUDGE: I have just one for *you*, Mr Hunter, and one for the good doctor. Bring me up to date: where did the British Medical Association hold its annual meetings in 1977 and 1978?

HUNTER: In Glasgow and Cardiff respectively.

JUDGE: Not over-exotic places?

HUNTER: Not over-exotic, judge.

JUDGE: Thank you. (*Hunter sits*) And doctor, how many of the young, starry-eyed doctors in the Lincoln Collective were making $100,000 a year, do you think?

JAEGER: Not one.

JUDGE: And will they?

JAEGER: You just wait, judge: in a few years from now they'll be raking it in like everyone else.

JUDGE: Thank you, doctor, for that very frank and informative answer; and on that note this court is adjourned.

REFERENCES—SESSION EIGHT

1. Aring, C. D., *Journal of the American Medical Association*, April 8, 1974, 1974, vol. 228, p. 177. (Copyright 1974–75, American Medical Association).
2. Round the World, *Lancet*, May 24, 1975, p. 1182.
3. Cameron, C. T. M., *BMJ*, October 1, 1977, p. 877.
4. Dunea, G., *BMJ*, March 15, 1975, p. 621.
5. Round the World, *Lancet*, July 19, 1975, p. 122.
6. Editorial, *JAMA*, February 16, 1976, p. 756.
7. Meyers, A. F., *NEJM*, June 10, 1976, p. 1348.
8. Editorial, *Lancet*, January 3, 1976, p. 23.
9. Editorial, *Lancet*, January 3, 1976, p. 27.
10. Dale, M. G., *JAMA*, July 8, 1974, p. 157.
11. Round the World, *Lancet*, December 6, 1975, p. 1140.
12. Round the World, *Lancet*, October 2, 1976, p. 734.

13. Jessee, W. F., *et al.*, *NEJM*, March 27, 1975, p. 668.
14. Brewer, L. A., *JAMA*, February 16, 1976, p. 725.
15. Dunphy, J. E., *NEJM*, November 8, 1973, p. 1045.
16. Gilson, S. B., *NEJM*, November 8, 1973, p. 1045.
17. Sade, R. M., *NEJM*, November 8, 1973, p. 1045.
18. LeMaitre, G. D., *NEJM*, November 8, 1973, p. 1046.
19. Spear, P. W., *NEJM*, August 7, 1975, p. 310.
20. Schroeder, S. A., *et al.*, *JAMA*, August 20, 1973, p. 969.
21. Fett, J. D., *NEJM*, January 1, 1976, p. 58.
22. Clark, B. P., *NEJM*, February 19, 1976, p. 449.
23. Rosier, R. P., *NEJM*, February 19, 1976, p. 449.
24. *The Times*, April 21, 1976, p. 6.
21. *Pulse*, February 28, 1976, p. 14.
26. In Australia Now, *Lancet*, March 6, 1976, p. 525.
27. Review Body Report 1977, *BMJ*, June 4, 1977, p. 1480.
28. BMA's Written Evidence to Review Body, *BMJ*, May 15, 1976, p. 1227.
29. Leading Article, *BMJ*, March 19, 1977, p. 737.
30. Bunker, J. P., *NEJM*, January 15, 1970, p. 135.
31. Schieber, G. J., *et al.*, *NEJM*, May 13, 1976, p. 1089.
32. Whisnant, D. E., *Lancet*, December 18, 1976, p. 1358.
33. Cooper, J. K., and Heald, K., *JAMA*, March 25, 1974, p. 1410.
34. Nickerson, R. J., *et al.*, *NEJM*, October 21, 1976, p. 921.
35. Ibid., October 28, 1976, p. 982.
36. Hauck, W. W., Jr, *et al.*, *JAMA*, October 18, 1976, p. 1864.
37. Editorial, *JAMA*, January 17, 1977, p. 267.
38. Vayda, E., *NEJM*, December 6, 1973, p. 1224.
39. Vayda, E., *NEJM*, February 28, 1974, p. 521.
40. Editorial, *NEJM*, December 6, 1973, p. 1249.
41. Bunker, J. P., and Brown, B. W., Jr, *NEJM*, May 9, 1974, p. 1051.
42. Bunker, J. P., *et al.*, *NEJM*, July 29, 1976, p. 264.
43. Editorial, *JAMA*, September 2, 1974, p. 1335.
44. Dyck, R. J., *et al.*, *NEJM*, June 9, 1977, p. 1326.
45. Sharpe, J. C., and Smith, W. W., *JAMA*, October 20, 1962, p. 114.
46. Vaillant, G. E., Sobowale, N. C., and McArthur, C., *NEJM*, August 24, 1972, p. 372.
47. Bittker, T. E., *JAMA*, October 11, 1976, p. 1713.
48. Simpson, M. A., *World Medicine*, September 24, 1975, p. 54.
49. Pearce, K. I., at 1975 Canadian Medical Association Annual Scientific Meeting, quoted in Landon, N. R., *Pulse*, August 2, 1975, p. 10.
50. McCormick, J., *Proceedings of the Royal Society of Medicine*, January 1975, p. 16.
51. Dublin, T. D., *NEJM*, April 20, 1972, p. 870.
52. Stimmel, B., *NEJM*, July 10, 1975, p. 68.
53. Mason, H. R., *JAMA*, July 22, 1974, p. 428.
54. Weiss, R. J., *et al.*, *NEJM*, June 20, 1974, p. 1408.
55. Ibid., June 27, 1974, p. 1453.
56. Medical Licensure 1973, Statistical Review, *JAMA*, July 22, 1974, p. 445.
57. Goldblatt, A., *et al.*, *NEJM*, January 16, 1975, p. 137.
58. Medical Education in the United States, 1974–1975, *JAMA*, December 29, 1975, p. 1355.
59. Ibid., p. 1357.
60. Round the World, *Lancet*, July 12, 1975, p. 72.

61. Medical Education in the United States, 1975–1976, *JAMA*, December 27, 1976, p. 2961.
62. Maxwell, R., *Health Care : The Growing Dilemma*, 2nd end, McKinsey and Co., Inc., New York, 1975.
63. Ronaghy, H. A., Cahill, K., and Baker, T. D., *JAMA*, February 4, 1974, p. 538.
64. Tavassoli, M., *JAMA*, May 13, 1974, p. 825.
65. Fendall, N. R. E., *BMJ*, April 26, 1975, p. 190.
66. Round the World, *Lancet*, December 25, 1976, p. 1400.
67. Charlton, E., *Pulse*, October 22, 1977, p. 34.
68. Dunea, G., *BMJ*, June 11, 1977, p. 1518.
69. Cox, J., *BMJ*, August 13, 1977, p. 444.
70. Round the World, *Lancet*, December 11, 1976, p. 1294.
71. Tank, K. M., *NEJM*, May 26, 1977, p. 1237.
72. Senewiratne, B., *BMJ*, March 15, 1975, p. 618.
73. Parkhouse, J., *Lancet*, September 11, 1976, p. 566.
74. Mayer, T. C., *Pulse*, June 26, 1976, p. 5.
75. Editorial, *Lancet*, September 20, 1975, p. 539.
76. Rhode, J. M., *Lancet*, August 9, 1975, p. 274.
77. McNamara, J. J., *NEJM*, July 27, 1972, p. 171.
78. Dunea, G., *BMJ*, July 10, 1976, p. 101.
79. Conference Reports, *BMJ*, April 22, 1972, p. 214.
80. Medical Practice, *BMJ*, July 7, 1973, p. 30.
81. Medical Practice, *BMJ*, May 11, 1974, p. 313.
82. Bradshaw, S., *BMJ*, June 1, 1974, p. 506.
83. *BMA News*, March 1976, p. 177.
84. Wilson, R. G., in Conference Report, *BMJ*, July 17, 1976, p. 157.
85. Supplement, *BMJ*, February 14, 1976, p. 410.
86. *BMJ*, 9 February 1974, advertisements, p. v.
87. Hart, C., *BMJ*, December 22, 1973, p. 741.
88. Garrett, A. S., *BMJ*, January 26, 1974, p. 161.
89. *BMA News*, March 1976, p. 177.
90. *JAMA*, September 26, 1977, p. 1355.

PSROs
Welch, C. E., *JAMA*, April 7, 1975, p. 47.

Inequalities in the British National Health Service
Morris, J. N., *Proceedings of the Royal Society of Medicine*, March 1973, p. 225.
Doll, R., *Proceedings of the Royal Society of Medicine*, August 1973, p. 729.
Townsend, P., *Lancet*, June 15, 1974, p. 1179.

Mental Illness in Doctors
Murray, R. M., *Lancet*, June 15, 1974, p. 1211.

Operation Rates
Roos, N. P., Roos, L. L., Jr, and Henteleff, P. D., *NEJM*, August 18, 1977, p. 360.
Editorial, *NEJM*, August 18, 1977, p. 387.
Bunker, J. P., Barnes, B. A., and Mosteller, F. (eds.), *Costs, Risks, and Benefits of Surgery*, Oxford Univetsity Press, New York, 1977.

Doctor Migration

Leading Article, *BMJ*, December 21, 1974, p. 674.

Senewiratne, B., *BMJ*, March 22, 1975, p. 669.

Alhtar, H., *The Times*, July 6, 1976, p. 14. (More than 50,000,000 rural Pakistanis have no basic medical services near their homes, yet in the last 30 years half the doctors qualifying in Pakistan have emigrated. The Pakistan government, which hoped to treble the output of doctors by 1978, imposed an almost total ban on doctor emigration in 1973. But see Session 17 as to whether the answer is indeed an increase in doctor output.)

Meskauskas, J. A., Benson, J. A., Jr, and Hopkins, E., *NEJM*, October 13, 1977, p. 808. (Report of a study showing that graduates of foreign medical schools, whether foreign nationals—mostly Asian—or US nationals, did worse than graduates of American and Canadian medical schools in the certifying examination of the American Board of Internal Medicine, the passing of which starts a doctor off on a career as a specialist general physician.)

Editorial, *NEJM*, October 13, 1977, p. 836. (Editorial on the last reference, on the whole opposed to the US relying at all in future on US nationals trained in foreign medical schools.)

Nassar, M. E., *NEJM*, January 19, 1978, p. 169. (The first of eight letters, all in one way or another critical of the last two references, with a reply from Dr. J. A. Benson, Jr, co-author of the last reference but one. This p particular letter queries whether the Board exam does, in fact, prepare people to become good doctors.)

Rosai, J., *NEJM*, January 19, 1978, p. 170. (Another of the eight letters, stating that the American government is now seeking to keep out graduates of foreign medical schools because graduates of American schools are having difficulty in finding jobs; to which Dr Benson replies that the American Board of Internal Medicine published in 1971 findings similar to those here at issue.)

HIGH TECHNOLOGY MEDICINE-FACTS

Enter Dr James Batt

HUNTER: You are Dr James Batt, lecturer in bio-engineering in relation to medicine at a new English university? You are a medical man, Dr Batt?

BATT: Yes, but I got a doctorate in physics first, then switched to medicine. There would be openings, I felt, for someone qualified in the two disciplines. I wasn't suddenly wanting to devote my life to suffering humanity. Nothing like that.

HUNTER: Would you agree that modern scientific medicine is an integral part of our modern western society in its principles, its methods, its aims and so on? A society dominated by science, by technology, by industry? (*Pause*) Well, as you hesitate: medical scientists are like other scientists in our society? They use the same principles, the same way of working, often the same apparatus, the same chemicals, even the same journals to some extent.

BATT: Yes – it's the industry and technology part I'm a bit less sure about.

HUNTER: Modern medicine relies on the pharmaceutical industry to supply it with drugs? There is an expanding industry for the manufacture of medical instruments, machinery, gadgets? Medicine has borrowed various techniques from industry? It is sometimes called 'the health industry'?

BATT: Yes, all right. A lot of the spin-off from the American space-industry program was medical too.

HUNTER: And surely there can be little dispute about technology, indeed high technology, being crucial to medicine. Much of modern medicine has been created by engineers, metallurgists, electronics experts, technicians and technologists of one kind or another who have invaded it in the last 30 years? Many of the technologists of the factory assembly line or the development laboratory would be perfectly at home in the modern hospital or medical research laboratory?

BATT: Oh, absolutely.

HUNTER: So that modern western scientific medicine *is* an integral part of modern western society? It cannot be viewed separately from the society of which it is a part? (*Batt nods*) In particular, you cannot have the benefits of the one without the benefits of the other? (*Batt hesitates, then nods again*) And it is the predominant kind of orthodox medicine today, indeed almost the only kind – at any rate in hospitals? Well now, when did modern scientific medicine – high-technology medicine – start?

BATT: I suppose some people would say – you know, the academic types, the medical historians – about 100 or 120 years ago, even earlier. But it really got into its stride only in the last half century, I'd say; and really only in the last 20 or 25 years, or thereabouts.

HUNTER: We established with Professor Larkin the other day that in general the expectation of life in western countries has increased very little, if at all, in the last couple of decades.

BATT: You're not saying that's the result of modern medicine, are you?

HUNTER: Professor Larkin indicated it was the effect of modern society, the society of which modern medicine is an integral part. He said too that hospitals have not played any major part in the saving of large numbers of lives, especially not in the last 20 or 30 years. Indeed, he said there had been an unfruitful emphasis on hospitals in that period.

BATT: Well, it's been a period of consolidation before we make the next big leap forward.

HUNTER: Then let us look at what has been consolidated, at the details of modern high-technology medicine. First, would you say that medical men use ordinary technological items as much as the next man in their ordinary lives? – I mean motor cars, planes, deep freezes, televisions, radios, cassettes, and so on?

BATT: Oh, yes. More so, I'd say, if anything.

HUNTER: They set no example in the way of doing without these gadgets?

BATT: Well, no. Why should they? And I wouldn't call them just gadgets. They're almost necessities today.

HUNTER: And yet for young people the car is the biggest single killing factor in all western countries.

BATT: Yes, you've got a point there. Still you could hardly expect doctors to – well, to cycle or walk, could you? We must be realistic.

HUNTER: And doctors use dictating machines, and telephone-answering machines, and radio car links from their cars to their offices? (*Batt nods*) And almost the most familiar sound in a hospital today is the bleep-bleep coming from the device in a doctor's pocket that tells him he is wanted and should go to the nearest telephone?

BATT: Well, naturally it is.

JUDGE: You feel, doctor, life would be unbearable without the bleeper and the telephone?

BATT: Well, no, not quite unbearable, judge, but almost impossible today. I mean here in the States millions of *non*-medical people will have pocket bleepers soon. We'll be the same in the UK in no time.

JUDGE: You see no drawbacks to such a technological spider's web?

BATT: No, it'll obviously be a great advantage to be able to keep in touch with everything all the time.

JUDGE: The spider's sentiments certainly.

HUNTER: Shall we move on, doctor, to disposable items in medicine? – Those made from plastic or aluminum or wood or paper. They have come in with high-technology medicine, and there is a great number of them?

BATT: Certainly – everything from disposable syringes to disposable proctoscopes; disposable sheets, tablecloths, knives, spoons, and plates and cups; disposable airways, disposable ashtrays, disposable scalpels, catheters, forceps, shrouds. It's marvellous, the range that's been developed.

JUDGE: Have shrouds not always been disposable, doctor?

BATT: Yes, I suppose they have, come to think of it. Yes.

HUNTER: You are aware that the same criticism has been leveled against medical disposables as against disposables in ordinary everyday life? That many of the items could perfectly well be in permanent, reusable form; that they consume resources – trees for wood and paper, oil for plastics, minerals – all of which are not inexhaustible, and the exploitation of which despoils our environment; that they are strange and alienating to the patient; that many disposable items, especially those made of plastic, are difficult or impossible to dispose of, and simply litter the earth, and may for generations to come?[1]

BATT: There are always cranks complaining about the price you pay for any progress.

JUDGE: High-technology medicine hasn't made disposable patients yet, doctor?

BATT: No, but bits of them certainly are.

HUNTER: To be replaced by mechanical items devised by high-technology medical people like yourself?

BATT: Or by transplants, of course. I'm only one member of one team, mind you. Still, when you think of the hardware we've got today – artificial hips and knees and shoulders, for instance. About 30,000 hip replacements alone every year in the UK,[2] and a number variously put at 75,000[3] and 150,000[2] here in the States. And there'll be a lot more in five or 10 years time.

HUNTER: 70 percent of them in people over 60? Costing, even a few years ago, about £750 a time, with a mortality of 1–2 percent, and a failure rate of 10 percent?[2] Or 20 percent for the earliest cases?[3] And often, if there is a failure, the patient is left a good deal worse off than if he had never had the operation?[3, 4]

BATT: You haven't mentioned the economic benefit, which is considerable, especially in those under 60.

HUNTER: I didn't mention either, doctor, the calculation that, to meet the demands for hip replacement in its ageing population would call for the construction of a new 300-bed hospital *every year* in Britain alone.[4] What would such a hospital cost? – £10,000,000? £20,000,000? (*Pause*) And the results are less good – are they not? – for replacements of most other joints? The elbow and shoulder, for instance, in which the replacement may end in disaster, in the shape even of an amputation as the only possible treatment.[5]

BATT: That's true, but that's being researched at this moment.

HUNTER: How many different types of artificial knee joint are there? Will you accept the figure of at least 25?[6] Does that not suggest that perhaps none of them is perfect, that perhaps all are highly imperfect? Especially as the two–three year failure rate after total knee replacement is 15–25 percent.[3]

BATT: To me it suggests people are pressing ahead to find a solution to the problem.

HUNTER: Do you know how many adults in Great Britain were estimated in 1968 to be handicapped or physically impaired by arthritis? Will you accept the figure of at least 800,000?[2] Suppose half of them – 400,000 – were before long to be regarded as suitable for a joint replacement operation, and that, as a very conservative estimate, each operation were to cost the £750 that each hip operation has been costing. What is £750 multiplied by 400,000?

BATT: £300,000,000. Around $600,000,000. A lot of pain and disability would be relieved though. And mind you, some of those 400,000 might not even want to have their joints replaced.

HUNTER: You said that some tens of thousands of hip-replacement operations are being performed each year here in the United States. Most of them will be in old people? Some of them males? Are you aware that in the American version of the high-technology society, the expectation of life for the male has been pretty well static, anyway for the older male, in recent years? And that the same applies to some other western countries?

BATT: I don't see what you're driving at.

HUNTER: You don't think the same process that, in the shape of high-technology medicine, produces hip replacement – excellent though it may often prove, viewed in isolation – may also in another dispensation sometimes reduce the life span, or prevent it increasing? – So that a man won't live long enough to have his hip replaced, or to enjoy the benefits of a replacement?

BATT: No, I don't see that at all.

HUNTER: You agree that some of the materials used in joint replacement have come from the American space program?[7]

(*Batt nods*) And that the space program was the great symbol of the high-technology life style that appears inevitably to lead to certain diseases, some of them lethal: coronary heart disease, obesity, lung cancer, and so on? So that the same life-style that in a sense cures also kills? You can't see that we give with one hand and perhaps take away more with the other?

BATT: No, I don't, I'm afraid.

HUNTER: Shall we move on to high-technology hearts? A purely mechanical heart is being investigated – for insertion into the human body? And heart pacemakers – to keep the heart beating properly are commonplace?

BATT: Yes, though we're a bit conservative back home about using pacemakers. And we're quite some way from a mechanical heart, though we'll make it one day.

HUNTER: And then you will be free of all the difficulties associated with transplanting a live human heart?

BATT: That's right: no rejection phenomena, no finding of donors . . .

HUNTER: No rapid development in the new heart of the coronary heart disease for which the old one was removed? You know that it did develop after a couple of years in the case of Dr Philip Blaiberg, the South African dentist who received a heart transplant? – In what was previously the absolutely healthy heart of a young man, the donor?[8]

BATT: Yes, and one day we'll learn how to prevent it developing.

HUNTER: The doctor concerned wrote that he had not in 40 years' experience seen such widespread atheroma of the coronary arteries as was found in the transplanted heart.[8]

BATT: That's right. Of course, it may just have been a rejection phenomenon, not atheroma, though perhaps the two are the same in a way.

JUDGE: Dr Batt, let me make sure I take you aright. You are agreeing that the late Dr Blaiberg was given a transplanted heart because the arteries of his own heart had developed atheroma. (*Batt nods*) Two years later he died, and it was found that the arteries of the new heart, perfectly healthy at the time of the transplant, had in that short time developed atheroma – presumably because of the continued presence in Dr Blaiberg of those factors that had produced the disease in his own heart. I am right so far?

BATT: And very clear, yes.

JUDGE: And you feel the answer is to seek some means of preventing the transplanted heart developing the atheroma? (*Batt nods*) But in that case the prevention could surely be applied to the original heart – the one the man was born with.

BATT: That's certainly one way of looking at it; but it might be a very expensive kind of treatment.

JUDGE: Might it not be better in that case to look for a cheap, generally-applicable means of prevention?

BATT: Oh, but that kind of prevention's a different scene altogether. Not yet proven either; and not my province if it comes to that.

JUDGE: Yes, Mr Hunter?

HUNTER: Dr Batt, the pancreas, or sweetbread, produces insulin; and it is insulin or the body's usage of it that is defective in diabetes? (*Batt nods*) In the normal person a rise in the blood sugar level makes the pancreas produce insulin which then causes the sugar level to fall; but this does not happen in the diabetic?

BATT: That's right, roughly.

HUNTER: However, is it not now possible to connect a diabetic to a machine that will supply his body with insulin as soon as the machine registers a rise in the blood sugar level?[9, 10]

BATT: Yes, and some people are working on its miniaturization. Then perhaps it could be inserted into the body of the diabetic and work for months. No daily insulin injections needed, nothing.[9, 10]

HUNTER: But insulin may be short by the end of the century?[10]

BATT: Yes. You see, you get it from animal pancreas, of which there is a limited supply; and by the end of the century countries that are poor now might not be so poor, and then they'd probably have some diabetes.[10]

HUNTER: Because diabetes is a disease of affluence? Probably a result in part of the diet consumed in our affluent society, the high-technology society? (*Batt nods*) So what is proposed?

BATT: It's possible to alter the genetic make-up of a bacterium to make it produce insulin.[11] You put into it some genetic material from a creature that does make insulin, and that teaches the bacterium how to, and it'll go on and on, a sort of insulin factory. You've got to feed it, of course. So far this has been done only for rat insulin; but if you can do it for rat insulin you can almost certainly do it for human insulin.

HUNTER: And then there'll be plenty for everyone? You are referring to a form of genetic engineering? (*Batt nods*) The fantasy of scientists one day producing some kind of Frankenstein aside, in 1974 and 1975 did not a large number of scientists express great concern about the possible dangers of bacterial genetic engineering?[12,13] And have the American National Institutes of Health not issued very stringent regulations to control work in this field, at any rate in their own laboratories, and banned certain types of work altogether?[14]

BATT: That's right. And there are absolutely fool-proof precautions against dangerous germs escaping. If there were any, I mean.

HUNTER: The strict precautions taken at Fort Detrick, Maryland, the American biological warfare center, have not always proved fully effective, have they? – In 25 years there have been 400 laboratory infections and some deaths.[15]

BATT: Yes, but we learn from our mistakes. We're learning all the time.

HUNTER: The dangers of someone accidentally – or perhaps even deliberately – producing a bacterium, by means of genetic engineering, that could cause a terrible epidemic, if it escaped from the laboratory, have been compared in the *New York Times* to those of the proliferation of nuclear weapons.[15]

BATT: Oh, journalists are always seeing dangers that scientists can't see.

HUNTER: The same comparison has been made in the even more sober pages of the *New England Journal of Medicine*,[16] which also spoke of the possibility of 'ecologic disaster'. You know too that Dr George Wald, professor of biology at Harvard, and a Nobel prize winner, is opposed to genetic engineering being practiced at the university?[15] He even doubts whether it should be conducted anywhere, whether we have any right to interfere with what has taken nature millions of years to evolve.[15]

BATT: Science is always interfering with nature. Think of the benefits we might get: insulin, hormones, perhaps a cancer cure.

HUNTER: What good will a cure for individual cancers be if a greater cancer is destroying mankind?

BATT: I think that's nonsense myself. Anyway, someone somewhere's going to do this research. In the end, if man knows there's some knowledge waiting for him to discover it, he'll find ways to discover it, rules or no rules.

JUDGE: You are merely saying that man is an ingenious and dangerous creature, doctor. Are the proposed regulations in this sphere adequate? Do we *know* they are?

BATT: We can keep animals germ-free for years. If we can prevent germs getting into creatures, we can prevent them getting out of laboratories – or else, if they do get out, spot them and kill them off pretty quickly. It's been possible, judge, to maintain a child germ-free for years: a boy in Texas who was found at birth not to have the normal immune response.

JUDGE: Meaning, doctor?

BATT: Meaning his body couldn't fight infections properly, so any infection might kill him. They suspected before birth he might be like that, so the delivery was germ-free, and he was put straight away into a transparent plastic chamber, isolated from all possible contact with germs. [17, 18]

HUNTER: And with humans?

BATT: Direct contact, yes. There are sleeves in the wall of the chamber, ending in gloves, and the nurses and his parents can put their hands in and touch him – with the material intervening between his skin and theirs, naturally.

JUDGE: This unfortunate child is still alive?

BATT: He certainly was when I last heard any news. [19] He was six then. He still hasn't got any immunity, so no one's quite sure what the next move should be. Actually a few germs have got inside – he isn't completely germ-free now. [19]

HUNTER: A similar technique can be used for leukemia patients [20] and for certain operations, [21] can it not? To prevent infections.

BATT: Yes, where you're putting in a new hip you can seal part of a big plastic envelope to the leg and blow it up. The envelope, I mean. It's got sleeves and gloves too, and the surgeons operate through these; and absolutely sterile air is run through the envelope all the time; and so germs simply can't get to the operation area.

JUDGE: Yes, do go on, doctor.

BATT: There's also a new kind of operating theater. It's got a hole in one wall, and a big long plastic bag has its mouth sealed all the way round this hole, and the rest of the bag sticks into the theater. If you're being operated on, you never properly get into the theater – you're simply pushed into the plastic bag from the outside. [22]

JUDGE: Yes, go on, please.

BATT: And to make doubly sure there'll be no infection the surgeons and nurses inside the theater wear a special sealed suit, with its own air-conditioning unit – so, even when they do start to operate through the plastic bag (they make a cut in it), none of their germs get to the patient.

HUNTER: A similar suit is used, I think, doctor, for some cancer patients who have been given anti-cancer drugs that lower their ability to fight infections. [23] Yes? (*Batt nods*) These suits are like those used by American astronauts during their quarantine period after returning to earth? [23]

BATT: That's right. High-technology society really showing what it can do.

HUNTER: And meantime in underdeveloped countries children die for want of food or pure water or a few tablets? (*Pause*) Shall we move on to another aspect of high-technology medicine – miscellaneous medical gadgets? Apart from those we've mentioned, there are jet injectors, and machines that will inject substances into a patient's vein automatically in response to a signal from some monitoring device?[9]

JUDGE: Monitoring? Watching, measuring . . . is that what is meant?

BATT: Yes, judge. Of course, the machine doesn't pick up a syringe and inject you. The needle's already in a vein, and the machine simply releases into the tubing leading to the needle whatever substance is to be injected.

HUNTER: There are dialysis machines, of course, to perform the kidney's functions; heart-lung machines; electronic thermometers and electronic blood pressure recorders; instruments to watch the pulse, the heart of the baby before birth, and the heart of the coronary patient (and a machine to shock it out of an abnormal rhythm), and to watch the breathing; what are called fiberoptic instruments – long and flexible – to be inserted into one or other orifice of the body so that the doctor may see for himself what is going on, either directly or by injecting a special material and then using X-rays. [24, 25]

BATT: Yes, the Japanese are very good with them. They can insert the tip of an instrument down through the esophagus – the gullet, judge – and stomach and duodenum, and into the common bile duct almost every time. [26] Mind you, it causes inflammation of the pancreas or the bile duct about once in every fifty times it's done. [27] Still, that's a small price to pay for actually seeing what's wrong.

HUNTER: Is it not true that each fiberoptic instrument costs about $10,000, and a doctor concerned with the stomach and intestines alone may need as many as seven different instruments; and they are all being made obsolete fairly rapidly? [26] It is also possible – is it not? – to insert a not dissimilar viewing tube into a woman's abdomen, and by inserting an operating instrument simultaneously at a different point to sterilize her? Or, if she is pregnant, to insert a viewing tube into the womb to see if the fetus is normal or not; so that, if it is abnormal, it may be aborted. [28] Doctors do seem to have something of a passion for peering into the human body. I wonder why.

BATT: Because you can trust the evidence of your eyes. Well, usually, not always.

HUNTER: I want now to deal with one field in which this passion they have for watching and controlling the body's processes has aroused some controversy. I mean the tendency to conduct more and more deliveries in hospital, and the correspondingly increased prevalence of what is called active management of labor: that is, control by the doctor instead of by nature. I believe at the moment, Dr Batt, some 90 percent of British women have their babies in hospital.[29] (*Batt nods*) But many obstetricians would like to see 100 percent hospital deliveries?[29, 30] And have two of them not said that, 'Experience has shown that labour is far from safe if left to the capricious whims of Nature'?[31]

BATT: Yes, and I go along with that every time.

HUNTER: Other experts are against this move towards active management of all labor in hospital,[32, 33, 34] or at best doubtful about it?[35]

BATT: 100 percent hospital deliveries is the best policy.

HUNTER: As I understand it, doctor, nobody disputes that many women should certainly have their babies in a hospital: it's that 100 percent and the possibility of excessive or unnecessary inter-ference – and the possible drawbacks and dangers – that some doctors are very doubtful about.

BATT: You get some people who'll criticize any change at all – simply because it's a change.

HUNTER: The main advantages to active hospital management of labor – do correct me if I am wrong – are said to be less pain, a shorter labor, and more convenience for the mother, and, most important, a lower perinatal mortality: that is, fewer babies either born dead or dying in the first week of life, when the death can often be due to a difficult labor. The perinatal mortality rate, judge – or PMR, as it is sometimes known – is crucial to the argument.

JUDGE: I am much obliged, Mr Hunter.

HUNTER: (*to Batt*): You agree with my summary of the alleged advantages of hospital delivery? (*Batt nods*) And what is involved, apart from bringing the mother into hospital, is often the inducing of labor – that is, starting the labor artificially at what is said to be the best time for the mother or baby[36] (or the most convenient for the doctors and nurses), routine monitoring of the contractions of the uterus, perhaps with the help of a computer, and the giving of intravenous injections of a drug called oxytocin automatically to improve them,[36, 37] routine monitoring of the baby's heart during the labor – before birth, that is – by means of electrodes fixed to its scalp,[38] and taking blood from the baby during labor for analysis;[39] the giving of pain-relieving drugs to the mother, and often a special kind of spinal anesthesia.[35] Sometimes, too, a forceps delivery or a Cesarean section delivery becomes necessary; and there is a special-care unit for babies who are born in poor condition for one reason or another.

BATT: That's a fair summary.

HUNTER: I put it to you that this 100 percent of hospital deliveries, with the possibility of interference, is at best merely expensive and of unproven value, and at worst positively harmful; that it indicates to a great extent that the obstetricians are so delighted with their newfound power to interfere that they have forgotten birth is usually a natural process that was conducted, commonly with success, by ordinary women and their husbands and friends and relatives long before the first obstetrician was ever heard of; that a big proportion of deliveries can take place quite safely and properly at home today, and that such a delivery, unlike many – probably most – hospital deliveries, is often a deeply enriching emotional experience for the mother, the father,[34, 35] and any other children there may be. I suggest to you that 100 percent active hospital management of labor is simply high-technology medicine rampant.

BATT: No, I completely disagree. Labor pain isn't enriching. Hospital delivery's safe for the mother; and for the baby too. You can't always tell beforehand when there will be some trouble in a confinement,[30] and anyway, even when family doctors agree that for certain types of pregnancy a hospital delivery is best, they may not stick to the rules when the time comes;[30] and if there is any trouble, by the time the mother is got to hospital or an emergency unit has got out to her it may be too late to save the baby. Or the baby – any baby – may develop some trouble soon after birth and only a hospital can deal with it.

HUNTER: And are you aware that one distinguished British obstetrician – who, of course, thinks that some deliveries should take place in hospital – has said that some women 'are terrified of hospitals and of modern obstetrical technology'?[40] 'They may,' he added, 'suffer as a result.'

BATT: Well, but what are tranquilizers for?

HUNTER: But are too many drugs not to be avoided when a woman is in labor? May not some of them harm the baby? Is not the best answer to terror to remove the cause?

BATT: That's all very well, but you've got to balance the risks.

HUNTER: You are aware that a survey of 336 women who had had a baby at home and a baby in hospital showed that 80 percent preferred home confinement;[30] and that a later survey of 65 women having a home confinement – of whom 28 were having a first baby, the other 37 having all had previous experience of hospital confinement – showed that 80 percent again said, *after* the home confinement, that they would prefer to have the next baby at home? In this second group almost half the fathers were present at the home birth.[34]

BATT: You're not telling me ordinary women know better than a doctor what's best for them?

HUNTER: Yes, I have the temerity to suggest that sometimes they do, doctor; and, perhaps more important, that their bodies belong to them, and so do decisions concerning them. However, my next point concerns induction of labor – the artificial starting of labor, in other words. Some obstetricians[36, 41] believe this should be done automatically, or very commonly, if a pregnancy has reached a certain very late stage or if what is called a toxemia has developed, and so on; but others[42, 43] believe one should be more selective – because in that way just as good results can be achieved and fewer Cesarean deliveries.

BATT: Yes, there are arguments both ways, so it's best to play safe and go for routine induction, I think.

HUNTER: But, doctor, are you aware there is published evidence[44] that in England and Wales between 1956 and 1968 there were more infant deaths associated with the birth period in those areas having a high home delivery rate, but that after 1968 there were *fewer* such deaths in areas having a high home delivery rate? – And, of course, labor is not induced in the home. Does that not suggest that the law of diminishing, and in the end of negative, returns operates in this field? Are you aware that increased hospital confinements in Cardiff between 1965 and 1973, complete with fetal monitoring, induction, and acceleration of labor, made little or no difference to such deaths?[37] That in Holland between 1960 and 1973 the proportion of hospital deliveries increased from 27.5 percent to 49 percent, and perinatal mortality fell from 25 to 16.3 per thousand; but that for home deliveries it fell during the same period from 14 to 4.5 per thousand?[32] Does that suggest home delivery is always undesirable? – Even though attempts have been made to explain away these figures with a variety of arguments.[45] Are you aware that the *British Medical Journal*, which in more than one leading article has come out in favor of hospital confinements,[29, 46] has also pointed out in a separate leading article[47] that the value of hospital-style monitoring of the mother and baby before birth is unproven, and so is the hospital monitoring of the fetal heart rate and so on during birth – although, so convinced are doctors that the latter is a good thing, equipment for it will, the article said, almost certainly be introduced, proof or no proof, into labor wards through the United Kingdom?[47] Are you aware too that Sweden has almost the lowest maternal death rate in the world, and that, although it has a high rate of hospital deliveries, the *main* factor responsible is thought to be that each mother has a midwife who looks after her right through the pregnancy and labor? Do you really still think that every single pregnant woman should have her baby in hospital.

BATT: Yes, I do. The Royal College of Obstetricians and Gynaecologists has been in favor of it for years.[48]

HUNTER: Is that College infallible, doctor? (*Pause*) Are you acquainted, Dr Batt, with a study of British births in 1970, and in particular with a volume dealing with the first week of life of the babies?

BATT: I've heard of it.

HUNTER: The perinatal mortality rates were shown in that study to have been 4.3, 6.1, and 27.8 respectively for home births, births supervised by the family doctor, and births supervised by hospital consultants.[49]

BATT: Yes, the consultants in hospital doubtless got all or most of the difficult cases.

HUNTER: You're sure that is the whole explanation?

BATT: It's pretty obvious to me, if not to a lawyer. You're not going to tell me a midwife at home or a family doctor at home or in hospital is as good as a consultant obstetrician with all the facilities of a tip-top hospital at his fingertips?

HUNTER: I have here a copy of the *Lancet* for April 3, 1976, in which there is a leading article[49] commenting on the report, and from which I extracted those figures. It says: 'In part the high PMR' – the perinatal mortality rate, you will remember, judge – 'associated with these hospital deliveries may be explained by selection of at-risk cases' – that is what you said, doctor: the difficult cases. However, the article went on: 'Unfortunately, it is impossible not to suspect that iatrogenic factors' – factors produced by doctors – 'have also contributed. Nor is it possible to ignore the fact that the deficiencies in perinatal care revealed in the report apply to a major extent to the hospital service.' As one example of these deficiencies the article mentioned that about one in four of the hospital babies were not examined in the first day of life; but of all the babies who *were* going to die in the first week three quarters died in the first 24 hours. As another example, only one in three infants were examined in the 24 hours before discharge from hospital. I could multiply the instances. It does look as though, not merely was there a high perinatal mortality for the babies delivered in hospital, but that some of it was due to the absence of the very factors you alleged made hospital delivery superior to home delivery. No?

BATT: Those figures are very surprising, I must admit. Very surprising.

HUNTER: Does it also surprise you to know that the report showed home confinements fell from about 36 percent in 1958 to about 12 percent in 1970; that induction of labor rose in that period from

13 percent to 30 percent; forceps deliveries increased from 4.7 percent to 7.9 percent and Cesarean deliveries from 2.7 percent to 4.5 percent; and that in 1970 by the tenth day after birth 70 percent of the babies were being bottle-fed, compared with a mere 15 percent in 1946?[49] High-technology medicine marching backwards or forwards?

BATT: No, joking and bottle-feeding aside – let's stick to the important issues – the answer to those perinatal deaths in hospital and the other deficiencies is to improve the hospitals: get more doctors, more laboratory facilities, more apparatus, better training. . . .

HUNTER: And if women then find hospitals even more cold and scientific and factory-like?

BATT: The answer is to improve the hospitals even more, isn't it?[30, 50, 51] I mean, *make* them more homely, camouflage them. Humanize them.

JUDGE: By means of a new type of medical ancillary, doctor – a humanizer? You do not feel that the nature of modern, high-technology medicine is such that it is a contradiction in terms to speak of humanizing a modern maternity hospital?[52] How does one humanize a computer? How does one humanize the process of routine monitoring of a baby's heart while the baby is still in the mother's womb? How does one humanize an automatic injection? How does one humanize a man in a mask? I am not saying these things are not sometimes, perhaps very often, highly desirable; but to humanize them. . . .

BATT: Well, one can try.

JUDGE: You do not think one perhaps takes high-technology medicine whole or not at all? – Its good points and its bad ones. That is the argument Mr Hunter deployed earlier regarding high-technology medicine in relation to the high-technology society, and you agreed with it.

BATT: Well, I'm afraid I don't agree with him now.

HUNTER: Has it not been suggested, Dr Batt, that education of mothers, proper preparation for childbirth, improvement in nutrition and health generally, and the better spacing-out of families, as in the case of the corresponding elements in relation to the general public health, have been the factors largely responsible for the improvement in the maternal and the perinatal and early infant mortality rates in western countries in the last few decades,[53] and that the increased rate of hospital deliveries has made a much smaller contribution? – And that such factors would do as much in future as 100 percent hospital confinements to improve the outlook for mothers and babies even further?[54]

BATT: They would have some effect, I daresay.

HUNTER: The report I have just mentioned[49] stated that the PMR for women in social class I was only 7.5 per thousand; for social class II women it was 15.8; and for women in classes IV and V it was 26.8. Some effect, or a very marked effect, do you think? Or are you going to deny that education, nutrition, general health, spacing of families, and preparation for childbirth are all better the higher the social class?

BATT: All right. Quite a big effect.

HUNTER: Thank you. And now isn't the truth of the matter that for every expert who is convinced of the desirability of 100 percent hospital delivery and active management of labor[31, 55, 56] there is another expert who takes a different view or thinks there is no firm evidence either way;[57, 58, 59] and that in a recent debate on this topic in the *British Medical Journal* the two contributions from experts who were not directly involved but who were experienced at assessing the type of evidence involved were in accord with those who find the evidence for 100 percent hospital deliveries unconvincing?[60, 61]

BATT: Oh, there's a debate. I admit that. But even a single baby dead or disabled is an argument against home confinements.

HUNTER: I dispute that, doctor. (*Pause*) Yes, doctor, I said that I dispute it. I think it is a typical fallacy of the high-technology mind to lay it down as axiomatic that any price is worth paying to avoid a single death. No one would dispute that many mothers should have their babies in hospital. It is that 100 percent and the *frequent total* active management of labor that sticks, I suggest to you, in the throats even of many doctors. What you are saying is that, to save perhaps one baby's life – at very best, it would probably be a great deal less – you would automatically subject 100 women, the majority of them against their wills, to the loneliness and alienation and inhumanity – yes, inhumanity – of a big hospital for what is perhaps the most intimate and important experience in a woman's life; and you would exclude the husbands and families therefore, or most of them, from the experience of the birth. Do you not think the many mothers and their babies who would be perfectly safe if *their* deliveries took place at home and only the difficult or doubtful deliveries were conducted in hospital – that they might lose something major, something irreplaceable, if *all* the births were to take place in hospital by medical fiat; perhaps something more important *in toto* than the life of one baby, however deplorable the loss of that baby might seem in isolation?

BATT: No, I don't. They lose nothing they wouldn't get back in a few days. And it's probably not just one in a hundred babies either.

HUNTER: I fear I have authority for that statement, doctor;[35] there is, for the present at any rate, what seems to be an *irreducible* minimum of one perinatal death per 100 births in the United Kingdom. Our present perinatal death rate is two per 100 births. Do you want me to go on with the arithmetic? (*Pause*) The article from which those figures are taken states, 'In such a situation it is very easy unwittingly to pass the point of optimum intervention and to end up causing more problems than originally existed in the first place.'[35] And the saving of that one extra baby in every 100 births would probably be secured, not merely by 100 percent hospital deliveries, but also by improved antenatal work, improved techniques for dealing with the difficult cases, improved nutrition and education generally. You admitted as much just now when we were discussing PMRs and social class. Correct?

BATT: Yes.

HUNTER: The 100 percent hospital deliveries would probably make only a minor contribution. Yes? (*Batt nods*) Well now, as to the mothers and babies losing very little from having confinements in hospital: you are aware that, in the case of some animals, if the mother is separated from the new-born for even an hour or two just after birth, she may refuse to look after it later, and may feed her own and other young indiscriminately?

BATT: No, I did not know that.

HUNTER: A sad thought? (*Batt nods*) I have here the *New England Journal of Medicine* for March 2, 1972 in which there is a report[62] on the effect of giving mothers, who had had their babies in hospital, more contact than usual with the babies. It is apparently the custom in hospitals here to give the mother a glimpse of the baby soon after birth, a brief further contact at between six and 12 hours; and then to give the baby to the mother for 20–30 minutes every four hours for the almost invariable bottle feeds.

JUDGE: Is a similar rigid schedule used in hospitals in the United Kingdom, doctor?

BATT: Well, yes, in quite a few. Something similar anyway. You've got to have efficiency after all. Otherwise you'd have anarchy.

JUDGE: I can imagine nothing pleasanter than some anarchical babies and mothers, but no matter. Yes, Mr Hunter?

HUNTER: Is there any hospital environment in which the mother would have the same freedom of access to her baby as she would enjoy at home?

BATT: I'd say not on the whole.

HUNTER: The workers who wrote the paper to which I just referred examined two groups of mothers: the first group had only the contacts with their babies that I have just described; the second group had an extra hour's contact within three hours of birth, and five extra hours each day for the first three days.

JUDGE: Not a surfeit?

HUNTER: No, indeed, judge, but more than the hospital norm. A month after the birth the two groups of mothers were examined in three respects: first, they were asked whether they picked the baby up if he cried when he was dry and had been fed (if they did, they got a high score), and whether they had been out since the birth, and, if so, had felt worried while out (if they had not been out, or had felt worried while out, they got a high score). Second, they were observed, while a doctor was examining the baby, to see if they stood and watched what was going on (if they did, they got a high score), and whether, if the baby cried during the examination, they tried to sooth him (if so, they got a high score). Third, they were observed for the amount of fondling they gave the baby, and the amount of eye-to-eye contact they had with the baby. On every one of the three tests the group of mothers that had had extra early contact with their babies scored higher than the other group – significantly higher, doctor. In other words, judge, it was unlikely to be just a chance finding.

JUDGE: Odd, what some scientists will investigate! My grandmother could have told them all that.

HUNTER: But Dr Batt likes scientific proof; and so I have given him scientific evidence for something that hundreds of thousands of mothers and babies in this and in other countries are losing every year, and will continue to lose – for the sake of saving the life of less than one baby in every hundred, perhaps a good deal less.·

BATT: There was no evidence about benefit to the babies.

JUDGE: I am not prejudging the larger issue, doctor, but there was no evidence of benefit to the mothers. Do you think we really need evidence that a baby and a mother benefit from looking at one another? From the one fondling the other?

HUNTER: In fact, judge, I can allay Dr Batt's anxiety about the babies. The authors of the paper stated – and I quote – 'Early and extended contact for the human mother may have a powerful effect on her interaction with her infant and consequently its later development.' Any comment, doctor?

BATT: Only that it's perfectly possible for hospitals to arrange for extended contact.

HUNTER: The *British Medical Journal* in a leading article[63] has said they should. It quoted the work I have just mentioned, said that the difference between the two groups of mothers persisted at one year and two years, and that babies separated from their mothers after birth more often become battered babies later or else fail for no obvious reason to thrive. The article described how much better a home delivery is in this respect than a hospital delivery. It said the mother should see and hold her naked baby soon after birth, and put it to the breast. This should be arranged in hospital. It said: 'There can be few more poignant tragedies than that of the baby whose life and future potential are saved by excellent technical . . . care but whose potential is never realised because our failure to promote parental attachment has resulted in neglect or abuse.' Sad that such an article should ever have to be written, do you not think? Perhaps it was especially sad in its title, which was 'Helping Mothers to Love Their Babies'. As though a mother needs to be *taught* to love her own child. Is there no end to the voracious appetite you high-technology doctors have for interfering with life's everyday natural processes?

JUDGE: I think if you move on, Mr Hunter. . . . That was a leading question; and Dr Batt seems not inclined to argue the case further. I have formed no judgment, doctor.

HUNTER: (*to Batt*): Is it true, doctor, that high scientific endeavor is going into the production of an entirely artificial milk that will exactly mimic human milk?[64]

BATT: Yes, and a jolly good thing too.

HUNTER: And that cows are being inoculated with certain germs so that their milk may contain the particular antibodies – to germs – that are present in all human milk?[65] The protein, sodium, and phosphate contents of cow's milk are reduced; vegetable fats are put into it instead of butter fat; all kinds of changes are made to bring it closer in composition to human milk, though human milk can be obtained in abundance from the human breast. Why cannot you high-technology scientists be content with what nature provides? What do you think the human breast is for?

JUDGE: You are not required to answer that question, doctor. Mr Hunter?

HUNTER: Some patients, for one reason or another, cannot or should not take any food by mouth. They can be fed – can they not, doctor? – with a wholly synthetic diet, given into the kind of artery-vein connection that is used for dialysis patients; and it is envisaged that some of them may have to be fed for life in this way.[66]

BATT: Well, and if it saves their lives. . . .

HUNTER: But, doctor, is it all worth it? Do you think all the effort, the worry, the dehumanization involved are justified? Is death always, at whatever cost, to be avoided for everyone? (*Pause*) A mouse has had all its blood removed – has it not? – to be replaced by a purely chemical substitute, and it has survived for a time.[67] This has not yet been attempted for man?

BATT: You can never be sure when something like that may not pay off.

HUNTER: Automation is now common in laboratory testing of blood, urine, and so on, is it not?[68] (*Batt nods*) And it is often cheaper to carry out a dozen tests routinely on every specimen than to use one's intelligence and carry out just the two or three tests for each person that will be quite enough?

BATT: Yes, but the machine does it all, so why worry?

HUNTER: One reason might be that it has been shown – correct me if I am wrong – that, if you carry out 20 separate tests on apparently normal people, only about one in three gives a normal result to every test.[69] Of course, few of the so-called abnormal results found in 'well' people mean any illness is present.[68]

BATT: Yes, I agree we need to refine our tests, and one day we shall.

HUNTER: But, doctor, does the testing not all cost money? And does it not perhaps cost one more than money to get into the way of thinking that machines can do everything for us? May we not become too dependent on machines, unable to adapt in time of crisis, bereft of old skills?

BATT: We can take that one when we come to it.

HUNTER: Do you know of a British investigation[70] of which factors were important to diagnosis by a specialist? – The family doctor's letter and what the patient said; the examination of the patient; or special investigations – laboratory tests, X-rays, and so on?

BATT: I don't just recall it off-hand.

HUNTER: Out of 80 patients the correct final diagnosis was made in 66 on the basis of the letter and the patient's history. In only six patients did examination make the specialist alter the diagnosis he had made after listening to the patient; and in only seven were special investigations needed to get at the final diagnosis. The authors of the paper felt that more time and facilities should therefore be devoted to taking the history and less on new laboratory services, and that medical students should be taught accordingly. There was no connection between the number of laboratory tests done on a patient and the certainty of the final diagnosis.

BATT: Yes, but you can't sit all day just listening to people ramble on.

JUDGE: That is the lot of most judges, doctor.

HUNTER: In England and Wales, doctor, did the number of laboratory tests performed not increase by 150 percent in the period 1961 to 1973?[71] While the cost in hospitals of laboratory investigations more than quadrupled?[71]

BATT: Well, high-quality medicine costs money, you know.

HUNTER: And do you know that here in the USA more than 2,000,000,000 laboratory tests are performed each year, costing more than $6,000,000,000?[72] – Ten tests for every single inhabitant. And that it has been estimated that the number of tests and the cost will have trebled by 1980?[72] Did you know that one American expert suggests that laboratory tests are sometimes requested by a doctor simply to show the patient or other doctors that he is doing something, even though an abnormal result to a test will not lead to any change at all in diagnosis or treatment. And that sometimes the doctor apparently doesn't even know when the result *is* abnormal?[72]

BATT: Well, yes, but that one'll be sorted out once we have enough computers.

HUNTER: To do the thinking for us? High-technology medicine does have some already, of course. Should you care to tell us about them?

BATT: There is a computer now that will analyze the results from an auto-analyzer[73] – the kind of routine testing machine you were just on about. And there's another kind that will take a preliminary history from the patient before the doctor comes into the picture at all.[74] And it's been suggested[75] it could then, especially if the results of certain examinations performed by paramedical personnel were fed into it – it could then suggest some extra investigations and even in the end come up with some preliminary suggestions on the diagnosis. Of course, a computer can help in diagnosis[76] if the patient's full history is fed into it, especially the diagnosis of some rare conditions;[73] and it can help in controlling drug prescriptions, and checking on reactions to drugs;[73] and in the storage and scrutiny of laboratory and hospital records.[73] Let me see – oh, yes, and in intensive care units to give early warning of some serious change in a patient's condition. And for keeping a birth-to-death record of certain characteristics of groups of people if you want to do some research.[73]

HUNTER: And is there not a suggestion that a computer could be used to give some kind of psychotherapy?[77] – To give words of welcome to a patient, to encourage him during a computer interview, and even to make jokes of a kind? What this computer can't yet comprehend, I believe, is the non-verbal information a patient can provide during an interview with a human.[77] Also the hope has been expressed that, even though information about a patient may be stored in a computer under a number allotted to him, his doctor will still refer to him by name, not by number. And is the most modern hospital in the world – at Riyadh in Saudi Arabia – not run by 14 computers?[78] (*Batt nods*) And then, of course, doctor, there is computerized axial tomography. Will you explain that for the court?

BATT: Yes, I forgot the cat scanner. It's a British invention, judge; a machine that passes X-rays through the skull and brain in a series of horizontal sections. You get about 30,000 records for each section, and a computer digests them all and comes up with half a dozen pictures covering the whole brain – six or so is usually enough.[79] It's being used for the body now too.[80] It's selling like hot cakes, especially here in the States.

HUNTER: Where some doctors have begun to question the need for the epidemic of purchases[81, 82, 83] – perhaps understandably as the average cost of a scanner is $500,000?[82] The US already has about 800 or 1000; and by 1980 it expects to have about 2500 at a total cost of $1,200,000,000 with an estimated annual running cost of $1,650,000,000.[82] And yet it's been pointed out[82] that, at the time of many of the purchases, the published evidence for their value was fairly limited. Needless to say, as this method is commonly used for examining the head, Washington, DC, has the highest installed-or-ordered concentration[83] in the US – one for every 60,000 people; and Kansas has the lowest – one for every million people. Of course, in our own country the National Health Service has been experimenting with the use of computers in hospitals,[84] though so far, despite the expenditure of millions of pounds, there is little positive to show. Indeed, the *British Medical Journal*,[84] no opponent of high-technology medicine and not given to hyperbole, has described the whole project as a 'grandiose shambles'. No comment, doctor? (*Pause*) Well, despite the computer even high-technology doctors still use books and journals, do they not?

BATT: Yes, of course. I suppose I read about 20 or so journals regularly.

HUNTER: Then you are very abstemious. You know the American journal, the *Annals of Internal Medicine*? (*Batt nods*) Did you know that in one 1973 issue it gave the views of some 2500 American doctors on what today's good doctor should be reading?[85] Perhaps you will take my word for it that it suggested a general physician should read at least 33 journals a month, and should have the latest editions of at least 36 books whose total cost would *then* have been $1162 and whose total number of pages was around 44,000. A truly dedicated physician, the article implied, would be able to put his hand on 250 books and 126 journals. One wonders whether he'd have any time to put his hand on a patient.

BATT: A doctor simply has to keep up to date.

HUNTER: With books of over 2000, even over 3000 pages, and costing 150 dollars each, or more? – There are plenty of such books, are there not? Each dealing with a single subdivision of high-technology medicine? (*Batt nods*) And would you know how many journals are taken by the library of the Royal Society of Medicine in London? Will you take my word for it that the number is about 2500?[86]

BATT: It's the most important medical library in Europe.

HUNTER: But 2500 individual journals, doctor, coming out every week or month or quarter. Do you really think that number is necessary?

BATT: Well, presumably someone must read them.

HUNTER: I am not criticizing the Society, doctor. It is doubtless the victim of a process that is a lot bigger than itself. But it is difficult to see the need for 2500 journals, no matter how many different kinds of doctor it is catering for. And the truth is – is it not? – that most doctors do not, in fact, read all the journals and books they *say* the good doctor should read. They just flip the pages over, a lot of them, if they even do that. (*Pause*) Medical writing now. It is lucid, doctor?

BATT: Oh, no. A man in one field simply can't understand most of what comes out in another field, often he can't understand papers on topics in his own field.

HUNTER: And is this due, do you think, to over-specialization, and to the corresponding growth of medical jargon, or to the use of plain bad English?[87]

BATT: I suppose both to some extent.

HUNTER: The jargon has grown but the health has ceased to?

BATT: Another thing that doesn't help, of course, is that most papers today are written by a number of authors. Six, seven, eight – ten or a dozen sometimes.

HUNTER: Just to back that point: I have here a copy of the *Lancet* for September 8, 1973. I could have chosen many other issues and articles, indeed specimens of many other journals. But now in this issue on page 530 to 534 there is an article[88] dealing with three patients having a condition of which only two cases had ever previously been reported in the whole world. There were eight authors: seven medical men, and one doctor of philosophy – or 1.6 of a doctor to every single known case in the entire world. The title of the paper was 'Neutrophil Dysfunction, Chronic Granulomatous Disease, and Non-spherocytic Haemolytic Anemia Caused by Complete Deficiency of Glucose-6-phosphate Dehydrogenase'.

JUDGE: (*writing*): You did say 'complete' deficiency, Mr Hunter?
HUNTER: Yes, judge. The immediately succeeding paper,[89] on pages 535 to 538, also reported on three patients. They were suffering from a separate condition of which only three other cases had ever been reported in the whole world. It had eight authors, all medical men. It was entitled 'Mesangiocapillary Nephritis, Partial Lipodystrophy, and Hypocomplementemia'.
JUDGE: These papers, though each dealing with a rare condition, communicated some discovery of great significance perhaps?
HUNTER: Apparently not, judge: at least of the six original articles[5] contained in that issue of the *Lancet* they were only number 5 and number 6.
BATT: You can't stop scientists extending the frontiers. You never know what may emerge.
HUNTER: Well, I am now, doctor, going to quote you some words from the *Lancet* of October 12, 1968, and I wonder if you can guess who spoke them: 'I do sometimes wonder whether the vast sums of money now being spent, in many countries, on research might not produce more rapid and spectacular improvement in world health if devoted to the application of what is already known'.[90] Well?
BATT: I haven't a clue.
HUNTER: They were spoken by the late Lord Rosenheim. He was then President of the Royal College of Physicians. Is that not just about the most prestigious position there is in the world of British medicine? (*Batt nods*) And he was also one of the most distinguished medical scientists of his time?
BATT: I wouldn't dispute it.
HUNTER: Finally, apart from jargon and multiple authorship and perhaps the need to appear very profound, could one reason for the very bad writing doctors themselves admit is extremely common in the profession's journals be that doctors read very little outside their own subject? – That their minds are, from an early age, concentrated on a narrower and narrower scientific and technological horizon?
BATT: I daresay, but that's the price of progress.
HUNTER: Did you know that only 60 percent of American college graduates read at least one serious book a year?[91] Or that the last editor of the *New England Journal of Medicine* recommended that, to improve their writing ability, doctors should 'set themselves a goal of reading annually at least six books of high literary quality'?[91] – I am quoting from the issue of the journal of March 4, 1976. Dr Batt, I put it to you that most doctors are culturally deprived, and that this is the price of their worship of high-

technology medicine; and that there has been no equivalent benefit at all – certainly not, as Professor Larkin told us, in the way of improved health for the people.

BATT: I keep saying it: you can't stop science and technology going forward. You can't stop our high-technology society going forward.

HUNTER: And one shouldn't try, even when it is blind and headed for the edge of a cliff? (*Pause*) No further questions.

JUDGE: Doctor, you are aware that this new type of X-ray apparatus – the computerized tomographic scanner – is now used in Saudi Arabia, Iraq, Jordan, and Iran, and is on order also for Dubai, Abu Dhabi, Qatar, and Libya; and that in Iran it is even used in the private practice of radiologists?[92]

BATT: I didn't know that, but I'm not surprised. They can all afford it with the oil revenue they have, so why not?

JUDGE: You do not think that, from the viewpoint of the health of the population of those countries, the money should be spent differently?

BATT: Perhaps, but then they want to catch up with us technically. It's a matter of national pride.

JUDGE: Do you know that the World Health Organization estimates that, of some $12\frac{1}{2}$ million children born in the eastern Mediterranean region each year – that is, very largely in these oil-rich countries – almost 2,000,000 die in infancy?[93] You take my word for that? (*Batt nods*) How many of those infant lives will be saved by these scanners, costing £250,000 each?

BATT: Very few, I expect.

JUDGE: Perhaps none.

BATT: Possibly, but people aren't always very rational when it comes to being one up on their neighbor; and now, with Concorde, these countries have the UK – even the USA – as their neighbors in a sense.

JUDGE: Are you aware that, of all the technical medical items of the kind that we have been discussing today, the biggest single item exported to those oil-rich countries is medical disposables,[93] many of which are made from oil?

BATT: I take your word for that, judge.

JUDGE: Are you aware that there has also been a large increase in mental illness in these countries of recent years?[93]

BATT: There's always some price to pay, progress always has side-effects.

JUDGE: High-technology medicine is not overmuch concerned with mental illness, is it? Or with psychosocial factors in disease causation, or with health education, or the work of the family doctor or even the nurse-visitor or the physician assistant?

BATT: No, that's true enough. Those fields are not really suitable for the kind of approach I have to problem solving.

JUDGE: In that connection I should like to raise two points with you. First, high-technology medicine, as you said, is underpinned by science, and presumably it therefore shares the central methodological principle of science, which is to objectivize, to split up the object of study the better to understand it.

BATT: Well, yes, that's specialization. It's essential.

JUDGE: For knowledge?

BATT: That's right.

JUDGE: And wisdom, and compassion?

BATT: I don't quite follow, you're talking about quite separate things.

JUDGE: Not perhaps made separate by science? Is not the danger of the fissiparous approach of science, doctor, that it may cause one to lose sight of the larger picture? – To see only the disease and not the patient who harbors it?

BATT: But then if you can cure the disease . . .

JUDGE: Is it not always a patient, a person, that you have to cure or care for? (*Pause*) Finally, doctor, would you agree that at the very heart of science and of high-technology medicine lies measurement – quantification, as it is sometimes called. (*Batt nods*) It is the life blood of science? Without it high-technology medicine could not exist? (*Batt nods again*) Do you agree also that what matters most to a patient, often the only thing that matters, is the quality of the care he receives?

BATT: Yes, I go along with that; but then patients don't understand always what's at stake. The doctor always has to be a few steps ahead.

JUDGE: On a different path? A high-technology path? Seeking a diagnosis? (*Batt nods*) But now this *quality* of care that matters to the patient: you cannot by definition measure true quality? To the extent that you bring in quantification and the tools that it requires, to that extent you necessarily diminish quality? One cannot measure anything of great human value?

BATT: I'm not a bedside doctor, but no, I wouldn't accept that at all.

JUDGE: You don't think the truth is that one can measure certain aspects of a quality – the number of times a doctor visits a patient, say, or how many training courses he goes to – but never the ultimate interchange between person and person that is the crux of the encounter between the healer and the sick?

BATT: I can't agree there's something there you can't measure. I mean, if it's there obviously you can measure it.

JUDGE: And if you cannot measure it, it is not there? (*Pause*) You can measure a mother's love for her sick child, a doctor's compassion for his dying patient?

BATT: There are always methods for anything if you think hard enough.

JUDGE: Similar to those used for measuring the strength of the relationship between a mother and her baby?

BATT: That's right, you've understood, you've got my position.

JUDGE: Yes, doctor. I have, I think. (*Pause*) I have to thank you. And this court is now adjourned.

REFERENCES—SESSION NINE

1. Bradshaw, S., *Lancet*, November 24, 1973, p. 1200.
2. Taylor, D. G., *Proceedings of the Royal Society of London*, B, January 20, 1976, p. 145.
3. Harris, W. H., *NEJM*, September 22, 1977, p. 650.
4. Freeman, M. A. R., *BMJ*, November 27, 1976, p. 1301.
5. Medical News, *JAMA*, March 29, 1976, p. 1313.
6. Editorial, *Lancet*, May 8, 1976, p. 1002.
7. The Environment, *JAMA*, January 18, 1971, p. 369.
8. Thomson, J. G., *Lancet*, November 22, 1969, p. 1088.
9. Leading Article, *BMJ*, October 26, 1974, p. 178.
10. Landon, N. R., *Pulse*, August 9, 1975, p. 8.
11. *The Times*, May 25, 1977, p. 7.
12. Medical News, *JAMA*, April 28, 1975, p. 337.
13. Medical News, *JAMA*, May 5, 1975, pl 473.
14. *The Times*, July 1, 1976, p. 7.
15. *The Times*, November 6, 1976, p. 8.
16. Editorial, *NEJM*, May 26, 1977, p. 1226.
17. Medical News, *JAMA*, December 13, 1971, p. 1631.
18. Gwynne, P., *New Scientist*, December 12, 1974, p. 829.
19. Medical News, *JAMA*, February 7, 1977, p. 521.
20. Trexler, P. C., Spiers, A. S. D., and Gaya, H., *BMJ*, December 6, 1975, p. 549.
21. McLauchlan, J., *et al.*, *BMJ*, February 23, 1974, p. 322.
22. Cox, R. N., Glover, D. D., and Lam, S. J. S., *Lancet*, April 13, 1974, p. 661.
23. Poplack, D. G., Penland, W. Z., and Levine, A. S., *Lancet*, June 22, 1974, p. 1261.
24. Equipment Supplement, *British Journal of Hospital Medicine*, May 1974, seriatim.
25. Ibid., November 1974, seriatim.
26. Editorial, *NEJM*, October 26, 1972, p. 879.
27. Silvis, S. E., *et al.*, *JAMA*, March 1, 1976, p. 928.
28. Mahoney, M. J., and Hobbins, J. C., *NEJM*, August 4, 1977, p. 258.
29. Leading Article, *BMJ*, January 10, 1976, p. 55.
30. Cox, C. A., *et al.*, *BMJ*, January 10, 1976, p. 84.

31. Beard, R. W., and Chamberlain, G., *Lancet*, April 24, 1976, p. 904.
32. Van Alten, D., Kloosterman, G. J., and Treffers, P. E., *BMJ*, March 27, 1976, p. 771.
33. Hudson, C. K., *BMJ*, January 24, 1976, p. 216.
34. Goldthorp, W. O., and Richman, J., *Practitioner*, June 1974, p. 845.
35. Dunn, P. M., *Lancet*, April 10, 1976, p. 790.
36. Coles, R. A., Howie, P. W., and Macnaughton, M. C., *Lancet*, April 5, 1975, p. 767.
37. Chalmers, I., *et al.*, *BMJ*, March 27, 1976, p. 735.
38. Edington, P. T., Sibanda, J., and Beard, R. W., *BMJ*, August 9, 1975, p. 341.
39. Filshie, M., *British Journal of Hospital Medicine*, July 1974, p. 33.
40. Arthure, H., *Journal of Obstretrics and Gynaecology of the British Commonwealth*, January 1973, p. 1.
41. McNay, M. B., *et al.*, *BMJ*, February 5, 1977, p. 347.
42. O'Driscoll, K., Carroll, C. J., and Coughlan, M., *BMJ*, December 27, 1975, p. 727.
43. Bonnar, J., *BMJ*, March 13, 1976, p. 651.
44. Ashford, J. R., and Forster, G., *BMJ*, March 13, 1976, p. 648.
45. Davis, J. A., *et al.*, *BMJ*, March 13, 1976, p. 648.
46. Leading Article, *BMJ*, October 1, 1977, p. 845.
47. Leading Article, *BMJ*, March 19, 1977, p. 734.
48. Leading Article, *BMJ*, November 23, 1968, p. 468.
49. Editorial, *Lancet*, April 3, 1976, p. 729.
50. Matthews, A. E. B., and Fox, J. S., *BMJ*, February 14, 1976, p. 395.
51. Rosen, M., *et al.*, *BMJ*, February 21, 1976, p. 458.
52. Stacey, M., *BMJ*, March 27, 1976, p. 771.
53. Ashford, J. R., *et al.*, *BMJ*, January 31, 1976, p. 279.
54. Slattery, J., *BMJ*, January 24, 1976, p. 216.
55. Campbell, A. G. M., *BMJ*, January 31, 1976, p. 279.
56. Crawford, J. S., *Lancet*, April 24, 1976, p. 903.
57. Dunn, P. M., *Lancet*, May 15, 1976, p. 1068.
58. Richards, M., *Lancet*, May 15, 1976, p. 1069.
59. Barry, C. N., *BMJ*, February 7, 1976, p. 341.
60. Campbell, H., Lowe, C. R., and Cochrane, A. L., *BMJ*, April 24, 1976, p. 1013.
61. Kirke, P., *BMJ*, April 24, 1976, p. 1014.
62. Klaus, M. H., *et al.*, *NEJM*, March 2, 1972, p. 460.
63. Leading Article, *BMJ*, September 3, 1977, p. 595.
64. Willis, A. T., *et al.*, *BMJ*, October 13, 1973, p. 67.
65. Wharton, B. A., and Berger, H. M., *BMJ*, May 29, 1976, p. 1326.
66. Scribner, B. H., *et al.*, *JAMA*, April 20, 1970, p. 457.
67. Geyer, R. P., *NEJM*, November 15, 1973, p. 1077.
68. Bailey, A., *Lancet*, December 14, 1974, p. 1436.
69. Holland, W. W., *Lancet*, December 21, 1974, p. 1494.
70. Hampton, J. R., *et al.*, *BMJ*, May 31, 1975, p. 486.
71. 'Information Service Sheet', No. 28, Office of Health Economics, London, March 1976.
72. Krieg, A. F., Gambino, R., and Galen, R. S., *JAMA*, July 7, 1975, p. 76.
73. Doll, R., *Proceedings of the Royal Society of Medicine*, July 1968, p. 709.
74. Bailey, A., *Proceedings of the Royal Society of Medicine*, March 1974, p. 180.

75. Lucas, R. W., *et al.*, *BMJ*, September 11, 1976, p. 623.
76. De Dombal, F. T., *et al.*, *BMJ*, March 2, 1974, p. 376.
77. Slack, W. V., and Slack, C. W., *NEJM*, June 15, 1972, p. 1304.
78. Wright, P., *The Times*, Supplement, May 13, 1975, p. I.
79. Menzer, L., Sabin, T., and Mark, V. H., *JAMA*, November 17, 1975, p. 754.
80. Leading Article, *BMJ*, May 10, 1975, p. 300.
81. Shapiro, S. H., and Wyman, S. M., *NEJM*, April 22, 1976, p. 954.
82. Creditor, M. C., and Garrett, J. B., *NEJM*, July 7, 1977, p. 49.
83. Fineberg, H. V., Parker, G. S., and Pearlman, L. A., *NEJM*, July 28, 1977, p. 216.
84. Leading Article, *BMJ*, February 12, 1977, p. 404.
85. Allyn, R., and Stearns, N. S., *Annals of Internal Medicine*, August 1973, p. 293.
86. Annual Report of the Council 1973–1974, Royal Society of Medicine, p. 21, 1975, London.
87. Crichton, M., *NEJM*, December 11, 1975, p. 1257.
88. Gray, G. R., *et al.*, *Lancet*, September 8, 1973, p. 530.
89. Peters, D. K., *et al.*, *Lancet*, September 8, 1973, p. 535.
90. Rosenheim, M., *Lancet*, October 12, 1968, p. 821.
91. Editorial, *NEJM*, March 4, 1976, p. 546.
92. Wright, P., *The Times*, November 24, 1977, p. 14.
93. Grainge, A., *The Times*, November 24, 1977, p. 13.

Arthritis as an Engineering Problem
Medical Practice, *BMJ*, November 18, 1972, p. 415.

Genetic Engineering
Leading Article, *BMJ*, May 10, 1975, p. 295.
Leading Article, *BMJ*, February 7, 1976, p. 302.
Gaylin, W., *NEJM*, September 22, 1977. p. 665.
Editorial, *NEJM*, November 24, 1977, p. 1176.
Greenberg, D. S., *NEJM*, November 24, 1977, p. 1187.

Effects of Induction of Labor
Fedrick, J., and Yudkin, P., *BMJ*, March 27, 1976, p. 738.

Infant Feeding
Addy, D. P., *BMJ*, May 22, 1976, p. 1268.
Bradshaw, J. S., *BMJ*, June 12, 1976, p. 1468.
Jelliffe, D. B., and Jelliffe, E. F. P., *NEJM*, October 27, 1977, p. 912.

Computers in Medicine
Pascoe, J. E., *Proceedings of the Royal Society of Medicine*, September 1974, p. 946.
Anderson, J., and Tomlinson, R. W. S., *Proceedings of the Royal Society of of Medicine*, September 1974, p. 948.
Rivett, G. C., *Health Trends*, February 1975, p. 5, 9.

Measurement in Medicine, Quantification
Bradshaw, J. S., *BMJ*, June 14, 1975, p. 611.

HIGH TECHNOLOGY MEDICINE - CONSEQUENCES AND SIGNIFICANCE

Enter Professor Joan Weskoff

JUDGE: You are Joan Weskoff, a Professor of Medicine here in the United States? You are being questioned initially by myself, professor, mainly because I want first to understand your thinking on some of Dr Batt's evidence. You deal with patients at an everyday clinical level, but you also carry out a great many experiments? (*Weskoff nods*) On humans?

WESKOFF: On healthy volunteers, and sometimes on patients; with all due precautions. Also, of course, on animals.

JUDGE: And you are a senior member of the staff of your medical school, and chairwoman of your hospital's ethical committee, and therefore fully cognisant of all the ramifications of high-technology medicine? (*Weskoff nods*) You were present throughout yesterday's hearing? Did you agree with Dr Batt's implicit thesis: that, although a small error may have been made here, or a wrong turning taken there, the broad sweep of medicine in the last two or three decades has been forward and to man's benefit?

WESKOFF: I went along with that. I agreed too on most matters of detail. I would have put a somewhat different emphasis here or there, that is all. I would not have accepted as readily as Dr Batt did, judge, the idea that high-technology medicine is a completely integral part of modern society, a kind of branch of it. Modern medicine is related to it, of course, and there is *some* traffic between them. I could not wholly accept either the notion that our high-technology society and high-technology medicine also constitute some kind of juggernaut, rushing onwards ever faster and faster; or that one cannot pick and choose among the good and bad elements in a society, or in a discipline such as medicine.

JUDGE: And what about the use by doctors of gadgets in their ordinary lives, their use of disposables, their borrowing of the fruits of other disciplines, their tendency to use automation or computers?

WESKOFF: That is simply to say that they are children of their time, not saints or fanatics. And then Mr Hunter chose to emphasize some examples from high-technology medicine that were so rare as to be completely untypical – such as the child in the isolator, or the computer that interviews people.

JUDGE: You do not feel, professor, that sometimes one may best see the real import of an argument or a trend by deliberately taking it to an extreme? – As, say, by imagining what would have happened if all doctors *had* been saints or fanatics? – As, say, by extrapolating the current growth rate of the American health industry which would, I am told, if continued, lead by the year AD 2000 to the entire American nation being engaged fulltime in delivering health care to itself.

WESKOFF: No, judge, because both those examples are really unthinkable.

JUDGE: But by thinking the unthinkable, by extrapolating to an extreme, may one not be led to take a right course of action?

WESKOFF: I don't see that one need go to the edge and look over.

JUDGE: Or to the desert – or Hiroshima and Nagasaki, say – and think? (*Pause*) Well, and what about the price for being able to replace joints perhaps being a loss in life expectancy?

WESKOFF: That was the perfect example of our not necessarily being stuck with every product of the high-technology society for ever. The fact that hip replacement and a small temporary drop in life expectancy for certain male age groups happened at more or less the same time in the States doesn't mean they had a common root, and that, if you get rid of one, you must get rid of the other too. We *can* pick and choose. We'll keep the artificial hip, *and* we'll put life expectancy up again for males – given a little time.

JUDGE: Did you agree with Dr Batt that the last 20 years have in one sense been years of consolidation for medical science, of a flexing of the muscles for a new step forward?

WESKOFF: I hesitate, judge, only because, while I agree in one way, I think that even in the last 20 years we've actually *achieved* a lot: we've enormously improved our ability to diagnose and to treat disease, and our general surgical ability; we've developed open-heart surgery, we've developed coronary care units – intensive care units generally – we've made kidney transplants a reality. We've taken a small step here and a small step there; and a lot of small steps make one big step.

JUDGE: Thank you, professor. Mr Hunter?

HUNTER (*rising*): I shall deal, first, Professor Weskoff, with the points you have just made. Transplants: how many people in the United Kingdom might benefit from a kidney transplant?

WESKOFF: I think the figure has been put at around 2000 a year. [1]

HUNTER: And how many people are killed on British roads each year? – It is around 7000, one third of them between the ages of 15 and 24. [2]

WESKOFF: I'd get your drift if all the accidents were caused by doctors rushing to hospital to give kidney transplants; but they're not.

HUNTER: You do not see that the abilities to build a modern automobile and to perform a kidney transplant are different branches of the same tree?

WESKOFF: Not at all.

HUNTER: The man who makes a kidney dialysis machine or operates one – would he not be quite at home in many parts of an automobile factory?

WESKOFF: I guess there's a grain of truth in that. Just a grain.

HUNTER: You do not see that the garage mechanic who does spare-part surgery on a car, and the kidney surgeon who does it on the car's owner, think along the same lines, could almost swop places in one or two respects?

WESKOFF: I rather resent your implied criticism of kidney transplant surgeons.

HUNTER: I have not said a word against them. I am merely trying to get *you* – and the court – to see their activities in full context. (*Pause*) Most donors of transplant kidneys have been – and probably will continue to be in the future – victims of road accidents. You agree? Which is the greater sin in a society – to kill a lot of young people with automobiles, or to let a lesser number of young people die from kidney disease?

WESKOFF: That's a completely false antithesis.

HUNTER: You will be aware that in 1973 no less than 18,000 young Americans, aged 15 to 24, died in motor-vehicle accidents – I am rounding off the figures – 5000 were murdered, and 4000 committed suicide. 700,000 American youngsters are injured in car accidents each year. The paper[3] in which these figures were given stated, 'For a considerable proportion of American children and youth, the "culture of violence" is now both a major health threat and a way of life'; and it ascribed much of this culture to television viewing. It quoted a figure of seven–eight hours of viewing a day by pre-school American children, and three hours a day by those aged 12 to 17.

WESKOFF: But what has this to do with kidney transplants?

HUNTER: You don't see television *and* the automobile *and* gratuitous violence *and* kidney transplant techniques as having grown up together?

WESKOFF: That doesn't mean one in any way causes the others.

HUNTER: Not as being all branches of the same tree? Siblings? (*Pause*) Very well. Secondly, you mentioned an improvement in diagnostic and treatment skills in the last 20 years. Some cases of hypertension – high blood pressure – can now be remedied by operation can they not? – A very small minority? An operation, very roughly speaking, on the kidney? (*Weskoff nods*) In order to detect this small minority of cases a series of complex tests must be carried out, and in certain centers, both here and in my country, those tests are carried out on all or most patients with a raised blood pressure.

WESKOFF: That is correct.

HUNTER: This is a product of high-technology medicine during the last 20 years? (*Weskoff nods*) The Johns Hopkins School of Medicine in Baltimore is one of the most distinguished in the world? (*She nods again*) I have here a copy of the *New England Journal of Medicine*[4] containing an article that reports a study of the medical management, among other things, of 113 patients with hypertension by doctors all of whom were Johns Hopkins graduates.

WESKOFF: I know, Mr Hunter: after five months 50 of the 113 patients still didn't have their high blood pressures properly controlled.

HUNTER: And yet it is possible today, with modern drugs, for any average doctor – or a nurse, or even a briefly-trained youngster – to control almost all patients with high blood pressure in a matter of weeks, is it not? – By following them up properly, and adjusting their drug dosage and so on.

WESKOFF: I accept that, but—

HUNTER: It was found that of those 50 'uncontrolled' patients 26 were not being followed up at all at five months, and of the remaining 24 no fewer than 19 weren't getting an adequate dosage of their drugs. And yet a lot of these patients had been put through that complex diagnostic process we just discussed – to see if they had hypertension of a kind that an operation would correct. How many such surgically remediable cases were found as a result, professor?

WESKOFF: None, but I want—

HUNTER: Not a single one. But it was even worse, was it not? – Because the study revealed that, when some specialists and super-specialists looked at what these John Hopkins doctors had been doing, the criticism they made was not just that the treatment was bad – which it certainly was – but that *not enough* investigations had been carried out. They said the work-up – I believe that is the term – was inadequate: only about one patient in six had, so they said, been properly investigated. Is that not so, professor? (*Weskoff nods*) The high-technology diagnostic procedures were quite fruitless (and yet there should have been more of them, the experts said); but the high-technology treatment – though most effective if properly applied, and what matters most to the patient – was simply *not* properly applied. And this, the authors of the paper said, was because today's doctors needed to be taught properly about simple things like seeing the patients regularly and altering their drug dosages. Do you number the facts about diagnosis and treatment revealed in this study as among the triumphs of high-technology medicine, professor, or among the facts that show the machine – the juggernaut, I think you rightly called it – has got out of the driver's control?

WESKOFF: I've been trying for five minutes to get a word in edge-ways. You can't generalize from a single study. You cannot ever generalize from a single study. Not being a scientist, Mr Hunter, you perhaps wouldn't understand.

HUNTER: No, I am only a lawyer, professor; but would a single study not tell one that cyanide was invariably lethal? (*Pause*) Well, now, one can work out – can one not? – the total cost of first screening all Americans with high blood pressure to see if they might have a cause for their hypertension that an operation would put right, and then performing a needed extra test, and then doing the operation when it was indicated? Four American medical scientists did their sums in this matter, did they not? What was the cost? – wasn't it $10,000,000,000 to 13,000,000,000?[5] – 10 percent of the total amount spent on health in the United States?

WESKOFF: A more conservative estimate put it at three to four billion dollars only.[5]

HUNTER: Only? – You'd sooner be sat upon by a hippopotamus than by an elephant, would you, professor?

JUDGE: I think the professor would give a good account of herself if either kind of animal made the attempt.

WESKOFF: I get by when men try it too.

HUNTER: Did not two of the same doctors, professor, establish that, if you didn't bother at all about whether or not surgery was possible but instead just went ahead and treated every high-blood pressure patient with drugs, your results overall would normally be every bit as good as if you spent three or four or ten or thirteen billion dollars on all that diagnosis and surgery?[6]

WESKOFF: Yes, there was such a paper, but again it's just one paper, and there were various ifs and buts to it.

HUNTER: Thirdly, you mentioned, as another achievement of high-technology medicine, open-heart surgery. In order to achieve exact diagnosis before attempting such surgery – and often for other reasons – a procedure called cardiac catheterization is often performed, is it not?

WESKOFF: Yes, it is.

HUNTER: A fine tube – the catheter – is insinuated into the heart via blood vessel, and certain measurement can then be made, fluids injected, and so on? (*Weskoff nods*) In a report[7] of such a catheterization in a woman patient who later died there was mention of the 'abject terror' that she had experienced during the procedure, and that was common among certain types of patient subjected to the procedure. In his reply[8] to a comment on this, both appearing in the *New England Journal of Medicine,* one of the doctors concerned said that in these patients, who have often been seriously ill for a long time – and I now quote – 'sudden death due to psychological stress alone may ensue.' During the procedure, that is. Death, in other words, from terror. He went on: 'The Catheter Laboratory team, although ultimately interested in such indexes of cardiac function as systolic upstroke time, must recognize the emotional impact of a totally foreign procedure performed in an awake patient in the hostile environment of a laboratory filled with electronic recorders, computers, resuscitation equipment, and a masked and gowned team of often unfamiliar faces.' (Do you see now why I use the term 'high-technology medicine,' professor?) 'Although every effort is expended, before and during the catheterization procedure, to dispel the "abject terror" . . . it is not always possible to do so.' He added that cardiac catheterization was, however, a necessary evil for the present; he hoped other techniques being developed would diminish the need for it. (*Pause*) This really is a new type of medicine – is it not, professor? – that induces abject terror in even a few patients although its practitioners are very well-intentioned, as this doctor clearly was. It is a little like, say, Concorde, is it not? – Magnificent, but terrifying.

WESKOFF: There is a very real dilemma. I recognize it. I should explain that often one can't for technical reasons anesthetize these patients or give them tranquilizers. But no one wishes to see terror inflicted.

HUNTER: That is what I am saying: that the machine has run away with the driver. (*Pause*) Now as to heart surgery itself, another triumph of high-technology medicine, you said; many patients who have undergone it suffer serious mental disorder afterwards?

WESKOFF: A temporary one, yes; some of them do. They may also be cured of their heart condition.

HUNTER: They may be grossly confused, hallucinated, deluded, paranoidal? One study[9] in your country showed that eight out of 12 patients who had undergone heart surgery but were all thought to be mentally normal after it had, in fact, suffered major mental disturbances, but had managed to hide the fact from the doctors. You accept that?

WESKOFF: The fact that mental upset—

HUNTER: Mental illness, please. Gross mental illness.

WESKOFF: Oh, very well – the fact that mental illness occurs is not surprising when one considers that heart surgery is major surgery which always means, even today, a gross interference with normal bodily processes.

HUNTER: I do not dispute it; but the patients feeling they had to conceal their illness from their doctors . . .?

WESKOFF: Also the patient will nearly always be in an intensive care unit after the operation.

HUNTER: A type of unit you also mentioned as a triumph of high-technology medicine – a unit where there is an atmosphere of great tension? – Where another patient may die at any moment, where oxygen tents hiss, and the heart monitors flash; where – as in many new operating theaters – there may be no windows at all so that, as there is then no daylight or natural darkness, the lights may have to be dimmed to simulate night and turned up to simulate day; where the patient may not be able to move, perhaps not able to speak, though still quite able to hear; where doctors and nurses are busy, on edge, expectant, full of guilt and insecurity? Where they often relieve their own anxieties by concentrating more on the machines than on the patients – because the machines are easier to deal with?[9, 10] – Where, indeed, the whole panoply of high-technology medicine is seen at its best, or worst?

WESKOFF: One is dealing with life and death: that is the price of saving a life.

HUNTER: One doctor has described an expression of 'frozen terror' on the faces of patients in these units after their heart operations.[10] You knew that? One has to be terrified to be saved? – As once with some religions?

WESKOFF: One can always give tranquilizers, or something stronger.

HUNTER: You echo Dr Batt, and Mr Buck: 'Emotional stress?' – 'Then put the patient out.' (*Pause*) You know, professor, that, in 1975, a day in an ordinary ward in a Boston hospital cost $250 while a day in an intensive care unit there cost more than $400?[11] (*Weskoff nods*) And yet the value of intensive care units for various conditions has been queried in your country,[11] has it not?

WESKOFF: Everything's queried some time or other by some self-styled consumer advocate.

HUNTER: The paper to which I referred was by a doctor. Anyway, you won't question that 12 percent of all America's nurses work in intensive care units? (*Pause*) No? And you won't dispute that one American *doctor* has written, 'A limited experience in the intensive care unit leads me to believe that one should not want to be among its clientele unless profoundly unconscious'?[12]

WESKOFF: You have said nothing that is new to me, Mr Hunter. Progress always carries some penalties.

HUNTER: You mean surely that high-technology medicine carries some? Whether or not it represents true progress is what we are here to decide, professor. You mentioned as yet another of its achievements – coronary care units. I put it to you that four out of five patients in such units suffer from anxiety, and three out of five from depression – one in six from a severe depression. [10] (*Weskoff nods*) And that half the patients treated in American coronary care units do not have the myocardial infarction – heart-muscle death, judge – that is the basic reason for the existence of the units. [13]

WESKOFF: Yes, I know. I know it all, and I am totally unrepentant. For every paper you can quote that criticizes coronary care units I could quote you one that praises them.

HUNTER: By a doctor who works in one? (*Pause*) I have now dealt with all the achievements but one, that you said had been produced by high-technology medicine in the last 20 years: kidney transplants, improvements in diagnosis and treatment, heart surgery, intensive care units, and coronary care units. The one exception is the improvement in general surgical ability that you mentioned. I accept it has occurred. I am less sure it is invariably beneficial. I take it you would agree with me that hemicorporectomy is one result of the 'improvement', so perhaps you will describe that operation for the court.

WESKOFF: It involves, where there is an advanced cancer affecting the lower half of the body, the cutting of the body in half at the waist, and then, after making suitable provision for dealing with the excreta, doing the best the surgeon can for the surviving person. [14]

HUNTER: The surviving upper half of the body? (*Pause*) Such half-men have lived for years? (*Weskoff nods*) You would describe hemicorporectomy as a triumph for high-technology medicine? – Taking the broad view now, not the narrow technical view.

WESKOFF: You might not be so critical, Mr Hunter, if you were the patient. And hemicorporectomy is rare, an extreme example.

JUDGE: I suspect Mr Hunter chose it for the reason I mentioned to you earlier, professor; and I think that what he implies is that, while one may admire the courage of the patients, or the enormous technical skill of the surgeons, one – well, I say it in all humility – some people perhaps might prefer death.

WESKOFF: And if *your* patient does *not* prefer death?

HUNTER: Yes, when the juggernaut has gone as far as it has, the dilemmas are impossible to solve – as I hope to illustrate shortly. (*Pause*) With Dr Batt we mostly considered the *matériel* of high-technology medicine; and so far, with yourself, we have discussed what you felt to have been some of the 'achievements' obtained with it. Here and there an ethical element has intruded; but I now want to look specifically at certain ethical aspects of high-technology medicine. Will you first, then, tell the court about spina bifida and developments in connection with it during the last 20 years?

WESKOFF: It is a condition in which part of the baby's lower bony spine is missing, and the spinal cord – composed of the nerves controlling the lower part of the body – or its coverings are often exposed to a varying extent, and perhaps not developed properly. Sometimes the baby will develop a hydrocephalus too: that is, colloquially, 'water on the brain'. There is a blockage to proper drainage of the fluid in and around the brain and spinal cord, and the baby's head gets bigger and bigger if the condition is not treated. There are one or two other neural tube defects, as they're called; but I won't go into that. These defects can be quite mild. Altogether there are around 2500 cases a year in the UK, and around 8000 in the USA.[15, 16] Not every one of those is a case of spina bifida, let alone a serious case, of course.

HUNTER: And what *used* to happen to the spina bifida babies? – The serious cases?

WESKOFF: Half used to die at or very soon after birth. Occasionally a surgeon would operate, but the majority of those who survived more than a day or two used eventually to die, mostly in the first few weeks or months.

HUNTER: They were allowed to die? No special steps were taken to keep them alive?

WESKOFF: Correct. Some survived, a minority into their teens.[17] There is often paralysis or weakness of the legs in spina bifida cases, bladder and bowel control may be imperfect, infection may occur, and so on. By definition those who did survive into their teens were the least affected.

HUNTER: But high-technology medicine has now intervened?

WESKOFF: Well, about a half still die at or soon after birth; but in the late 1950s a method was developed for treating hydrocephalus which was quite effective; and following that, in the early 1960s, some surgeons in your country began operating on spina bifida very early. Many of their colleagues in other countries soon started to do the same.

HUNTER: They began operating on all the spina bifida cases who didn't die at once or almost at once? (*Weskoff nods*) And the end results?

WESKOFF: Well, from the point of view of survival, the results are better if you operate on all cases at once than if you do nothing, but quite often there is some paralysis of the legs, no matter what is done, and lack of bladder or bowel control, complete or partial; and not infrequently there is mental defect. And there may have to be further operations to straighten the legs, or an extra operation on the spine, or a repeat operation for the hydrocephalus; or operations in connection with the lack of bladder or bowel control. Often the child will have to wear callipers on his legs, or be confined to a wheelchair.

HUNTER: But how exactly did the results from this aggressive surgical approach – I believe that is the term – compare with the previous results when little or nothing was done?

WESKOFF: I'm afraid I don't carry any truly reliable figures in my head. This is not my sphere of special interest, you understand.

HUNTER: I understand. But I am now going to quote you figures from a *Lancet* article,[17] dealing with some cases treated in the United Kingdom. Old-fashioned, non-operative treatment: 17 out of every 100 survived into their teens, eight with minimal handicap, and five in wheelchairs; operative treatment for all cases: 50 out of 100 surviving, 15 with minimal handicap, and 27 (I repeat – 27) in wheelchairs. In other words, the price of those extra seven patients with minimal handicap was 22 extra wheelchair cases.

WESKOFF: I accept those figures; but it was soon realized that some of those operated on would not survive for very long, and some would have a very, very poor quality of life; and so most surgeons began to operate only on selected cases.

HUNTER: And some surgeons continued with the 100 percent operation procedure? (*Weskoff nods*) And others have recommended euthanasia for some cases? (*Weskoff nods again*) And yet all the doctors concerned are intelligent, dedicated, conscientious men and women, wanting to do what is best?

WESKOFF: Naturally.

HUNTER: However, selecting spina bifida patients for operation is now the most usual procedure? In the selection process the doctor has to consider the nature of the family? – Some families respond very well to the presence of an extra, handicapped child, other families do not – other children of the family may suffer, there is often a divorce as a result of the tensions involved? There is a very painful decision to be made?

WESKOFF: Very painful indeed, especially as it should be taken fairly quickly, and the parents may be deeply upset by the birth of a deformed baby, and in no state to make a valid decision.

HUNTER: So sometimes the surgeon has to make it?

WESKOFF: The surgeon and the nurses and everyone else involved; and it's not easy for them. You may have a child who you *feel* has a reasonable chance of a decent life, and yet you judge the family would not give him much support. On the other hand you may have a perfect family but a child whose life, no matter what you do, will probably be a misery. There's every gradation in between. What do you do?

HUNTER: Doctors differ here as well? – On the guidelines to use? (*Weskoff nods*) Can you give me any idea of the financial cost of keeping these children alive? – In your country?

WESKOFF: One 1976 estimate put the cost for life-time care of a child with what is called open spina bifida at $100,000–250,000.[16]

HUNTER: And this whole, difficult, agonizing, and expensive position has been created – this is the immediate point of my questioning – by what seemed perfectly natural, proper developments in high-technology medicine?

WESKOFF: You don't stop going ahead because you run into one or two difficulties.

JUDGE: Professor, what happens to any babies who are not operated upon?

WESKOFF: The practice varies, judge; but, in general, the doctor simply refuses to go to extreme lengths to keep the baby alive. If there's an infection, he perhaps won't use antibiotics, and so on.

JUDGE: And so the baby and the unfortunate parents are put out of their misery? – In time? (*Weskoff nods*) Are drugs ever given that might accelerate death? Sedative drugs? (*Pause*) I think you should answer, professor.

WESKOFF: Yes, they are occasionally, but in good faith.

JUDGE: I do not dispute that. Tell me, are the junior doctors who may be involved in the prolonged surgical treatment of these children in the USA or UK sometimes from underdeveloped countries? (*Weskoff nods*) And in the countries of origin of those doctors children who, with some fairly brief, simple, and cheap medical treatment, would grow up into perfectly normal human beings die for want of such treatment? (*Weskoff nods again*) And now do you happen to know how many therapeutic abortions are performed in the UK and USA each year?

WESKOFF: Yes, it's around 150,000 in the UK, and just over 1,000,000 in the US.

JUDGE: Most of the fetuses, if they had not been aborted, would have grown into physically and mentally normal human babies?

WESKOFF: Yes.

JUDGE: Thank you, professor. Mr Hunter?

HUNTER: (*to Weskoff*): Some experts see a possible answer to spina bifida, I believe, in what is called amniocentesis – that is, the withdrawing of fluid from the uterus – in mid-pregnancy, and the testing of it for a substance called alphafetoprotein, the level of which is commonly high if the fetus has a spina bifida deformity. The mothers could in that case be offered an abortion. Such an amniocentesis would be performed only if a preliminary test on the mother's blood had shown a high level of alphafetoprotein in it, and an ultrasound test had excluded the possibility that it was due to the mother carrying twins or triplets.[15, 16, 18, 19]

WESKOFF: Yes, this is one very hopeful approach.

HUNTER: But there are difficulties to it? (*Weskoff nods*) First, in Britain, for example, 20–30 percent of pregnant women leave their first doctor visit too late for the tests to be carried out?[15] – The taking of the mother's blood, its testing, the ultrasound test (which helps to locate the placenta and confirms the duration of the pregnancy), the amniocentesis, the testing of the withdrawn fluid, and the abortion, if one is indicated, should all be carried out roughly in the 16th to the 20th week of pregnancy?[18] (*Weskoff nods*) The test on the mother's blood or the amniotic fluid is not an easy one, and yet an error in the second test can mean either that a mother with an abnormal fetus will be told it is normal, or a mother with a normal one will be told it is abnormal? Neither test is yet perfect?

WESKOFF: Correct; and even in the best hands you miss out on about one in five open spina bifida cases,[15, 18] the most serious kind; not to say the 10 percent that are minor in degree;[15, 16] and you also get a very small proportion of what are called 'false positives'.

HUNTER: In which case the doctor might advise an abortion for a mother who was carrying a quite normal fetus? (*Weskoff nods*) It has been calculated that this testing might leave in the United States 1000 cases of open spina bifida – the more severe kind – undetected each year?[15] The mothers in question would be just as upset as any who were mistakenly aborted when carrying a normal fetus, or perhaps normal twins? There are far more false positives in the test on the mother's blood than in the test on the amniotic fluid?[18] – So that quite a few mothers would suffer great unnecessary anxiety between the two tests? (*Weskoff nods*) And, of course, the assumption underlying the whole procedure from the start is that women undergoing it *must* be prepared to have an abortion if the testing suggests the fetus is abnormal? What's more, even though in expert hands the small operation of amniocentesis carries very little risk of itself inducing abortion,[16] that would almost certainly not be true if the operation were to be performed on the 60,000 American women[15] and the 12,000 or so British women[19] who, it's been calculated, would need it? It might then induce abortion in 1–2 percent of them,[19, 20] some, of course, carrying quite normal fetuses?

WESKOFF: You certainly do your homework, Mr Hunter.

HUNTER: I have done one extra piece, professor: if the amniotic fluid were withdrawn, it would be difficult to refuse to test the fetal cells in the fluid for what are called chromosomal abnormalities or metabolic disorders:[15, 19, 20] that is, conditions such as Down's syndrome (mongolism, as it was once called), phenylketonuria, and so on. You agree?

WESKOFF: I certainly can't disagree.

HUNTER: With 3,000,000 women pregnant in the USA every year, and about 600,000 in Britain, all of this, if it is adopted, will be very costly?

WESKOFF: But cheaper, in the case of spina bifida, than the cost of looking after the handicapped children who would otherwise be born.

HUNTER: Is not the position that no one is quite sure?[15, 18] – That in fact, there has been a good deal of debate on the matter? (*Weskoff nods*) No one has yet drawn up a psychological balance sheet in any case? The testing is probably to be introduced in the UK, but it is not, for various reasons, to be generally adopted in the USA for the time being?[15] (*Weskoff nods*) What *is* absolutely sure is that high-technology medicine has in this case presented doctors and mothers and fathers with a whole series of very difficult questions to answer, some of them deep ethical questions – in the case of all pregnancies. Every pregnant woman in our two countries – almost 4,000,000 women every year – may soon have to say to herself, 'Should I be willing to have my child aborted if the doctors tell me that it would very probably be abnormal?' A mixed blessing?

WESKOFF: To me the benefits seem to outweigh the drawbacks. I think most people would feel that way.

HUNTER: It is a fact – is it not, professor – that spina bifida is only one of a number of abnormalities that can affect the newborn child, any one of which would, 20 or 30 years ago, have usually led to an early death whereas today some of the affected babies – pending the widespread use of this new kind of preventive approach with all its drawbacks – can be treated and kept alive thanks to developments in high-technology medicine?

WESKOFF: That is what medicine's about – in part. That is progress.

HUNTER: I repeat: we are here to decide if it *is* progress, professor. These children may be treated in intensive care units, with repeated operations, with drugs, with intravenous feeds, with artificial respiration, with the kind of elemental diets the astronauts have . . . And this may cost the parents deep emotional distress?

And may cost them or society tens of thousands of dollars per patient? And yet at the end of it all a child may die? Even if he lives at home, he can often never have anything resembling a normal life, and just as often he will spend his life in an institution? You know that two doctors in America have said, 'We may, as a society, scorn the civilizations that slaughtered their infants, but our present treatment of the retarded is in some ways more cruel?'[21]

WESKOFF: The answer is to improve the institutions, isn't it? – Not to let the babies die.

HUNTER: But, aside from whether life *anywhere* would be worthwhile for these babies, you know money won't be switched from the intensive care unit to the institution for the mentally subnormal, do you not? I will now quote what a distinguished English doctor has said[22] in the *British Medical Journal* on this topic: improvements in the routine services of the National Health Service, he said, are low priority, 'but we can look forward to the expansion of the accident and emergency services, intensive treatment centres, haemodialysis units, organ-transplant facilities, etc. They are very expensive, claim very high prestige, and are the pride of their mother-hospitals. The work is demanding, is a high challenge to everyone engaged in it, and provides a basis for advancing knowledge. But from the point of view of cost-effectiveness it is uneconomic. In deploying the limited resources available in these fields for preference we are tackling the most difficult rather than the most rewarding problems.' Exactly the same could be said about developments in your country, could it not?

WESKOFF: I'd sooner not speculate on what might be said, Mr Hunter.

HUNTER: Well then, here are some things that *have* been said in your country. I quote again from that article in the *New England Journal of Medicine*:[21] one doctor to another about a baby of the type just mentioned – 'For this child don't you think it's time to turn off your curiosity so you can turn on your kindness?' The article was quoting what had actually been said. It stated also that some people in your country have felt that very defective children shouldn't just be left to die – because that would mean the loss of 'teaching material'. It also said, about the decision not to persist with treatment when the prospect of a meaningful life for a child was poor or hopeless, that 'The awesome finality of these decisions, combined with a potential for error in prognosis, made the choice agonizing for families and health professionals.' Does the fact that high-technology medicine has created all these problems, especially these ethical problems – does it not worry you deeply, professor?

(*Pause*) May I give you another quotation then, this time from the Harvard Professor of Psychiatry? – 'At long last we are beginning to ask, not *can* it be done, but *should* it be done?'[23]

WESKOFF: Look, Mr Hunter, automobiles kill some people, but you don't therefore abolish them.

HUNTER: And yet, aside from whether the internal combustion engine has not done more harm than good, you do call a halt somewhere: you have a speed limit for automobiles.

WESKOFF: We have restraints in the ethical field too: restraints, not abolition of all new procedures. The best of them is the conscience of the individual doctor, caring for a patient or carrying out an investigation. There's also a restraint implicit in the fact that doctors know their fellow doctors are watching what they do – in the wards, in the operating theater, the laboratory or wherever it may be. And as a last resort – doctors know the editors of medical journals won't publish the results of research if the ethics of it are suspect.[24] The whole medical institution is geared against unethical practices.

HUNTER: Those three types of restraint are not invariably effective, are they? You must, at one extreme, have heard of doctors being involved in the infliction of torture.

WESKOFF: You refer to a tiny minority who would be abnormal no matter what jobs they were in.

HUNTER: But high-technology medicine does give doctors unusual opportunities to deploy any immorality that is in them – or amorality, which is worse – does it not? (*Pause*) High-technology medicine now insists on definitive proof of the value of a new drug or device or operation or diagnostic procedure before it is generally used? And proof is obtained by tests, in the end on human beings? Often the test is of no conceivable diagnostic or treatment value to the person subjected to the test?

WESKOFF: Correct. I have conducted many such tests myself, and taken part in quite a few as a subject.

HUNTER: You are an intelligent, informed woman, professor; obviously not one to submit to any kind of pressure or persuasion? (*Weskoff nods*) Would you say the same of all those who have been subjected to certain of the tests of the types just mentioned? – Of mentally subnormal people, say, or poor people, black people, children, even ordinary sick people in a hospital; old people, or people near to death?

WESKOFF: It is for them that we now have, as well as the restraints of conscience, one or two extra formal safeguards.

HUNTER: These formal safeguards were not much debated before the mid-1960s, were they? (*Pause*) You have heard of the late

Dr Henry Beecher? (*Weskoff nods*) He was a distinguished American doctor who in June 1966 published a paper – described as a landmark – in the *New England Journal of Medicine* that cited 22 studies involving medical experiments on humans that he judged to be unethical?[25] (*Weskoff nods*) You have heard of Dr Maurice Pappworth?

WESKOFF: The English doctor who wrote a book called *Human Guinea Pigs*?[26]

HUNTER: Yes. His book was published in 1967, and it had much the same theme as Dr Beecher's article but was wider in scope? (*Weskoff nods*) And do you know that it was in that year that the Royal College of Physicians of London issued a report[27] on the ethics of clinical research investigations? – From a committee appointed twelve months previously following receipt of a letter by the President of the College from a number of its Fellows, setting out the concern that had been expressed on this matter over the years by lay people and doctors, and in particular quoting Dr Beecher's 1966 article? I wonder why they had not written earlier. After all, they were practicing doctors, who would, so you said, be watching what their colleagues did, and unethical practices clearly did not begin in 1966. (*Pause*) The report of this committee was against formal codes, and 'rigid or central bureaucratic controls', but suggested that every hospital or institution where clinical research investigations were conducted should have a special ethical committee to oversee the ethics of all such proposed investigations.

WESKOFF: Yes, and that's the system we have here in the States.[28]

HUNTER: Because in 1967 – notice the year, professor, a panel appointed by the President's Office of Science and Technology recommended the taking of suitable precautions in all institutions receiving government research funds?[29] – And something similar for other medical institutions? And then in 1971 didn't your Department of Health, Education, and Welfare issue a guide laying down exactly when the consent of a person to a research investigation could be described as 'informed'?[29] And in 1974 your Congress set up a National Commission for the Protection of Human Subjects of Biomedical and Behavioral Research?[30] It has already reported[31] on the ethical aspects of research using the fetus, or prisoners, and also on psychosurgery? It has still to report on research involving children or the mentally infirm in institutions? And it has been proposed in your Senate that the Commission should be succeeded by a permanent, more powerful body, the National Advisory Council?[30, 31] This does look very much like those central bureaucratic controls that the Royal College of

Physicians was very much against, not to say some doctors in your country.[30] No? And hasn't all this happened, professor, because the restraints on research that you thought most important – the consciences of doctors in one form or another – were thought by government not to have been strong enough?

WESKOFF: No, it means an extra safeguard or two; and politicians getting in on the act.[30]

HUNTER: The elected representatives of the people? It is, of course, the bodies and minds of the people that the doctors experiment with? That was the case in the secret experiments conducted by your Defense Department and CIA, was it not?[30, 32] The Rockefeller Commission found that the CIA had studied ways, including the use of drugs, of influencing human behavior – in 'unsuspecting subjects within the US'.[32] It also studied the effects of 'radiation, electric shock, psychology, psychiatry, sociology, and harassment substances'.[32] And individual medical men were involved?[32] – It was, in fact, this affair that led your Senate to propose the setting up of the permanent National Advisory Council to succeed the National Commission I mentioned just now?[30]

WESKOFF: Yes, and all this over-reaction, over-regimentation has been criticized.[30]

HUNTER: By American doctors? (*Pause*) But now the position in Britain: in 1970, following some disquiet on the part of the public, the UK Department of Health and Social Security set up an Advisory Group to look at the use of fetuses for research purposes. It reported in 1972.[33] Also I have here a circular[34] – HSC (IS) 153 of June 1975 – from the Department of Health and Social Security, calling the attention of Regional and Area Health Authorities and Boards of Governors of Teaching Hospitals to, first, the Report on fetal research just mentioned; second, the 1973 up-dated Report[35] of the committee of the Royal College of Physicians already mentioned; and third, an extract from the 1962–3 Report[36] of the British Medical Research Council, setting out its views on clinical research investigations on children and the mentally handicapped. What I wish to stress again at this point is the source of the circular – a government department. It looks – does it not, professor – as though you and the Royal College of Physicians have lost this particular battle against anyone but doctors being involved in ethical decisions?

WESKOFF: Nothing is finally decided yet. For a variety of reasons we have been through a bad time.

HUNTER: The doctors have, you mean?

WESKOFF: Politics has crept in; but after all the dust has settled, we'll find, I think, that the consciences of individual doctors, and of their colleagues, and of medical-journal editors will still be the most important shield against abuse.

HUNTER: You know that doubts about the effectiveness of that shield have been expressed by doctors themselves,[32, 37] and by a professional philosopher?[38] (*Pause*) Now, at the heart of this whole controversy lies the matter of informed consent? – That is, whether the person involved – the patient, the prisoner, even the normal healthy volunteer – really understands what it is proposed to do to him, and why, and what the consequences might be. (*Weskoff nods*) And you know it has been said that, even in the intelligent ordinary patient, fully informed consent to research is almost impossible? – He can't be told every single thing that *might* happen or he'd be scared out of his wits. He can't understand some of the medical information he does receive. He can't imagine exactly what he will, in fact, experience. The editor of the *New England Journal of Medicine* wrote: 'Incapacitated and hospitalized because of illness, frightened by strange and impersonal routines, and fearful for his health and perhaps life, he is far from exercising a free power of choice when the person to whom he anchors all his hopes asks, "Say, you wouldn't mind, would you, if you joined some of the other patients on this floor and helped us to carry out some very important research we are doing?".'[39]

WESKOFF: Yes, but the doctor simply does the very best he can in the circumstances.

HUNTER: Best for whom, if research is involved? (*Pause*) It seems he hasn't always done so – because the editor in that same article also said, 'The procedure currently approved in the United States for enlisting human experimental subjects has one great virtue: patient-subjects are put on notice that their management is in part at least an experiment. The deceptions of the past are no longer tolerated.' 'Deceptions of the past', professor? (*Pause*) Where were the consciences and the colleagues then? – Well now, suppose we move from ordinary people to prisoners. The National Commission laid down in 1976 very strict rules indeed to govern their participation in research,[31] the essential upshot of which will probably be a minimal use of prisoners in the US in future. But perhaps we could look back briefly to see why the Commission had to look at this matter. In the past prisoners sometimes received money for 'volunteering' to take part in medical research (and might have no other source of money); their willingness – or unwillingness – to do so might be revealed to parole boards and would certainly be known to their jailers; they could get a little extra freedom and comfort out of the research, it would add a little interest to their lives? And prisoners might look upon the doctor who wanted to do the research as a potential friend – perhaps as an only friend. Well? A lot of concern on this topic has been expressed in your country over the years, has it not?[40, 41]

WESKOFF: Yes, naturally there were problems. There could also be real benefits to the prisoner, as one or two people[42] who disagreed with the critics – including at least one prisoner[43] – pointed out. A prisoner might *want* to help his fellow men.

HUNTER: None the less the National Commission seems on the whole to have sided with the critics? (*Pause*) Well, now, from generalities to particulars. The Sloan-Kettering Cancer Center in New York has an international reputation?

WESKOFF: It certainly has.

HUNTER: In the early 1960s two doctors, working in a Brooklyn hospital on a research project of the Center, supervised the injection of 22 old and seriously ill patients with live cancer cells? They did not tell the patients they were being injected with cancer cells, what they did was no part of diagnosis or treatment of their patients' conditions, and some of the patients were in any case incapable of giving consent? Correct so far? (*Weskoff nods*) The New York newspapers gave the matter a lot of coverage in 1964? (*She nods again*) An official investigation decided that the so-called consent of the patients had been fraudulently obtained, and that the two doctors were guilty of 'unprofessional conduct' and of 'fraud and deceit in the practise of medicine'?[44, 45] No comment, professor? Where were the doctors' consciences then? (*Pause*) Well now, does the name 'Tuskegee' mean anything to you?

WESKOFF: It is the name of a town in Alabama which has been attached to a study of untreated syphilis in poor blacks. This study started in 1932, the fact that they were not to be treated and the risks of the study were not explained to the men involved, nor was their consent to the study obtained. Even in the 1940s, when penicillin, as a very effective treatment for syphilis became available, they were not treated. Quite apart from the ethical aspects, the study was badly designed; and nothing was ever learnt from it.[46, 47]

HUNTER: And how many men were involved?

WESKOFF: It was about 400,[47] I think. They didn't all have syphilis, in fact – some were just controls; and of course, a lot of them have died since 1932. The study was terminated in 1972.

HUNTER: On the recommendation of a panel set up to investigate the matter?[46] (*Weskoff nods*) And it was proposed to compensate the survivors who had had syphilis and the control subjects and the families of any of the men involved who have died?[47]

WESKOFF: It is an episode of which no one is proud; and all I want to say in extenuation is that it started in 1932 when we were not nearly as conscious as we have since become of our ethical duties in the research field.

HUNTER: But it continued, professor, until 1972 – through the 1950s and 1960s, through the era of high-technology medicine's birth and development. Whatever one may think about such work in the 1930s and 1940s – even then it was clearly unethical – its later continuance, presumably with the knowledge or connivance of a number of doctors, is the point at issue now. I am saying that, despite all you have told us about doctors' individual consciences, and those of their professional colleagues, and so on – despite it all, high-technology medicine failed over a period of many years to put right a very obvious wrong. (*Pause*) This Tuskegee affair in fact led to the setting up of the National Commission?[46] (*Weskoff nods*)

JUDGE: Was this Tuskegee research a private investigation, professor?

WESKOFF: No, it was a United States Public Health Service study.

HUNTER: This next matter does not involve a research investigation; but I wonder, professor, if you know who said these words, and when: 'There is uncontroverted evidence in the record that minors and other incompetents have been sterilized with federal funds and that an indefinite number of poor people have been improperly coerced into accepting a sterilization operation under the threat that various federally supported welfare benefits would be withdrawn unless they submitted to irreversible sterilization,[48] Well?

WESKOFF: They were said by a judge in Washington, Judge Gesell, in 1974.

HUNTER: Correct me if I am wrong in any particular, professor: some 150,000 poor people had been sterilized each year over a period of years, many black, some mentally defective. The judge ruled that new regulations brought in by the federal authorities to remedy the situation – after it had received some publicity – did not provide sufficient safeguards against coercion by doctors or others. He said that ordinary adults must be told clearly from the start that, even if they failed to accept sterilization, any federal benefits they were receiving would continue; and he forbade sterilization of minors, no matter what the circumstances – at any rate under the statute in question.[48]

WESKOFF: That is absolutely correct. Again nobody is proud of the situation. However, as you said, it was not a research matter.

HUNTER: But it was an ethical matter? It did involve a situation in which doctors' consciences might have been expected to be active, and in which a number of doctors was involved and about which many doctors knew; and yet neither the doctors' consciences nor the surveillance of their colleagues seem to have been in the least effective?

WESKOFF: As I say, nearly all hospitals today have their own ethical committees to oversee proposed experimental work.

HUNTER: That is not an answer to my question. Do you deny these committees have varying procedures, varying powers, varying criteria on what shall and shall not be submitted to them for approval?[37] – And all are heavily weighted with the expertise of their doctor members? – Hardworking, well-meaning, but narrow-minded and biased doctors.[38] Biased in favor of investigation, in other words, in favor of other doctors, in favor of *not* showing disapproval of a colleague. (*Pause*) I put it to you, professor, that the Sloan-Kettering affair, the Tuskegee study, and the business of sterilizing the poor are typical products of the minds, not of evil men, but of doctors imbued with the ideas and ideals of high-technology medicine, men who did these things with muddled good intentions; and that these examples may indicate merely the tip of an iceberg.

WESKOFF: You have no right to imply that such practices are widespread.

HUNTER: Very well: perhaps you will now uncover a little more of the iceberg. Will you tell us, professor, what you know about Willowbrook?

WESKOFF: Willowbrook is – or rather, was – a very large state school on Staten Island, near New York, for mentally defective children. There was a good deal of infectious disease there of various kinds, including one called hepatitis B – or serum hepatitis – which is a virus infection of the liver.

JUDGE: It is common, professor?

WESKOFF: Common enough, judge. There may be some 80–100,000 cases a year in my country and about 10 percent of the patients die. The disease tends to be less severe in children. Also nearly all the children who went to Willowbrook got the disease within 12 months. There is no vaccine against it, but work has been going on for more than 30 years to try and find one.

JUDGE: Backed by?

WESKOFF: By the United States Army Medical Service. As one part of the work, it was decided, the consent of the parents having been obtained, to give material containing the virus – by mouth or by injection – to children, aged three to nine, newly admitted to Willowbrook, and then to make certain observations. The doctors concerned argued that they had the parents' consent, that the children would almost certainly get the disease anyway; that as a result of what was done they would have a mild infection with subsequent immunity; and that they would be nursed after receiving the virus material in a special, isolated, well-equipped and well-staffed unit – whereas the general run of children at Willowbrook who got hepatitis were often exposed at the same time to other infections. Some very interesting and useful information has emerged from all the work.[49, 50, 51, 52] In fact, a vaccine against hepatitis is within sight.[50]

JUDGE: When we are considering the ethics of a particular action, the question of whether or not benefit results from it is irrelevant; at any rate in a case of this kind. That is clear to you, Professor Weskoff?

WESKOFF: Surely; but while the Willowbrook hepatitis study has been criticized by some doctors,[53, 54] it has been defended by others.[55, 56]

JUDGE: Having been told by Mr Hunter what might be discussed today, I took the precaution of reading the 1963 statement[36] of the British Medical Research Council on the legal aspects of this matter, to which it still adhered as recently as 1973.[57] It reads in part: 'In the strict view of the law parents and guardians of minors cannot give consent on their behalf to any procedures which are of no particular benefit to them and which may carry some risk of harm.' It applies up to the age of 12.[36] As regards the USA, again it does seem that there is no legal ground for the belief that consent by parents – even if other conditions are satisfied – justifies a doctor in carrying out non-beneficial research on children, and *par excellence*, of course, mentally defective children.[58] It has been suggested that doctors and parents who take part in such an activity might lay themselves open to legal action.[28] It has been said in an American court that parents are free to make martyrs of themselves, but they are not free to make martyrs of their children.[58] That appears to be the legal position, although I am bound to add that its validity has been queried in both countries; and of course, legal and ethical considerations are not always identical.

WESKOFF: The Dr Henry Beecher we've already mentioned took the view that the attitude of your Medical Research Council was unreasonable.[59] He thought that research in children that won't benefit them is permissible if it has firm medical support and justification, and if the results may prove valuable to mankind and there is no discernible risk.

HUNTER: None the less, professor, he found that the Willowbrook study did *not* qualify on that score?

WESKOFF: Yes.

HUNTER: As regards the ethical aspect, professor, I should like to quote some authorities. First, the relevant section of the 1973 up-dated Report on the ethics of research, produced by a committee of the Royal College of Physicians of London reads: 'If advances in medical treatment are to continue so must clinical research investigation. It is in this light therefore that it is recommended that clinical research investigation of children or mentally handicapped adults which is not of direct benefit to the patient should be conducted, but only when the procedures entail negligible risk or discomfort and subject to the provisions of any common and statute law prevailing at the time. The parent or guardian should be consulted and his agreement recorded.'[35]

WESKOFF: That could be interpreted as 'pro' or 'con' the Willowbrook work.

HUNTER: The World Medical Association Draft Code of Ethics on Human Experimentation stated that 'Persons retained in mental hospitals or hospitals for mental defectives should not be used for human experiment'[60] conducted solely for the acquisition of knowledge. The Association has also laid it down[61] that 'Under no circumstances is a doctor permitted to do anything that would weaken the physical or mental resistance of the human being except from strictly therapeutic or prophylactic indications imposed in the interest of the patient.' It is difficult to reconcile the Willowbrook work with adherence to these two statements. There *is* a major ethical – and of course, legal – question involved.

WESKOFF: No argument, though the final version of that particular Code – the Declaration of Helsinki[62] – did not contain the words you quoted.

HUNTER: You miss my point, professor: in 1970 the Willowbrook doctors themselves stated[63] that, since its start in 1956, their work had conformed to the *Draft* Code. (*Pause*) Well now, to come to my main point as concerns Willowbrook: which would you say is the best general medical journal in the world?

WESKOFF: The *Lancet*.

HUNTER: I have here the issue of it for April 10, 1971. A letter[64] on page 749 indicates that there had been three *Lancet* leading articles referring to the Willowbrook study during the previous two years, and only in the third article was the least ethical doubt about the work expressed. The writer of the letter condemned the ethics of the Willowbrook work and said the *Lancet* should review its own position on the matter. In a footnote to the letter the editor of the *Lancet* himself very creditably admitted that the writer had raised a question 'it ought to have faced long ago. The journal's eagerness to discuss all the events in the elucidation of the spread of hepatitis left it exposed to these criticisms, which we accept . . .'

He added that the possibility of the work leading to a method of prevention of hepatitis 'could not justify the giving of infected material to children who would not directly benefit.'

WESKOFF: That simply means there is another doctor, albeit editor of a distinguished journal, who disapproves of the Willowbrook work on ethical grounds.

HUNTER: But you said earlier that doctors were in part deterred from performing unethical experiments by the attitude of editors of medical journals to publicizing results. Here now is what you agreed was the best general medical journal in the world, which only at the third attempt examines carefully what could properly – you have agreed – be regarded as an unethical study. The work had *not* been subjected to the editorial scrutiny you mentioned, and perhaps that applies to other studies. Not one of your safeguards seems to work: the individual consciences, the surveillance of colleagues, the editorial scrutiny. Is that not, indeed, why the state is intervening in this country, and is beginning to intervene in my country?

WESKOFF: I would point out to you, Mr Hunter, that the *New England Journal of Medicine* disagreed editorially with the *Lancet* on this matter[61] of the ethics of the Willowbrook work, and continued to publish the results of it.

HUNTER: That in no way alters the fact that the *Lancet* had apparently not in the first place considered the ethics of Willowbrook at all; and in any case, are you not aware that five of the six letters[65, 66, 67, 68, 69] on the topic that the *New England Journal of Medicine* subsequently published disagreed with the editor's view, and only one[70] gave it a qualified approval? If the editor had had letters wholly favorable to the view he had expressed he would have published some of them?

WESKOFF: Surely. He is an honorable man, as publication of those letters shows.

HUNTER: Professor, I am not impugning the excellent intentions of any of those involved in the Willowbrook matter. I am suggesting what is more frightening: that they did – or supported the doing of – what was probably the wrong thing, either for what they felt to be the best of reasons or without even realizing that anything needing an ethical judgment was involved. Yet again, I am suggesting high-technology medicine over-reached itself.

WESKOFF: And high-technology society has the answers?

HUNTER: No, but it has realized there are questions to be answered – by society, not just by the doctors. And yet many doctors disagree: one has said of pressures to be applied to doctors in the matter of the ethics of research: 'Policies concerning these pressures should be determined by the profession rather than by the public, who are inclined to give an emotional rather than a rational opinion.'[71]

WESKOFF: I go along with that.

HUNTER: And yet it is, after all, the bodies and minds of members of the public or of their children that are to be the subject of the doctors' experiments. Do they no longer have the right to help decide the larger issues involving themselves? (*Pause*) Well, I will now quote to you an American *doctor* – from Yale University School of Medicine. He has said, 'I am no longer certain that it is proper for the physician to ask his own patients to participate in studies that he is carrying out.'[37] We are back – are we not? – to what the judge questioned Dr Batt about yesterday: the inescapable conflict between the objectivity, the quantification of the high-technology medical scientist, carrying out an experiment, and the compassion of the medical man looking after a patient? Now, questions of the same kind as those we have been discussing, all posed by high-technology medicine, could be posed in respect of various other matters, could they not? – That of turning off the respirator, as it is described; the question of when to attempt to resuscitate a very old person whose heart has stopped; of psycho-surgery for aggression; of providing the pill for minors without their parents' knowledge; of experiments on the fetus; of fertiliza-tion of a human egg in the test tube; and so on, and so on? – Dozens of ethical problems that would not exist but for high-technology medicine.

WESKOFF: And where is all this getting us now, Mr Hunter?

HUNTER: To the deeper implications of all that we have been dis-cussing about high-technology medicine in the past two days. I want you to think back – to doctors as everyday users of gadgets, to medical disposables, to mechanical hearts and mechanical joints, to the little boy in Texas, living in a plastic tent, to those surgical isolating techniques; to the fiberoptic instruments, to monitoring machines, to computers, to automated laboratory testing, to all the refined diagnostic techniques doctors now have; to the artificial blood and the artificial human milk to maintaining life for years with intravenous feeding, to heart and kidney transplants, to the use of an artificial mechanical pancreas and the genetic engineering of a bacterium to make it produce a plentiful supply of insulin, to machines that will inject automatically, to 100 percent hospital confinements, to the abject terror cardiac catheterization can sometimes induce, to open-heart surgery and intensive care units and coronary care units (and the mental disturbance they may all cause), to operations on spina bifida babies, to hemicorporectomy, to the resuscitation of old people, to looking upon the patient as an object, to measurement as the be-all-and-end-all, to the concentration on an organ or a disease rather than a person, on the body not the mind, on the rare and intellectually challenging rather than the common and preventable disorder; to the Brooklyn doctors injecting cancer cells into people, to the Tuskegee blacks left with their syphilis untreated for years, to the sterilization of poor, mentally defective people, to Willowbrook. I want you to think back to all these, to try and link them together, to take a holistic view, and to ask yourself whether they do not – whatever the benefit, medical, economic or social, of one or other might be, regarded in isolation – whether as a whole they do not clearly spell out a mechanistic view of life in doctors, and above all a terrible passion for the achievement of complete knowledge and complete power by every available means. In a word, the doctors, like a lot of other scientists, are playing in earnest at being God. Is this not what high-technology medicine is all about?

JUDGE: Professor? You wish to answer Mr Hunter's question?

WESKOFF: I am a doctor, judge. I have devoted my life to research. I see an element of truth in what he is saying. I cannot give a plain 'Yes' or 'No' to it just like that. I need time to think.

HUNTER: I am almost finished, professor. I should like, however, to revert briefly to a point you disputed earlier in the day – that high-technology medicine and high-technology society are inextricably linked. Broadly speaking, the same engineering and chemical skills that go to produce the cigarettes, the foods, and the automobiles that help to produce coronary heart disease also produce the machines and drugs and instruments used in the coronary care unit? Or the tablets the coronary survivor will take? Or the exercise machine a man will use at home in order to try and avoid a coronary?

WESKOFF: At any one time in history men have a particular way of tackling their problems. All their problems.

HUNTER: But might doctors not now – at this unique time in history – discard both the answers and the problems? Say 'No'? Try a completely new way? Become saints or fanatics? (*Pause*) The very elements – technological, industrial, scientific elements – that, when used by medicine, may cure disease and prolong the length of a life may also, when present in society, diminish the quality of life. Yes? The steel that makes the scalpel also makes the car that hits the man the scalpel saves. The old man's hip prosthesis is made from a material found in Concorde against the noise of which he shuts his ears.

WESKOFF: Every drug has side-effects.

HUNTER: But need one think only of another *drug* as the answer? Must doctors be so completely – what was your phrase? – children of their time? (*Pause*) Should they not set an example? The same chemical industry that makes drugs and insecticides with which doctors save lives also pollutes the environment – for instance, with insecticides – and makes chemicals with which to treat the pollution; and makes fertilizers to help produce more food for the people it has helped to keep alive, and a 'pill' to prevent yet more being born? And napalm to help soldiers kill some who have been born?

WESKOFF: Every coin has two sides to it. You know that, Mr Hunter.

HUNTER: Yes: who, do you happen to know, was the greatest benefactor to British medicine between 1930 and 1960?

WESKOFF: Lord Nuffield, I guess.

HUNTER: Will you accept that between 1930 and 1956 the amount he gave to the Oxford hospitals and medical school was some £3,500,000[72] – which is, of course, the equivalent of far, far more today? (*Weskoff nods*) The late Lord Nuffield – I am not, of course, criticizing him as a person – made his money from what source?

WESKOFF: From making and selling automobiles.

HUNTER: Which kill people directly, and help to make them fat, and put up their pulse rates . . . Do I make my point? The automobile helps to put them into hospitals where they are treated with the aid of money gained from automobiles.

WESKOFF: I am not convinced.

HUNTER: You use radioactive elements in medicine for treatment and diagnosis? (*Weskoff nods*) You would not have them but for the atom bomb and the thermonuclear weapon, would you? Which gives the greater good in that case? Is it perhaps today, professor, that we have a coin of which both faces are tarnished? One face, it is true – that of high-technology medicine – means the saving of some lives, and it once meant the lengthening of men's lives, though even that trend seems now to have been halted or reversed; and in practice it has, in any case, other important negative aspects to which I shall return at a later session of the court; the net total effect being negative. And the other face is not merely a loss of quality in life, and possibly even the death of *man*, but very often sickness and death for men. Has not medicine, which should be devoted to the saving and succoring of individual lives and their easing into death, become part and parcel of a high-technology society, which seems, wittingly or not, directed towards the destruction, perhaps of all life itself, and certainly of individual lives?

WESKOFF: You cannot turn back the clock, Mr Hunter.

HUNTER: But one might look away from clocks altogether. No? (*Pause*) It would, I think, be appropriate for us to end with quotations on high-technology medicine from four very clear-sighted high-technology doctors. What the first of them said appeared in the *Journal of the American Medical Association.*[73] He was admitted to a university hospital, and he said that, while the technical care he received was excellent, true human contact, especially with nurses, was almost absent. Only one nurse actually visited him during his entire stay although – I now quote – 'Nursing aides and assistants, technicians from the laboratory, and dietitians came regularly and frequently to measure my blood pressure, weigh me, administer drugs, draw blood, and talk about my diet.' The nurses seemed always to be in their ward offices, writing or giving an assistant the drugs to be distributed to patients; though each morning, as the day nurses took over from the night nurses, the two groups would walk along the corridor with the various aides and mutter about the condition of individual patients, though never entering the rooms.

JUDGE: Is this typical, professor?

WESKOFF: Well, it's not untypical, judge; and in your country too.

HUNTER: The second doctor said in the same *Journal of the American Medical Association*[12] that 'large hospitals have become disquieting places, as anyone who has recently been a patient there can testify . . . the patient is usually low man on the totem pole in an organization that is largely for the convenient of others'. Obsolescence, he said, has extended to patients – the hospital or a ward wishes to be rid of certain patients, especially if their condition is uninteresting. Care has become task-centered, not patient-centered, communication often poor, noise common, a 40-hour week the aim of many of the staff. The third doctor wrote in the *New England Journal of Medicine,*[74] and, as in the Dr Jaeger session and for the same reasons, we shall see what he said projected on to the screen against the back wall of the court. *The quotation is projected.*

Technologic advances, commercialization of medical care, and money-changers have separated doctor and patient and promise to reduce the physician – not entirely without his complicity – to mere practitioner of rational science and operator of sophisticated instrumentation . . . Healing or making whole requires that the whole person be addressed wholeheartedly . . . There are already indications that Technique is fragmenting the community's common humanity . . . Technique is related to every aspect of life. It runs the gamut: food, population, agriculture, vocation, education, economics, surveillance, and control, the state, all our institutions, recreation and amusement, mass man, totalitarian man, and, ultimately, the dissociation of man . . . Although technicians themselves have tried and continue to try to control the future of technological evolution, their formula is predictable and limited. 'A technical problem demands a technical solution' . . . Not only does the medical profession function within and interact with broad social and political realities, but every aspect of human existence is of medical interest and concern. Therefore the climate of the larger scene is of immediate relevance to the practice of medicine and to the care of the patient.

Technological thinking has been particularly manifested by the selection of medical students. Intellectual keenness, mathematical prowess and scientific objectivity (with an attendant material acquisitiveness) assumed disproportionate importance in the choices made . . . these ascendant philosophies of specialised medical science over holistic care of the patient in his environment will continue . . . Technical aids were once mere adjuncts to clinical judgment. Today, new tests have become per se indispensable, too often for irrelevant and inappropriate reasons . . . Some physicians, though skeptical of the merits of extended survival without meaningful life, too often temper their best judgment in the care of a patient in compliance to the conventional pattern of the day . . . Others . . . become so absorbed in the narrow technical aspects of a case presentation or case study as to lose sight of its broader consequences . . . The present dictates of our teaching, training and practice direct us then to use costly techniques to seek for the unusual. We shun the prime need of a sick, soft, self-indulgent, anxious and driven people, their crying need for a sensible, sensitive and concerned doctor . . . Cockeyed, we study the cold scientific data, one eye on our peers, on the literature, on the clock; the other turned inward, focusing on our own deeper insecurities. The patient suffers by our distraction, feels more alone, is made more anxious by our 'absence' . . .

There has developed a coercive and irrelevant pattern of health care . . . The physician is becoming the victim of technology, and the instrument of the health industry. Technique is self-destructive. Technique in medicine at best is a mere attenuation of death. Tomorrow, it will be worse.

JUDGE: *(after pause)*: And your final quotation, Mr Hunter?
HUNTER: Again and for the same reasons I should like it to be projected, judge. It comes from an article in the *New England Journal of Medicine* of August 17, 1972 by a Dr Chad H. Calland.[75] He was writing, not on the basis of his own experience alone but on that of some 40 or 50 fellow patients. The 'nephrologist' to whom he refers means 'kindney specialist'. *The quotation is projected.*

The physician is more often a voyeur than a partaker in human suffering. I am a physician who has undergone chronic renal failure, dialysis, and multiple transplants. As a physician-partaker, I am distressed by the controversial dialogue that separates the nephrologist from the transplant surgeon, so that, in the end, it is the patient who is given short shrift. I have observed that both nephrologist and transplant surgeon work alone in their own separate fields, and that the patient becomes lost in a morass of professional role playing and physician self-justification . . . If the nephrologist could only know what goes on within his patients' lives, which he cannot, he would pay more attention to the quality of life and less attention to the quantity of life and to the disparities of the blood-brain barrier . . . the nephrologist has devoted his attention to his patients' biochemical findings rather than to his patients . . . The transplant surgeon has . . . accumulated data on graft survival and patient survival; when reporting his statistics, he does not mention his patients' fractures, infections, bleeding, and other problems . . . To many patients, the point that is most important is the quality of life, whether by hemodialysis or by transplantation. There are some data that cannot be quantified in years, dollars, kilograms or any other numbers, but are gathered in the often intangible experience of life . . . The primary reasons, I hope, that we became physicians were to love and help our fellow man. But the polemic that exists among physicians 'doing their own thing' does not help anyone . . . I have seen both sides of the fence, and I want to make proper commentary before more patients suffer.

JUDGE: (*after a pause*): You wish to comment, professor? (*Weskoff shakes her head*)
HUNTER: I think it should be said, judge, that Dr Calland died just three days after that article appeared.
JUDGE: I apologize, professor. Do forgive me . . . Mr Hunter? (*Pause*) Thank you, Professor Weskoff, for having endured a very long day of most arduous questioning with courage and understanding. This court is now adjourned.

REFERENCES—SESSION TEN

1. British Transplantation Society, *BMJ*, February 1, 1975, p. 251.
2. Mant, A. K., *BMJ*, August 3, 1974, p. 334.
3. Somers, A. R., *NEJM*, April 8, 1976, p. 811.
4. Brook, R. H., and Appel, F. A., *NEJM*, June 21, 1973, p. 1323.
5. McNeil, B. J., *et al.*, *NEJM*, July 31, 1975, p. 216.
6. McNeil, B. J., and Adelstein, S. J., *NEJM*, July 31, 1975, p. 221.
7. Harthorne, J. W., and Castleman, B., *NEJM*, June 14, 1973, p. 1290.
8. Harthorne, J. W., *NEJM*, August 30, 1973, p. 484.
9. Blacher, R. S., *JAMA*, October 16, 1972, p. 305.
10. Baxter, S., *British Journal of Hospital Medicine*, June 1974, p. 875.
11. Hiatt, H. H., *NEJM*, July 31, 1975, p. 235.
12. Aring, C. D., *Journal of the American Medical Association*, June 10, 1974, vol. 228, p. 1393. (Copyright 1974–5, American Medical Association)
13. Bloom, B. S., and Peterson, O. L., *NEJM*, January 11, 1973, p. 72.

14. Editorial, *JAMA*, April 20, 1970, p. 471.
15. Medical News, *JAMA*, October 3, 1977, p. 1441.
16. Milunsky, A., and Alpert, E., *NEJM*, July 15, 1976, p. 168.
17. Laurence, K. M., *Lancet*, February 23, 1974, p. 301.
18. Editorial, *Lancet*, June 25, 1977, p. 1345.
19. Harris, R., Jennison, R. F., and Barson, A. J., *BMJ* April 5, 1975, p. 34.
20. Leading Article, *BMJ*, June 4, 1977, p. 1430.
21. Duff, R. S., and Campbell, A. G. M., *NEJM*, October 25, 1973, p. 890.
22. Slater, E., *BMJ*, December 18, 1971, p. 734.
23. Eisenberg, L., *Science*, April 14, 1972, vol. 176, p. 123. (Copyright 1972, American Association for the Advancement of Science)
24. Editorial, *Archives of Diseases in Childhood*, September 1973, p. 751.
25. Beecher, H. K., *NEJM*, June 16, 1966, p. 1354.
26. Pappworth, M. H., *Human Guinea Pigs*, Routledge and Kegan Paul, London, 1967.
27. Supervision of the Ethics of Clinical Investigations in Institutions, Report of the Committee appointed by the Royal College of Physicians of London, *BMJ*, August 12, 1967, p. 429.
28. Levine, R. J., *JAMA*, April 21, 1975, p. 259.
29. Romano, J., *Archibes of General Psychiatry*, January 1974, p. 129.
30. Editorial, *JAMA*, January 19, 1976, p. 286.
31. Editorial, *NEJM*, January 6, 1977, p. 44.
32. Mufson, M., *NEJM*, July 7, 1977, p. 63.
33. Leading Article, *BMJ*, June 3, 1972, p. 550.
34. Supervision of the Ethics of Clinical Research Investigations and Fetal Research, Department of Health and Social Security, London, June 1975.
35. Supervision of the Ethics of Clinical Research Investigations in Institutions, Committee on the Supervision of the Ethics of Clinical Research Investigations in Institutions, The Royal College of Physicians, London, July 1973.
36. Medical Research Council, Report for the Year 1962–3, HMSO, London, p. 21.
37. Spiro, H. M., *NEJM*, November 27, 1975, p. 1134.
38. Fletcher, J., *NEJM*, September 30, 1971, p. 776.
39. Editorial, *NEJM*, August 31, 1972, p. 465.
40. Bach-Y-Rita, G., *JAMA*, July 1, 1974, p. 45.
41. Medical News, *JAMA*, February 2, 1976, p. 461.
42. Lasagna, L., *JAMA*, September 23, 1974, p. 1720.
43. Hatfield, F., *JAMA*, September 23, 1974, p. 1720.
44. News and Comment, *Science*, February 7, 1964, p. 551.
45. News and Comment, *Science*, February 11, 1966, p. 663.
46. Curran, W. J., *NEJM*, October 4, 1973, p. 730.
47. Medical News, *JAMA*, January 20, 1975, p. 233.
48. Curran, W. J., *NEJM*, July 4, 1974, p. 25.
49. Medical News, *JAMA*, May 15, 1972, p. 908.
50. Editorial, *NEJM*, April 12, 1973, p. 790.
51. Krugman, S., *Lancet*, May 8, 1971, p. 966.
52. Giles, J. P., *Lancet*, May 29, 1971, p. 1126.
53. Shapiro, S., *Lancet*, May 8, 1971, p. 967.
54. Pappworth, M. H., *Lancet*, June 5, 1971, p. 1181.
55. Willey, E. N., *Lancet*, May 22, 1971, p. 1078.
56. Pasamanick, B., *Lancet*, May 22, 1971, p. 1078.

57. Porter, A., *BMJ*, January 6, 1973, p. 46.
58. Medical News, *JAMA*, January 7, 1974, p. 13.
59. Curran, W. J., and Beecher, H. K., *JAMA*, October 6, 1969, p. 77.
60. World Medical Association Draft Code of Ethics on Human Experimentation, *BMJ*, October 27, 1962, p. 1119.
61. Editorial, *NEJM*, April 12, 1973, p. 791.
62. World Medical Association Declaration of Helsinki, *World Medical Journal*, September 1964, p. 281.
63. Krugman, S., and Giles, J. F., *JAMA*, May 11, 1970, p. 1019.
64. Goldby, S., *Lancet*, April 10, 1971, p. 749.
65. Nixon, R. K., *NEJM*, June 7, 1973, p. 1247.
66. Callie, A. S., *NEJM*, June 7, 1973, p. 1247.
67. Baumslag, N., and Yodaikes, R. E., *NEJM*, June 7, 1973, p. 1247.
68. Huskins, D. G., *NEJM*, June 7, 1973, p. 1247.
69. Szul, M., *NEJM*, June 7, 1973, p. 1248.
70. Shine, I., Howieson, J., and Griffen, W. O., Jr, *NEJM*, June 7, 1973, p. 1248.
71. Raine, D. N., *BMJ*, May 19, 1973, p. 402.
72. Doll, R., *Proceedings of the Royal Society of Medicine*, August 1973, p. 729.
73. Editorial, *Journal of the American Medical Association*, February 11, 1974, vol. 227, p. 647. (Copyright 1974–5, American Medical Association)
74. Boardman, D. W., *NEJM*, September 5, 1974, p. 497.
75. Calland, C. H., *NEJM*, August 17, 1972, p. 334.

Medical Ethics
Duncan, A. S., Dunstan, G. R., and Welbourn, R. B. (eds.), *Dictionary of Medical Ethics*, Darton, Longman, and Todd, London, 1977.

Patients with High Blood Pressure—Paucity of Positive Results from Special Investigations
Bailey, S. M., Evans, D. W., and Fleming, H. A., *Lancet*, July 12, 1975, p. 57.

Mental Illness in Intensive Care Units
Kiely, W. F., *JAMA*, June 21, 1976, p. 2759.

Ethics in Relation to Grossly Handicapped Children
Shaw, A., *NEJM*, October 25, 1973, p. 885.
Editorial, *NEJM*, October 25, 1973, p. 914.
Venes, J. L., and Huttenlocher, P. R., *NEJM*, February 28, 1974, p. 518. (The first of a series of nine letters in this issue of the journal, all commenting on one or other of the two previous references and reference 21.)
McCormick, R. A., *JAMA*, July 8, 1974, p. 172.
Lachs, J., *NEJM*, April 8, 1976, p. 838. (A defence of the humane putting to death of the non-human hydrocephalic child. In fact, as the next reference was to make clear, what the non-medical author had in mind was the hydranencephalic child. The latter is, indeed, by any ordinary standard, non-human: the hydrocephalic child may be a quite intelligent human being.)
Venes, J. L., *NEJM*, July 8, 1976, p. 115. (The first of five letters, all of which were critical of the case presented in the last reference, though at least two of them were based on the belief that Professor Lachs had indeed meant hydrocephalus, not hydranencephalus.)

Research on Children, Prisoners, etc.
Editorial, *NEJM*, January 18, 1973, p. 158.
Medical News, *JAMA*, March 17, 1975, p. 1123.
Campbell, A. G. M., *BMJ*, August 3, 1974, p. 334.

Spina Bifida—Cost, etc.
Lightowler, C. D. R., *BMJ*, May 15, 1971, p. 385.
Shurtleff, D. B., *et al.*, *NEJM*, November 8, 1974, p. 1005.
Forrest, D. M., *Proceedings of the Royal Society of Medicine*, April 1977, p. 233.
Zachary, R. B., *BMJ*, December 3, 1977, p. 1460.

Doctors and Torture
Sagan, L. A., and Jonsen, A., *NEJM*, June 24, 1976, p. 1427.

THE MEDICAL INSTITUTION

Enter Sir Guy Chumley

HUNTER: *(rising)*: Sir Guy Chumley? You are a consultant physician, a professor of medicine in England, a doctor very much involved in the various decision-making bodies of the British medical profession? *(Sir Guy nods)* You are, in fact, very much at the top of the medical tree, you have an overview of the whole field of medicine in various countries, you are a leading member of the world medical establishment?

SIR GUY: It is hardly for me to say that.

HUNTER: You would prefer someone else to say it for you?

SIR GUY: One learns to be indifferent to what people may say about oneself.

HUNTER: You are President, Sir Guy, of the Society of Physicians in Europe? – This is one element in what has been called the medical institution.

SIR GUY: I am not quite sure what the medical institution is.

HUNTER: It is the organized body of medicine with all its knowledge, beliefs, values, habits, methods, and the material structures that give them expression and enable them to be exercised. There is an international medical institution, and there are also national institutions, which are very like one another. In most western countries the institution has four elements: first, the medical schools and other medical educating bodies; second, the hospitals and other places of clinical and research medical activities; third, bodies such as, in the United Kingdom, the General Medical Council and the British Medical Association – regulatory and protective bodies, that is; and fourth, the miscellaneous fringe elements—medical societies, libraries, insurance bodies, and so on. There is some overlap, of course; but you recognize it now?

SIR GUY: I recognize the elements. I suppose there is a kind of loosely-knit structure.

HUNTER: I put it to you that the medical institution is a tightly-knit body, run mainly by and for doctors, and that in many ways it is not merely unrelated to health, but is now often antagonistic to health in the widest sense; that it is rigid, narrow in its outlook, hierarchical, self-satisfied, self-regulating, self-perpetuating, paternalistic and monopolistic.

SIR GUY: I do wonder that it has survived for so long.

HUNTER: An institution tends to survive if it has a legalized stranglehold on the only thing that could destroy it—in this case the ability of the individual man in society to stand on his own two feet as concerns his health.

SIR GUY: Such as when he has a broken leg, Mr Hunter?

HUNTER: I did not imply there were no occasions when doctors were needed. It is their right to define what is health and what is sickness, and their exclusive right to deal with them in a particular way that I am criticizing. First, then, the educational element. The thirty-odd medical schools in Britain, and then the bodies controlling and serving the interests of the different specialities—the Royal Colleges of Physicians, and of Surgeons, and of Obstetricians and Gynaecologists; and now of Psychiatrists, of Pathologists, of Radiologists, and of General Practitioners, the last four Royal Colleges all established in the past ten years or so. The standard process of establishing these institutional edifices goes like this, does it not, Sir Guy?—First, a small collection of people with an interest in one small field of medicine meet together; then they form a society, and elect one another members or fellows; then they will admit others only if they pass an examination; and finally they get themselves a special building, a coat of arms, royal patronage, a chain of office for the President, and so on and so on.

SIR GUY: That is how most good organizations start and progress.

HUNTER: An almost exactly similar progression, with the exception of the royal patronage, has been described as existing here in the United States, has it not?[1]

SIR GUY: I shouldn't be at all surprised.

HUNTER: Do you know how many specialties there are in the United States?—There are 65;[1] and it could well be 85[1] (or even 105) in another decade. Not self-perpetuating? And 90 percent of American medical graduates try to specialize.[2] Are you aware that it has been said again and again by doctors that this corresponds, not with the needs of the American people, but with the desires of the American doctors? Are you not aware that there are, for example, far too many American heart specialists, both physicians and surgeons,[1] but a gross shortage of family doctors? —Men who will look at the whole person, be friends and counsellors as well as technicians? And that often the training the specialist gets is much too complex in relation to what he will have to do later? Do you know that in 1976 the American government did what many doctors had over the years suggested it should do— passed an act, the Health Professions Educational Assistance Act of 1976 (PL 94–484), designed to increase the number of American doctors practicing family medicine; but that there is evidence that the doctors will manage to circumvent the intention of the act, and still specialize unnecessarily?[3] Specializing is more lucrative. They take up residencies in the family practice fields of internal medicine, pediatrics, and obstetrics and gynecology, but more than half of them have managed, in fact, to get themselves into subspecialties; that has been the case in the recent past, and will doubtless be the case in the future despite the act.[3] Do you want me to give you medical chapter and verse for all I have said?[1,2,3,4]

SIR GUY: No, Mr Hunter. I'm sure, being a lawyer, you've explored all the options. The fact that some doctors agree with you doesn't make you right.

HUNTER: The same preference for specializing has applied to a considerable extent in the United Kingdom, has it not?—Except when the remuneration of family doctors began to rival that of consultants? Tell me, Sir Guy, to start at the very beginning: what kind of students do the British medical schools admit today?—Most of them?

SIR GUY: A certain ability at science and maths helps.

HUNTER: It is essential in nearly all the schools, is it not?—Just as in the USA, and to the exclusion of any wider learning? And until relatively recently there used to be a strong bias, not so much to the entrant who was good at science, as to the young man rather than the young woman, to the products of what we British call our public—that is, our private, select, fee-paying—schools, and to those who could play rugby football, was there not? By that method of selection—which, I am told, still holds true unofficially to some extent—the medical institution made certain that doctors would on the whole stay middleclass, conformist, and male. Yes?

SIR GUY: You said something of the kind to Dr Batt and Dr Jaeger.

HUNTER: Because it is crucial. Something similar prevails here in the United States too, does it not?—Except that here until recently there has been an extra bias in favour of the white Anglo-Saxon rather than the black student, who is educationally disadvantaged before he even reaches medical school?

SIR GUY: We live in a very imperfect world, Mr Hunter. Even the Americans do. You will find bias, injustice, inadequacies in any trade or profession if you look carefully enough, and in any country. Medicine is no worse than any other profession; and I think there has been much done to put things right recently.

HUNTER: Plastic surgery? The students in most medical schools still have a very traditional education, do they not? Most of the training is centred in hospitals rather than in the community, although it is in the community that patients live and get their diseases, and to it that they have to return; and it is in the community that family medicine has to be practiced, not hospitals? A few students rebel; but most of them, their selection having ensured that they are conformists, allow themselves to be spoon-fed, do they not? Those who do really well as doctors in the truest sense do so despite their training, not because of it? (*Pause*) Everything I have said, Sir Guy, has been said by a doctor, usually by a number of doctors; a small number alas! And the result of the process is medical men who are quite good if a grave emergency is involved, or an episode of an acute illness, especially if it is uncommon and physical, but not good at all at dealing with people on a continuing, comprehensive basis?—As persons, that is, and with the great majority of illnesses and worries that afflict mankind.

SIR GUY: I do wonder that people go to doctors so often.

HUNTER: Is it surprising when the medical institution has a legalized monopoly of various aspects of healing? And are you really unaware of how often people go to unorthodox healers?—And that they go because they are dissatisfied with what doctors have done for them? No wonder: in teaching hospitals, such as yours, it is rare conditions that you prefer, and research, and the teaching of the latest advances, is it not? And even in the ordinary hospitals, where common conditions are seen more often, there is the same preference for treating disease at a late stage or injuries when they have occurred rather than preventing the occurrence of either. Is that not true?

SIR GUY: My dear Mr Hunter, prevention is not the job of hospital doctors.

HUNTER: Who says it is not?—Who split medicine, like the patient, into compartments?—Doctors did. And by favoring the activities that go on in hospitals you take the available money away from those few doctors who are going all out for prevention of common conditions. And attacking symptoms is not all that you do in hospitals, is it? Aside from the fact that you neglect the *person* who has the symptoms, you attack things you've found wrong in the patient's blood or urine, or in a tracing of the electrical activity of his heart or brain. Is that not so?

SIR GUY: Most abnormalities should be treated, I believe – with the patient's consent, of course, and with due regard for his dignity.

HUNTER: His dignity? Is that why you put all hospital patients to bed? – Out of regard for their dignity, and irrespective of whether or not they can walk around perfectly well? And is that why hospital patients are woken at an unearthly hour, and prodded by students, and never told why or when or how things are to be done to them, and generally treated like children? – And why in the United States there are now patient advocates and consumer advocates, so-called, whose job it is to explain to the patient what is being done, and why, and to communicate the patient's worries and complaints to the doctors?

SIR GUY: That sounds a very interesting and useful development, especially in hospitals.

HUNTER: Because they are largely run by the doctors and for the doctors? – The very temples of high-technology medicine, where its rituals are celebrated by the high priests – the consultants, that is – assisted in Britain by a hierarchical string of students, housemen, registrars, and senior registrars?

SIR GUY: And nurses too. Don't forget the nurses.

HUNTER: One would find it difficult: between 1949 and 1973, when the population of England and Wales increased by about 12 percent, the number of nurses in hospitals increased by rather more than 100 percent, and so did the number of doctors; and professional and technical staff increased by over 150 percent[5] – the biochemists, and physiotherapists, and occupational therapists, and dietitians, and radiographers. And then there are the secretaries, and record clerks, and administrators, and finance officers. They all, one way or another, figure in the medical retinue, do they not?

SIR GUY: I must say I haven't noticed many administrators in the retinue that comes on my ward rounds.

HUNTER: Nor, I daresay, do you find many of the higher-grade nurses. Why not? – Because in the United Kingdom after years of subservience both categories have at last taken a leaf out of your medical book, and established their own complicated institutional hierarchies. And much to your annoyance this has proved – because it is now less easy for you to control the top people in them.

SIR GUY: Oh, well, medicine happens in wards and operating theaters, you know, not in administrative offices.

HUNTER: And should it not mainly be happening in life rather than in either of those types of location? And have not you and the administrators and the nurses and everyone else involved in the hospital business got a vested interest in seeing that such places *do* remain the scenes for the action? – Quite aside from the occasions when they are appropriate? (*Pause*) Now – the third element in the medical institution: in the United Kingdom the General Medical Council, which, by its monopolistic control of the licensing – or registration, as it is called there – of health practitioners ('only doctors need apply'), and its supervision of medical education and medical ethics, reinforces the self-regulating, self-perpetuating element.

SIR GUY: But, my dear Mr Hunter, the General Medical Council is a statutory body, set up under the aegis of government.

HUNTER: Run by doctors, and largely run for doctors. I suggest to you that only someone who believed strongly in paternalism would think that government backing somehow guaranteed the Council's relevance to the health of the people, and its effectiveness. It has always taken a punitive moralistic line with doctors who went to bed with their patients, has it not? But in the 1960s, when much more damage was being done by doctors' overprescribing of amphetamines and barbiturates, it did very little. Nor for years did it face up to the problem posed by the immigration of large numbers of foreign medical graduates.

SIR GUY: You forget the Merrison Report of 1975, which recommended certain changes in the General Medical Council and its functions.

HUNTER: I have it here, [6] and I now quote from its recommendations concerning the Council's future composition: '. . . evidently a lay regulating body would labour under a substantial disadvantage. It is the essence of a professional skill that it deals with matters unfamiliar to the layman, and it follows that only those in the profession are in a position to judge many of the matters of standards of professional competence and conduct which will be involved. We are in no doubt that the community will indeed be best served by a professional regulating body.' In other words, its composition should stay much the same as that of the already existing Council – because of whose failings the Merrison Committee was convened.

JUDGE: Perhaps this court should at once disband itself. I am surprised that the lay members of the Merrison Committee did not see fit to resign *en bloc*, having put their names to that statement. They would appear to have indicated that the laity is incompetent to deal with everyday medical matters. Why then, when on the Merrison Committee, should lay people be thought to be competent to deal with very large matters of principle involving medicine? – The greater surely subsumes the less.

SIR GUY: The committee, judge, recommended various changes in the functions of the Council.

HUNTER: But the changed functions are to be carried out by the same kind of people who had failed the public previously? – The number of lay members of the Council is to be increased from three to ten; but against them, the Committee suggested, those ten will find arrayed 88 medical members (instead of the previous

43). How many of those 88 did the Merrison Committee specify should be young?

SIR GUY: You have me at a disadvantage.

HUNTER: Eight – eight out of 88, one in 11. And why should the profession not be subject to lay control, at least in large part? Who are the patients? Who supplies the money for health care? Whose health, whose sickness, whose lives are at stake when the doctors are practicing their skills or concealing their lack of them?

SIR GUY: The Merrison Committee was made up of intelligent, well-informed, experienced people, and had a lay majority.

HUNTER: Of one. And are doctors not so adept at mystification that they can brainwash even the most capable of lay people into meekly accepting that only doctors can possibly understand what doctors do? – Self-satisfied, self-perpetuating, self-regulating, Sir Guy? (*Pause*) Rigid, narrow? And now what about the British Medical Association?

SIR GUY: The BMA? – A professional organization, publishing learned journals, holding clinical and scientific meetings.

HUNTER: Yes, we have heard about those. A high-class trade union, a political pressure group, a money-negotiating body for doctors, an uptight conservative sphinx with nothing worth being sphinx-like about; hierarchical in structure, elephantine in movement, Byzantine in manoevre, minuscule in innovation.

SIR GUY: Very good, Mr Hunter. Of course, all big professional organizations are like that. The American Medical Association is just the same.

HUNTER: Except that it has been accused of being over-friendly with the Pharmaceutical Manufacturers' Association, has it not? And now the last and fourth element in the medical institution, Sir Guy, is the huge miscellany of societies, associations, unions, clubs, journals, nursing homes, private hospitals, and clinics, insurance organizations, councils – advisory, research, consultative – boards, panels, committees . . . You do not think that the medical institution – which began, reasonably enough, as a loose organization devoted to doing what it could to help people through sickness and even death (if that was inescapable) – that it got bigger and bigger, just as industrial society and other institutions, within it, have, and more and more interested in itself and the scientific approach, and less and less interested in what happened to the people to whom it ministered until what it deprived people of, directly or indirectly, began to outweigh any benefits it brought to them? – And that now it has completely outgrown its usefulness?

SIR GUY: The profession has defects certainly, but its virtues – the benefits it provides – are in my view far greater.

JUDGE: Am I right in thinking from what you said a moment ago, Sir Guy, that you have some specialized knowledge of the American medical scene?

SIR GUY: A very modest acquaintance with it, judge.

JUDGE: Nevertheless, you might just care with Mr Hunter's help to touch on the differences between the British and the American institutions.

SIR GUY: Well, I would say that educationally the United States is quite similar to the United Kingdom. There are specialty boards instead of our Royal Colleges, and so on, though many so-called American specialists are not board-certified at all. Their period of hospital training for specialists tends to be rather less than in our country. There are, of course, relatively far fewer general practitioners than we have – about 55,000 out of a total of some 300,000-odd doctors[7] in practice. In Great Britain we have some 26,000[8] family doctors out of a total of some 70,000 doctors in active practise.

HUNTER: If I may intervene, judge, between 1931 and 1971 the number of family doctors has in the USA dropped from 120,000 to 56,000 – while the population increased from about 120 millions to about 200 millions. Specialists correspondingly increased in number.

SIR GUY: Yes, the American public do seem rather taken with high-technology medicine despite all your strictures, Mr Hunter. And the American family doctor, judge, goes in for more tests and special examinations than his British opposite number, and tends to focus more on finding physical rather than 'nervous' or mental disease. And doctor visits to the home, which we still have, are now almost unknown here in the States.

JUDGE: And American hospitals?

SIR GUY: Oh, our housemen are called interns, and our registrars are called residents, and our consultants are called specialists. And of course, whereas the great majority of our hospitals are in the National Health Service most American hospitals are voluntary though non-profit-making, and a number of them belong to government, local or central, though there is also a substantial number of private, profit-making hospitals.

HUNTER: The doctors having a major say in the running of all types? They sometimes have a financial interest in American hospitals, as thousands of them do in drug stores? No? (*Pause*) And is it not the case that often an American hospital – in which a doctor may have a financial interest – will not admit a patient, no matter what his condition, unless it is satisfied that he will be able to pay the very large costs involved?

SIR GUY: Most Americans are insured against medical costs.

HUNTER: With a bias towards hospital costs – because the hospitals and insurance companies are in league with one another? And people prefer to go into hospital for minor conditions or simple investigations, knowing they would not be reimbursed if they were treated outside?

SIR GUY: I have heard that is sometimes the case. Of course, old people in America are covered financially by the government's Medicare scheme, and the underprivileged are covered by the government's Medicaid scheme.

HUNTER: Which works very unsatisfactorily? You have not heard of doctors working in the same building who on some trumped-up medical pretext or other send Medicaid patients to a succession of their colleagues so that they may all claim for giving different bits of attention to the same patients? Or of the doctor who will quickly walk past 30 or 40 Medicaid patients in a hospital, and then claim for attention given to each and every one?

SIR GUY: You seem remarkably well informed, Mr Hunter. Better than I am.

HUNTER: And is it not the case to your knowledge that there are many millions of Americans who are not poor enough to qualify for Medicaid, but not well enough off to be able to afford insurance premiums; who, if they get a serious illness, may have to run up bills that will take a lifetime to pay off, and who will sometimes wish, if they are to have a serious illness, that it may be a quick and fatal one rather than long-drawn-out – because that would mean financial ruin for their families? Is that news to you, Sir Guy?

SIR GUY: No, but I do hope I am not expected to be the keeper of America's conscience. If I may continue: the third element in the American medical – er – institution consists partly of the American Medical Association, which we have already mentioned. There is no equivalent to our General Medical Council: ethical matters here are mostly dealt with at local level; and instead of our system of registration the Americans have one of licensure, run federally and by the individual states. Fourthly, there are, of course, societies, journals, and the various other elements Mr Hunter mentioned in relation to the United Kingdom.

HUNTER: And there is a very powerful American Hospital Association too? Often to be found acting in harness with the American Medical Association? And there are the American medical insurance bodies? And there is the American Association of Medical Colleges, which you did not mention.

SIR GUY: Yes, it is what its name suggest, a coordinating body as

regards medical education, and often advisory to the government.
HUNTER: It extracts a good deal of money from the government?
(*Pause*) Would you not agree, Sir Guy, that, although doctors in
the United Kingdom are far from averse to money, and that a
great deal of money changes hands in connection with our health
service, the main difference between British and American medicine is the *enormous* central importance money has in the latter? –
for everyone involved?
SIR GUY: I suppose, Mr Hunter, you could say that.
HUNTER: Even in relation to medical research? There is very
great competition for government research money, is there not? –
Even cancer research being involved in it? A 'cure for cancer' was a
political issue in the early 1970s in the United States, was it not?[10]
SIR GUY: I don't study American politics, Mr Hunter.
HUNTER: And not even American medical journals?
JUDGE: The various mentioned differences aside, Sir Guy, would
you say that otherwise British and American medicine face the
same problems?
SIR GUY: Yes, broadly speaking, judge. Of course, we have a
national health service: the Americans have a very hybrid system,
although they seem to be moving gradually towards some form of
universal health insurance.
HUNTER: To which a lot of American doctors are violently opposed.
(*Sir Guy nods*) Ostensibly because they say they would be swamped
by a sudden upsurge for medical care – although the evidence
from Britain and from Quebec[11] and elsewhere is that, while
there would be some increase in demand, it would *not* be huge?
(*Sir Guy nods*) The real reason is that these American doctors do not
want government controlling their right to make as much money
as they can out of sickness, or any extra power to check the quality
of the care they are giving?
SIR GUY: Neither motive would be utterly dishonourable, though
I am less sure of their existence than you are, Mr Hunter.
HUNTER: The second reason for their antipathy would doubtless
vanish if the American doctors were convinced their money-
making powers would not be at all restricted or might even by
increased, by the further entry of government into the health
arena? (*Pause*) Now, Sir Guy, the number of doctors in a country
affects the size and power of the medical institution? (*Sir Guy
nods*)
JUDGE: Are you suggesting, Mr Hunter, that an increase in
numbers increases or lessens the power?
HUNTER: There is strong evidence, judge, against the operation of
normal market forces: if there are more doctors, they simply

provide new, extra items of service, especially if there is some kind of health insurance, and the cost per item goes up. The cost of providing health services depends on the number of doctors more than on any other single factor. Our Canadian cousins have learnt this lesson.[12]

JUDGE: You mean the doctors look for a new organ to remove, or a new test to perform, or a new drug to prescribe?

HUNTER: Yes, judge, you have described the position correctly. Now, Sir Guy, the size of the medical institution. You are aware that the number of doctors per 100,000 of the American population went up from 119 in 1950 to 152 in 1971?[9] That the number of medical students in the United States increased by about 50 percent between 1968 and 1974?[7] That while the population has been increasing by 1 percent a year the number of doctors has been increasing by 3 percent? (*Sir Guy nods*) And was not the main – perhaps the only – beneficiary the medical institution? Is this not a perfect instance of its self-perpetuating character? (*Pause*) Do you know that the Americans are expecting to have in the 1980s a total of well over 400,000 doctors as compared with some 300,000-odd in the mid-1970s? And do you know what the increase in junior hospital staff was in Great Britain between 1966 and 1974? (*Pause*) There was an increase from 13,000 to 19,000.[8] Do you know that in the late 1960s the Todd Commission on Medical Education recommended that the number of doctors in Britain, after discounting any population increase, should rise by 1.5–2 percent a year? – the corresponding rate of increase between 1911 and 1961 having been 1.25 percent a year. To keep up a growth rate of even 1.3 percent a year the number of doctors in Britain would probably have to increase from 78,000 in 1975 to 120,000 in 1995? You look incredulous, Sir Guy: I am quoting from a paper in the Proceedings of the Royal Society of Medicine for August 1975.[13] It indicated that, according to the Todd Commission, the output of UK medical graduates should increase from a figure of 2350 in the early 1970s to 4500 in the early 1990s – almost a doubling in 20 years. One last point: it indicated that in 1966 the Commission reckoned there would be a shortage of 10,000 doctors in the UK in 1976. Was there, Sir Guy? Was it not, in fact, being prophesied in 1976 – by doctors – that unemployment was looming up for the profession?[14] And might the shortage figure suggested not equally have been 5000 or 15,000? – Because, as we have already heard there is no correlation after a certain point between the density of doctors and the health of the people they serve. This enormous growth is related to the needs of the medical institution, not of the people – is it not, Sir Guy?

SIR GUY : If I may say a few words, judge, on this complex question of medical manpower, of how many doctors we need now, or shall need in five or ten or twenty years time. It is almost impossible to answer, there are so many factors involved. First, there is the population of the United Kingdom: will it increase or decrease? How many foreign graduates will enter the country? How many will leave, and how soon? How many of our own doctors will emigrate – to North America, to the old Commonwealth countries, to Europe? How many woman doctors shall we have? And how many babies will they have? Is there going to be an increase in the number of consultant posts, or of training posts in hospitals? – In other words, is the National Health Service going to expand? Will the state of the country's economy permit an expansion? Are we going to use paramedical personnel to do some of the work traditionally done by doctors? Are we going to have a flood of technical advances that will call for a lot more doctors, or perhaps allow us to manage with a lot less? These matters have been debated again and again, always with different answers. They have been debated recently,[15, 16, 17, 18, 19, 20] and there are usually as many different answers as there are doctors in the debate. Some say we need many more doctors, some say we need many fewer. There is no unanimity, no infallible prophet, and certainly no sinister intent to increase the number of doctors at all costs.

JUDGE: Thank you, Sir Guy; but we must concern ourselves with facts, not with debates. Mr Hunter, is this increase in the numbers of doctors a universal phenomenon in western countries?

HUNTER: The Maxwell book, to which Professor Larkin referred, indicates a similar situation in all the Scandinavian countries, in the Netherlands, Belgium, Luxembourg, France, Italy, Spain, Portugal, West Germany, Austria, Russia . . .[21] The medical institution, wedded to high-technology, is growing almost everywhere, but is nowhere productive of more health *pari passu* with its own growth.

JUDGE: Is any country trying to reverse the trend?

HUNTER: Yes, judge – Canada is taking steps to counter all the undesirable tendencies that have been mentioned here today: by some restriction on immigration, by controlling the numbers of students entering medical schools and the types of doctor they produce; by financial inducements to doctors to work in under-doctored areas and by limiting the numbers who can work in over-doctored areas – in particular, by active encouragement of the budding family doctor.[22] The whole matter is being debated there; but then as far back as 1971 they already had about 150 doctors for every 100,000 people.[21]

JUDGE: As compared with how many in the United Kingdom, say?

HUNTER: About 130 for every 100,000 people in the same year.[21]

JUDGE: Why have the Canadians chosen to go against the general trend?

HUNTER: Because they believe the health of the people can be better served, judge, in other ways.

JUDGE: As Professor Larkin indicated to us? Tell me, Sir Guy, in what ways are all these extra doctors purportedly employed in most western countries, leaving aside the mere creation of work?

SIR GUY: New technical advances, judge, absorb the activities of some of them. And, of course, there is the research that leads to the advances. But the main reason is the ever-increasing demand of the laity for more and more health..

HUNTER: The ever-increasing dependency upon doctors, Sir Guy, which is not necessarily synonymous with the receipt of health.

SIR GUY: I do not know what else it would be synonymous with.

HUNTER: Then I shall mention three things: unnecessary interventions, operations, procedures; the receipt of a prescription for a tranquilizer; the receipt of an account.

SIR GUY: My dear Mr Hunter, I really do think you are paranoidal about the profession and its activities.

HUNTER: Then I am in good company – good medical company. I have here the issue of the *Lancet* for April 3, 1976. That one issue, taken almost at random, contains at least three items – two articles and one letter – all from doctors, that support my thesis in the strongest possible terms. An article[23] on page 737 stated: 'Doctors have missed the opportunity to consider fundamental social, philosophical, and thus political matters hardly less important to our work than the scientific and technological research we so greatly value . . . Almost every patient who arrives in hospital after a head injury will have his skull X-rayed . . . Yet those films rarely influence subsequent treatment.' They are taken, the doctor indicated, just in case there might be a malpractice case. On page 736 another doctor[24] said, 'It is general practitioners and not patients who use hospitals. If this is true for new outpatient attendances, follow-up appointments must be created by hospital staff . . . In 1973 there were 46,674,000 attendances' – at hospital out-patient and accident and emergency departments in England – 'for a total population of 46,425,000. These numbers are staggering . . . Reform of several aspects of clinical care is now essential as well as desirable.' And third, in a letter[25] on page 740 appeared this: 'It might be found that the endless hours spent by patients and doctors in out-patient clinics are often wasted, that many of the consultations are totally unnecessary or could be done more

economically by a member of the primary health-care team . . .
The rationale for many standard procedures is ill founded. The
drugs that are prescribed both in hospital and general practice are
often not taken or are given for conditions which would do equally
well or better without. Much of the work done by general practitioners would be done better by ancillary workers. Many of the
screening programmes set up for well babies, schoolchildren, and
healthy adults have been inadequately researched.' Well, Sir
Guy? – There are three of your own professional colleagues,
writing independently of one another in a *single* issue of *one*
journal. Is this not a picture of an institution grown to monstrous
and ridiculous proportions, unproductive – in fact, positively
counter-productive because the money involved could be better
spent elsewhere?

SIR GUY: You will be alleging next, Mr Hunter, that doctors
control the whole of people's lives.

HUNTER: Well, they do already control the fields of conception,
contraception, and sterility, do they not? They supervise the
progress of pregnancy. They induce labor, and watch its progress,
and interfere if they have a mind to. They tell mothers how to feed
their babies. They run post-natal clinics and well-baby clinics and
clinics for pre-school children – and, of course, they keep an eye
on schoolchildren. They manage the lives of old people, calling it
geriatrics. They manage women at the change of life. They manage
health at work. They say who is mad and who is criminal. They tell
governments to vaccinate a nation – against influenza, say – and
the government does what it is told. They certify you as fit for
work or not fit for work, fit for military service or not fit. They
pontificate on a hundred topics, and people often think they are
infallible – and they often think so themselves. The medical
institution does already play a major role in the total running of
society – does it not, Sir Guy?

SIR GUY: We play some part, as responsible citizens. Medicine is a
learned profession.

HUNTER: Not an esoteric religion? – Whose highest priests never
even see a patient? – That has various other institutions – nursing,
administrative, that of the media, that of the drug and the medical
instrument industries – working alongside it to a great extent? –
Despite internecine disagreements now and again? That is
nearly always in unspoken collusion with government, that
responds to the symptoms of a healthy aversion to life in a factory
or mine by calling them sickness and prescribing a tablet (thus
preventing any movement for social change), that decides if we are
fit to be allowed to be born, and if so when we shall be born; and

when we shall die, and what shall be written on our death certificates: 'cancer', say, instead of 'profit to the cigarette manufacturer'; 'diabetes', say, instead of 'obesity from eating too much sugar and chocolate'; or 'coronary heart disease', say, instead of 'cigarettes, and cars, and too much fatty food, and too little roughage, and the stress of life in an industrial society'? That is the medical institution – is it not, Sir Guy? A church, a religion, a way of life and a way of death.

SIR GUY: Your eloquence, Mr Hunter, is flawless, but not your reasoning.

HUNTER: I am truly sorry you should think me concerned with words, and not with the human condition. (*Pause*) No further questions. (*Sits*)

JUDGE: Sir Guy, you wish to add anything?

SIR GUY: Thank you, judge. There is nothing sinister in what Mr Hunter has described as the medical institution. Very similar to it in western countries are your own legal profession, the educational profession, and the higher civil service, for example. None of these constitutes a conspiracy against the public. As to its being self-satisfied and so on: if the medical profession did not have a reasonable confidence in itself, it might not be very successful with patients. Self-regulating? – Well, surely it is better that a profession, whose prime responsibility is to its clients or patients, should regulate itself than that it should be regulated by government. Self-perpetuating? – If a profession does not hand on its knowledge, its wisdom, its traditions – through its educational system – then who will provide people with the service it offers? – The answer, of course in the case of medicine is a host of quacks and charlatans who already trade upon the gullibility of ordinary people, often very cruelly on the gullibility of people for whom no doctor – no person – in the world can do any good because they suffer from what is an incurable illness: multiple sclerosis, for instance, or a paralysis due to a stroke, or a cancer (though some cancers *are* curable – by doctors). Often, of course, the disease is not just incurable, it is going to kill the patient. *That* is why medicine needs a monopoly, at any rate of many aspects of the healing art – those in which life and death may be involved.

As to our being rigid: the court has already been told, I think, of the enormous technical changes there have been in the practice of medicine in the last few decades, and how it is becoming more and more specialized. Careful and cautious – but not rigid. As for the corresponding shortage of family doctors in some countries, and their maldistribution, and the migration of doctors from underdeveloped countries mentioned in other sessions – it is doctors themselves who have been most active in drawing attention to these matters, and very often in propounding solutions. Hierarchical? – Yes, I admit that unashamedly. But as to the increase, real or proposed, in the numbers of doctors, this surely indicates that the public *wants* more doctors. The same applies to what Mr Hunter described as our paternalistic attitude: the public wants it, the public wants to be reassured, encouraged, guided, even told what to do. I would describe Mr Hunter's medical institution as the figment of his imagination, and his attack on my profession as nothing more than an emotional tirade.

JUDGE: Thank you, Sir Guy. I have some questions myself. As regards the competence of lay people to form judgments on clinical matters: you are aware that in 1977 a select committee of the British House of Commons recommended that, where there was a complaint, such matters could properly be considered by the Health Service Commissioner – or Ombudsman, as he is known?[26] You do not wish to comment? Second, it has been calculated that in the United States the money spent on health care will increase from $130,000,000,000 in 1976 to twice that amount in 1981.[27]

SIR GUY: That is certainly a massive amount.

JUDGE: The original or the increase, or both? (*Pause*) And you have not denied that in the west generally the numbers of doctors have been increasing, that there is maldistribution of them, and increasing specialization, but no increase in health. (*Pause*) You are an intelligent and honest man, Sir Guy. But so is Mr Hunter. And – I do hope he will not mind me saying this – his questioning of you was very astringent; far more astringent than his questioning of any other witness we have seen. Would you entertain the possibility that, being inside the medical institution, indeed in a very high position within it, you fail to notice many of the faults it may have, you unconsciously have a bias to the maintenance of the *status quo*? – Mr Hunter, however, being a detached observer of it, can see faults; and his astringency merely reflects his frustration, his incredulity when faced with someone he recognizes, whatever he may have said today, to be intelligent and honest but who refuses to acknowledge faults that to himself are as plain as day?

SIR GUY: I am fallible. We are all fallible. I am certainly not immune to the common weaknesses of humanity. You may be right, judge. However, I say in all honesty that the picture of my profession that Mr Hunter has painted is one that I simply do not recognize except in one or two particulars. I always want the truth. If I am blind, I hope that my blindness may be remedied – for if Mr Hunter is right, then my profession is deeply in the wrong.

JUDGE: I am sure Mr Hunter would wish to join me in thanking you for the honesty and humility of that answer, Sir Guy. And the court is now adjourned.

REFERENCES—SESSION ELEVEN

1. Chase, R. A., *NEJM*, February 26, 1976, p. 497.
2. Levit, R. J., Sabshin, M., and Mueller, G. B., *NEJM*, March 7, 1974, p. 545.
3. Wechsler, H. W., Dorsey, J. L., and Bovey, J. D., *NEJM*, January 5, 1978, p. 15.
4. Boardman, D. W., *NEJM*, September 5, 1974, p. 497.
5. Klein, R., *BMJ*, January 3, 1976, p. 25.
6. *Report of the Committee of Inquiry into the Regulation of the Medical Profession*, HMSO, London, 1975.
7. Stimmel, B., *NEJM*, July 10, 1975, p. 68.
8. *Health and Personal Social Services Statistics for England* (with summary tables for Great Britain), Department of Health and Social Security, 1975, p. 30, HMSO, London, 1976.
9. Cooper, J. K., and Heald, K., *JAMA*, March 25, 1974, p. 1410.
10. Greenberg, D. S., *NEJM*, May 27, 1976, p. 1245.
11. Enterline, P. E., *et al.*, *NEJM*, May 27, 1976, p. 1245.
12. Baltzan, M. A., *Canadian Medical Association Journal*, January 6, 1973, p. 101.
13. Ellis, J., *Proceedings of the Royal Society of Medicine*, August 1975, p. 495.
14. *The Times*, March 29, 1976, p. 2.
15. Parkhouse, J., *Proceedings of the Royal Society of Medicine*, November 1976, p. 815.
16. Doran, F. S. A., *BMJ*, November 20, 1976, p. 1272.
17. British Medical Association, Report of Council to the Special Representative Meeting, Submission of Evidence, Royal Commission on the National Health Service, *BMJ*, January 29, 1977, p. 299.
18. Leading Article, *BMJ*, February 19, 1977, p. 465.
19. Hospital Junior Staffs Committee and the West Midlands Regional HJSC, Report of Council to the Special Representative Meeting, Submission of Evidence, Royal Commission on the National Health Service, Proposed Amendment, Present and Projected Numbers of Medical Students and Doctors, *BMJ*, March 5, 1977, p. 659.
20. Shrank, A. B., *The Times*, October 4, 1977, p. 18.
21. Maxwell, R., *Health Care: The Growing Dilemma*, Table 13, McKinsey and Co., Inc., New York, 1975.
22. Evans, J. R., *Health Manpower Problems: The Canadian Experience*, Lecture at the Institute of Medicine, Washington, D.C., May 9, 1976.
23. Norcross, K., *Lancet*, April 3, 1976, p. 737.
24. Loudon, I. S. L., *Lancet*, April 3, 1976, p. 736.
25. Strube, G., *Lancet*, April 3, 1976, p. 740.
26. *The Times*, December 2, 1977, p. 5.
27. Ginzberg, E., *NEJM*, April 7, 1977, p. 814.

Medical Students
Simpson, M. A., *Lancet*, March 9, 1974, p. 399.
Bennet, G., *Lancet*, August 24, 1974, p. 453.

McCormick, J., *Proceedings of the Royal Society of Medicine*, January 1975, p. 16.
Hundley, R. F. and Anthony, L. B., *NEJM*, May 27, 1976, p. 1241.
Cramer, S. F., *NEJM*, May 27, 1976, p. 1242.

The Medical Institution
Members Handbook, British Medical Association, London, 1970.
Evans, B., *World Medicine*, January 28, 1976, p. 17.
Annual Report for 1975, General Medical Council, London, 1976.

Medical Specialization
Calendar—with Section Programmes 1977–8, Royal Society of Medicine, London, 1977.
'Medical Education in the United States 1975–76', *JAMA*, December 27, 1976, p. 2971–92.
Aring, C. D., *JAMA*, April 26, 1976, p. 1849.

American Medicine
Editorial, *JAMA*, December 24–31, 1973, p. 1563.
Petersdorf, R. G., *NEJM*, August 29, 1974, p. 440.
O'Donnell, M., *World Medicine*, January 29, 1975, p. 15.
Ibid., February 26, 1975, p. 15.
Spiro, H. M., *NEJM*, April 10, 1975, p. 792.
Tuck, J. N., *World Medicine*, August 13, 1975, p. 17.
Simpson, M. A., *World Medicine*, November 5, 1975, p. 95.
Marsh, G. N., Wallace, R. B., and Whewell, J., *BMJ*, May 29, 1976, p. 1321.

Numbers of Doctors
'Medical Manpower: III—Policies', *BMJ*, January 17, 1976, p. 134.
News and Notes, *BMJ*, July 17, 1976, p. 185.
Clarke, C. A., *The Times Higher Educational Supplement*, January 21, 1977, p. iii.

A DOCTOR

Enter Dr John Aldam

HUNTER (*rising*): You are Dr John Aldam, a British family doctor, practicing in a rural area in the west of England? And you are how old, doctor?

ALDAM: 73. I've done 50 years in the same practice. Qualified when I was 22.

HUNTER: You have a partner in your practice?

ALDAM: Mmh, five years ago, when the pressure of patients was getting to be a bit too much, I took on a young man straight from hospital. He'd done a year as a medical registrar but he couldn't see any chance of becoming a consultant – he was no good at politics, you know – so he joined me.

HUNTER: It was your age made you take him on?

ALDAM: No, not just that. I'm still fairly fit, thank God! No, it was mainly that my patients were bringing me more and more complaints or troubles. Some other doctors have had the same experience, though quite a few say *their* numbers have started to fall off a bit. Of complaints and troubles I mean, not patients on their lists else the doctors would be up in arms. Out of pocket, you see, then. Their patients are going to hospital direct, I think, or else to some quack. Get as much from a quack as from some doctors, come to that.

HUNTER: And this young partner in the practice has perhaps introduced you to a lot of new ideas and methods?

ALDAM: Well, quite a few technical things, you know, some of which I don't fully understand. Not that I'm sure he always does himself, mind you. But things that really help the patients – no, not really an enormous amount. I may be wrong, of course.

HUNTER: He has made a big difference to your practice?

ALDAM: Some difference. Most of the patients like him. He got out of hospital in time, you see. Only just. He's been able to adapt, he's young enough. A few patients – I think it's only a few, mostly the younger ones – much prefer him to myself, they think he's more scientific, which is true. But he wanted to make all kinds of organizational changes, and I wasn't having any of that.

HUNTER: Such as?

ALDAM: Well – do you know? – he wanted me after 50 years to start appointment systems. This patient at 14.30 hours, the next at 14.40 hours – that kind of thing. Half-past two, I call it, or twenty to three. Anyway, I said I'd always seen patients as soon as I could after they came to my surgery or after I'd heard they were ill at home, and I wasn't going to change at my age. If you have an appointments system, it's more like a business, and half the time it works and half the time it doesn't; so I'm still doing what I've always done: first come, first served. (They know, they space themselves out for arriving.) That's except for emergencies, of course. If you have a nice, tidy appointments system, the emergency patients may take themselves off to hospital. Don't want mine doing that. Anyway, a lot of my patients like sitting around in the waiting room, they have a good natter. Often they do more for one another than I can. Some don't like it, of course; but you can't please everyone. Life wasn't meant to be a bed of roses for everybody. Some get the roses, some get the thorns.

HUNTER: And what else did your new partner want to introduce?

ALDAM: He wanted an automatic telephone-answering system. You know: 'Dr Aldam is off-duty. In case of emergency call Dr Bob's-your-uncle. Otherwise record your message – NOW.' I know what message I'd be recording if I was on the other end. So I said, 'Wait till I'm dead.' He's still waiting. And the same for these deputizing services – strange chaps turning up at 2 o'clock in the morning to see my patients in bed: the patient never clapped eyes on them before. Or they on the patients. No. I do it all myself with the help of this young man. Night calls too: I grumble but I get up. Same with holidays. Always off on holidays, these new chaps. Or else courses to bring themselves up to date. Sometimes both together. They must be as good as everyone else in the rat race: cars, wives, the lot. They're impatient. They can't wait for anything to mature. Today's wonder drug, they've forgotten it tomorrow. And yet they're often lax, I find, in the obvious things. Where was I? – Yes, what's more, he thought, did this young man, that my receptionist, who's been with me 30 years, should start asking patients who'd ring up about a visit from me just what their symptoms were and so on. Made her get out her smelling salts for the first time in years. But I said, 'If they want me to go, then I go; and if it's a wasted journey, then it's a wasted journey, and they get a piece of my mind into the bargain.' *And* to let her deal out repeat prescriptions on request. 'Spreading the work load through the health-care team' they call it: I call it not doing your job. I scotched that one too. I don't believe in simply repeating prescriptions, even when I'm seeing the patients. At first he thought I was a complete old fool. Now he just thinks I'm a bit of an old fool. Oh, I know most family doctors are doing fewer home visits now. We'll soon do none at all, we'll be like the Americans:

sickness forbidden in this home. Not me, I'll be dead. We're like them enough as it is. Not that I've anything against Americans. In small doses. The capitation system's half the trouble in this country: if you get so much, fixed, for every patient and what you want is cash, obviously you don't particularly want to see them. In America the doctors *do* want to see them – but only in their offices. More money for them in that. You know what's been said: 'American patients hate their doctors; British doctors hate their patients'?[1] I hope I don't hate mine, or they me. My young man – yes, he got it all from that teaching hospital he was at, you know. He sent half the patients to hospital at first – till I taught him different. No wonder we're not admired the way we were 50 years ago, even 30-odd years ago, when we could do much less for the patients. Less technical stuff anyway. No wonder they go in for nature cures and macrobiotic diets and other bits of nonsense. Some of them. Not mine, or if they did, they'd take damn good care to do it on the quiet. I'm talking too much.

HUNTER: No, do go on, please.

ALDAM: Well, in hospital they take all your clothes off and put you to bed, doesn't matter how ill or well you feel; then they give you a number and a little locker – no key, mind you, oh no – and then you're on the conveyor belt. 'Where am I going this time, nurse?' – 'I'm not sure, I think it's X-ray, I'll ask staff on the way out.' I know, I've been in a couple of times myself – as a patient, I mean. Otherwise I keep out of those big places as much as I can. I'm in and out of the local cottage hospital, mind you, seeing my patients. Just a little place, 40 beds. They tried to do away with it a few years back, but we soon scotched that one. Then they called it a community hospital, and that seemed to satisfy them. Now they can't have enough community hospitals. It's a *cottage* hospital, I'm in a cottage industry. The hospitals are factories, especially the teaching ones. Mind you, they're very good for *some* things. So are factories for making motor cars. Doesn't mean they're good for anything else, though, does it? Men aren't motor cars. Where do you go for a good suit – to a factory or a tailor's attic?

HUNTER: Do you see any unifying principle or principles to what goes on in the big teaching hospitals?

ALDAM: Principles? – I'm not much good at principles. Except moral ones. Not much good at those sometimes either. Let me think. Well, yes, they talk nowadays – do you know? – about giving the best available treatment to everyone, whatever condition he has. In hospital, of course. Now to my mind that's a lot of sentimental drivel. In this country, in the world, for any one condition there's just one man who's the very best for a particular operation or treatment or type of diagnosis. Any doctor knows that. Then there are a few excellent men, then maybe 20 or 30 very good men, and then, apart from a few incompetents' there's the mass of also-rans–perfectly capable but not in the same class as the number-one man. Technically, that is. But he's got only 24 hours in his day, the same as you and me, so there's a limit to the number of people he can see. That's quite aside from the *cost* of the very best treatment for everyone. You just can't have it, by definition. Good, sensible, competent treatment – that's what you can ask for, yes; but the best for everybody, my foot – it's impossible. Aside from the men, it's not possible to afford the machines they've got today. I mean, afford them for everyone. What else? – Yes, do you know it's often occurred to me that in the teaching hospitals they want to make the patients into machines, to make doctoring into a matter of nuts and bolts, all clean and certain and automatic? And it isn't: it's messy and human, and no one knows all the answers. Certainly not the doctor – he's human too. And they want to hold the patient at arm's length, at a distance. I think in hospitals they're really afraid of the patients as human beings. Some of the young doctors are. Afraid of them dying anyway. That proves the patient's human – 'Look, he's dead.' They'd do anything to stop a patient dying. It's because they think of the patients as machines. I say to them, 'Don't you see? – It'll happen to *you* one day, it's yourself you're treating,' but they can't follow that. When I see patients in these plastic tents, surgical isolators, and so on, all wired up, little tubes going in here, big tubes coming out there; and half a dozen machines round them, and three nurses and two doctors . . . They have legs, that's how you tell them from the machines. Yes, and none of them actually *saying* anything to the patient, or squeezing his hand to give him some hope – oh, no, that wouldn't be sterile, we only touch when we want to put another needle in a vein . . . Where was I? – Well, yes, when I see that I feel they're playing at being God, only they're keeping well away from the patient, which is something God would never do. And if God wants to come and take him, He'll get through all the tubes and wires and plastic, and He'll take him, won't He? I think, after a certain point, you can't have modern hospital medicine, all this controlled-trial stuff and research on patients and sort-of looking at them down a microscope – you can't have all that *and* deal with people as human beings, which means subjectively. Only after a certain point, mind you. If I have an operation, I like a good anesthetic. And I believe in immunizing people – though not against *everything*. We'll be immunizing them against the sneezes next. I'd like an antibiotic if I had a bad chest infection – so long as I wasn't so old and decrepit I was past it. When I'm past it, which perhaps won't be so long, I hope someone'll say, 'Well, he's past it, so let him go quietly.' I don't want to walk through the golden gates with tubes sticking out of every bit of me. I'm making fun, but you know what I mean. I think dignity's often more important than death.

HUNTER: Dr Aldam, you seem to be saying that after a certain point we began to lose more from modern medicine than we gained.

ALDAM: Yes, I believe that.

HUNTER: At what point in time would you say that happened?

ALDAM: I've thought about this, do you know? I feel it was in the early fifties. When I started at medical school there was damn all – I beg your pardon, judge – very little you could do for most patients. I mean in the way of prescribing for them and so on. You could give them sympathy and understanding, which is still the half of it. The bigger half. And you could do quite a lot of operating. And, of course, we had pure drinking water and all that sort of thing. But diabetes, tuberculosis, diphtheria, pneumonia, pernicious anemia – for these you couldn't do anything much. And for another 50 conditions just as bad, though not so common. They were terrible diseases. Well, all that changed during the next 30 years or so. I remember insulin coming in when I was a student in the early 1920s, and liver treatment for pernicious anemia came just as I qualified; and then the sulfa drugs in the thirties, and then penicillin and all the other antibiotics and drugs for TB in the forties; and in the fifties cortisone and the tranquilizers and the first good blood-pressure drugs, and so on. But after that, after about 1955, or so, we seem just to have been mopping up here and there. Mind you, we've learnt to do some marvellous *little* things, and a few big things – like artificial hips, though they're a mixed blessing in my personal view. Well, other people can do them, in hospitals, not me, my hand's not steady enough and I'd hardly know one end of an artificial hip from the other. But there are some really big killers now for which we've got nothing or very little. 50 years ago we had tuberculosis and all the other infections: today we've got lung cancer and coronary thrombosis. I'm supposed to call it ischemic heart disease now, I believe. I dunno, they change the names every few years but the diseases are there just the same. I sometimes think they believe if they give them a new name they'll become clearer or else go away – it's like calling a cottage hospital a community hospital. Makes things tidy. Doesn't make the patients any tidier or better though.

HUNTER: So there was some kind of watershed in treatment in the mid-1950s? (*Aldam nods*) And what other changes have you noticed in medicine?

ALDAM: Yes, there is something else. I suppose it started in the 1950s, maybe the forties. Science, half-baked science very often, but still science, started to come into general practice. It came in quite quickly: 1939 – you know, when the war started – hardly any science; 1950, bags of science. I got bitten myself. We all started testing for this and testing for that, and sending people to hospital just to see if they mightn't have the other. And we started prescribing – for everything. I mean for everything. It was the drug industry, some people say; but the drug industry's just a part of medicine really. It was the drug industry *and* the doctors *and* the patients, especially the patients. They began to think there was a pill for everything. I don't know who taught them, whether it was us or the newspapers or the drug firms, or whether they just worked it out for themselves. I think it was because they'd stopped going to church myself. The scientists destroyed religion, so they had to invent the tablets. No holy communion, no mumbo-jumbo from the vicar, so you got some mumbo-jumbo from the doctors instead – you got a drug.

HUNTER: Forgive me interrupting, doctor. You are aware that substantially more is spent in the UK National Health Service on drugs than on the family doctors who mostly prescribe them?

ALDAM: That doesn't surprise me.

HUNTER: I have here a document of the British Department of Health and Social Security, published in 1976, and entitled, 'Priorities for Health and Personal Social Services in England'.[2] Figure 3 on page 21 reveals that in 1970–71 the general medical services in England – family doctors' services, in other words – plus expenditure on health centers, prevention, and family planning cost £210 millions, and the pharmaceutical services £250 millions. The estimates for 1975–6 were respectively £250 millions and £310 millions; and the projected figures for 1979–80 respectively £290 millions and £380 millions. All rounded-off figures. In other words, the bias towards expenditure on drugs rather than on family doctors was expected to get more marked.

ALDAM: Of course it was. It's the pills they want, not the peddlers. Anyway, as I was saying, the patients started coming along years ago for their little parcels of health, and the paper the parcels were made up with was mostly prescription forms. Nowadays we've got all these plastic bags and wraps, so it's not just tablets, it's syringes and testing kits and contraceptives and needles for this and dressings for that. You know, all done up in little transparent bags. Touch me not: it's like those patients in hospitals in their tents. And wigs, and cosmetics to disguise some scar or other. What's the matter with a good healthy scar? – Not so long ago people used to be proud of their scars, not ashamed of them. They meant you'd been through it.

HUNTER: You said, doctor, that people have begun to think there's a pill for everything. Should you like to expand on that?

ALDAM: I seem to be doing a lot of talking. I apologize, judge.

JUDGE: On the contrary, doctor: I am vastly interested; and what you are saying is highly relevant to our enquiry.

ALDAM: When you get to my age you do one of two things: talk a lot or shut up a lot. I shut up a lot when I'm with patients, they've usually got plenty to say, all they need's an ear; you can sometimes have a sort of wide-awake nap till they're finished; and when I'm not with them I talk a lot. Anyway – yes, when I was young people used to come only when they really were ill or else were very much afraid they might be. Nowadays they come along for anything. Half the time it isn't sickness at all. I feel sorry for them. Not half as sorry as they feel for themselves, mind; though actually they're not so badly off, most of them. No, that's not right: there isn't the poverty there was but there's as much wretchedness as in the old days.

HUNTER: But is all this increased demand not simply the consequence of a free National Health Service, doctor?

ALDAM: Not simply. I used to think so, but I don't any longer – because it's getting worse and worse all the time, and we've had the National Health Service for 30 years now. In my practice it's getting worse anyway. And I'm told it's just as bad in other countries, even where patients have to pay out of their own pockets – those who *can* pay, that is. People have this huge appetite for doctors, for someone to take their decisions for them: they just can't have enough, they think the doctor's God Almighty. So does he sometimes. He's largely to blame for it all, as you told Sir Guy Thingummy. But I mean, most illnesses are small, and they get better anyway, no matter what anyone does for them – they don't need a doctor really. But people come to you with their little illnesses. And if they have a row with the wife, or they've got a complaint about the job, or the tax man's getting on their nerves – off to the doctor and tell him we want a tranquilizer, *and* we can let off some steam too. Mind you, they don't say that's the trouble, not at first. There's a way of doing these things. They say, 'I've got indigestion bad, doctor,' or 'My back's bad,' or 'Headaches,' and five minutes later you discover it's none of these things – it's mother-in-law, or the kids, or the chap above them at the office. In the old days people just got on with it, or else they changed their job or hit hubby with the rolling pin and then had a good cry about it, or they went round to mum, or the padre, or the pub or club, or the next-door neighbour – or the doctor now and again. But nowadays people don't seem to have any endurance or patience or – or guts. And they don't seem to have neighbours. The technologists with their motorways and high-rise buildings and so on destroyed *them*. Or families to rally round. And no rolling pins, they buy pastry ready made: add water and heat, serves six. And of course, they don't go to church. And so they come to the doctors instead.

HUNTER: And then what happens? – What do the doctors do?

ALDAM: Mostly in this country the doctors do one of three things. They perhaps rely on appointment systems, *and* a tough receptionist, *and* a telephone-answering system, and so on – to keep the patients away. They put a fence round themselves, in other words, and then they say, 'Where's the problem?' They're cowards, and they know it deep down; or else they're lazy and after the money. There's another kind sits there, five minutes to every patient, and a prescription to every patient, often three or four items on it, repeat as necessary – which is simply conveyor-belt medicine. 80 patients a day. 80 prescriptions. Ear plugs. *They're* nearly always money-grubbers. A lot of doctors combine those two systems. But it's the third kind that's really the worst, I think: the holier-than-thou brigade. They sit listening and listening, trying to solve every problem for every patient; then they write letters full of righteous indignation to the medical journals saying the Health Service is starved of money or how the clinical iceberg's coming up out of the water. They should try once or twice pushing the damned iceberg down again the way I do.

HUNTER: You mean you have little time for people with personal problems, doctor? I thought you had indicated—

ALDAM: No, I don't mean that. I know they have troubles. I sympathize with them. I have a go at everything from threatened divorce and near-murder to – to grandma's toenail clippings being on the floor. But I mean I have only 24 hours in my day, and I can never do the impossible anyway. My patients understand me by now. I always see them if they're ill, any hour of the day or night; and if it's only me can give a helping hand with some family or work problem, that kind of thing, then I do everything I can. But with a few patients nearly all the time, and with nearly all patients every so often, it's best – best for *them*, best for their problems – to say, 'No: *I* can't help you; go away and deal with it yourself, or let your wife or your boy friend help you to deal with it;' or else, 'Well, why couldn't you just have taken a couple of

aspirins, and gone to bed? – Things'll look different tomorrow.'
Anyway – though naturally I don't tell them this when they're
down – life isn't meant to be a bed of roses, as I think I said. If
you're alive, you suffer, you get aches and pains now and again,
you feel miserable sometimes.

HUNTER: Why do you say that third kind of doctor is the worst?

ALDAM: Because I think they're conceited. They attempt the impossible, they try to make a Garden of Eden for everybody, and
they don't like to admit it's impossible. They want their patients
to think they're God. They think it themselves. Must have a God.
They'll never say, 'No, I can't help you,' or 'No, go and help
yourself', – which I think is what God says, except *He* gives them
grace, not tranquilizers and empathy, so called.

HUNTER: But would the patients not go to unorthodox healers if
the doctor were to say 'No'?

ALDAM: Yes, they would, some of them, and they do. I know they
do. What's so wrong with that? At least these unorthodox people
listen, which is about all the doctor can do most of the time. He
can't perform miracles. I know. We've always had these problems,
only we used to have better ways of dealing with them when
society was healthier. Psychosocial problems, the professors call
them, as though they'd invented the things. I'd sooner go to some
of these unorthodox healers than to a lot of what we have today –
social workers. Paid do-gooders. Very mixed up themselves, quite
a few of them. And others are just well-meaning youngsters. A lot
have no qualifications – except something like a divorce. Some of
those who have a qualification think they're God, like those
doctors. Mind you, they're training them by the thousand now.
Relevant training. We'll see. How do you *train* someone to be
helpful and kind and understanding? – All they need to be taught
is a few addresses and a little elementary psychology and they
should have picked up that for themselves anyway. More important's a big heart in the right place, and a good stiff dose of common
sense. But, I don't know, if *I* want kindness, if *I* want advice, I
don't go to a social worker, a professional kindness-provider – I
go to my wife, or to a friend, or to a priest, or I just sit and think and
sleep on it. As often as not I decide I'd deserved whatever it was
I'd got. People have forgotten all that. I'm old-fashioned. No,
they haven't forgotten, it doesn't exist at all for most people any
longer, more's the pity, poor creatures! But social workers are like
paid keeners at an Irish wake. I prefer the real thing; or else I'll
grin and bear it, thank you.

HUNTER: You don't believe much in professional counsellors,
doctor?

ALDAM: No, I don't. Why, today, if your marriage is going wrong, there are people who claim to be able to teach you, not just how to love and how to make love – that's bad enough – but even how to quarrel with the person you're married to! They use a computer to show you how to have a row with the wife. Damned stupid nonsense! I'd lock the lot of them up for six months and tell them to have a good love-in or row-in or whatever stupid word they've got for their method of conning people – conning them into thinking, if you give up responsibility for your own life, you've gained something. You haven't of course. You've lost something. Something big. Everybody's a bit of a doctor at heart; but today they're afraid to admit it. Only the doctor or the nurse understands these things, they're so complicated. And a bit of a philosopher, or a bit of a stoic; but only the doctor or the social worker can *know* about that side of life. That's what our society, our high-technology medicine, as you call it, tells people.

HUNTER: But what about really serious pain, and really serious depressions? What about death? Has people's attitude to those too been altered by high-technology medicine, by the high-technology society?

ALDAM: Yes, it has. When a patient really is ill, when he's really suffering or in bad pain, or has a melancholia, then naturally I'd do anything I possibly could think of for him. But, first, I can't cure everything, and yet people seem to think I should be able to because I'm a doctor. We've all got to get old, we've all got to die some day. And anguish, suffering, I mean actually experiencing pain and grief and guilt – well, we all have these now and again. The only escape from them is to blot oneself out: perhaps permanently, and that's what a lot of people do – they commit suicide, or more often they make a half-hearted attempt, hoping someone will save them, bring them round, and then get rid of the cause of the suffering for them; or else temporarily with drink or a really powerful tranquilizer or sedative. I'm sorry for these people, I try and help them, of course; but in the end they still have to wake up and themselves help to deal with whatever was causing the suffering. And maybe there is no way, maybe they just have to endure whatever it is. But people shirk their responsibility, they won't face up to life. I can relieve pain nearly always, and soften distress; but I don't think life with pain is jet black and life without pain is pure white, and that my job is always to rub out all the black: the white hasn't got any meaning without a bit of the black, without our at least knowing it exists and *sometimes* has to be borne and sometimes is better borne – if the price of relieving it is not a price we want to pay. Getting better often involves pain or distress.

And that way you learn how to face up to it next time. Being well doesn't always mean having no pain at all – you may just have to learn to live with it. I heal people, I don't work miracles.

JUDGE: Are you really saying, doctor, that life *is* tragic? – That it is robbed of dignity, of grandeur, if we try always, and automatically, to get rid of the terrible elements in it, to pretend it can be all sweetness and light?

ALDAM: Am I? – Yes, I suppose I am. Yes, I'm sure I am. I simply put it in a different way, a medical way.

HUNTER: You are not talking, doctor, about the ennobling effect of pain?

ALDAM: Not at all. It is ennobling – occasionally. But it can be degrading, and it should always be relieved if the patient wants it relieved. *If* he does. I'm talking about real pain now. And I'm saying that pain and suffering are an integral part of life; and our modern medical attitude to them is to deny that, to pretend they are some kind of cancer that must be cut out of life the moment it appears. Never a part of being fully human. The same thing applies to death.

HUNTER: Yes, go on, doctor.

ALDAM: Well, life is meaningless, I feel, without death at the end of it. No one healthy wants to die. But an eternity of *this* life would be intolerable, unthinkable. And yet a lot of doctors today, especially younger, scientifically-minded doctors – I'm repeating myself again, it's my age – they look upon death, just as they look upon pain and anguish, as an enemy to be vanquished at all costs. *I* won't struggle with death to the bitter end; I do all I reasonably can, but I want it to be a person who dies, not a machine, when I'm looking after a patient. I think death's . . . death's a sort of cousin who lives with us whether we like it or not – sometimes to be put in the spare bedroom and forgotten about, sometimes to be greeted as one among a lot of cousins, sometimes to be . . . well, embraced; and always to be learned from. I must sound very flowery. It is difficult to express what I mean; but it is what my life as a doctor has taught me. In 50 years I have seen many people born, and grow up, and marry, and have children, and die. I've brought them in, and I've seen them out.

JUDGE: Go on, doctor.

ALDAM: This new attitude to pain and death and suffering is a product, I think, of scientific medicine, and most lay people have caught it from their doctors: 'Stop the pain – now, at once.' No alternative's considered. 'Don't let me suffer – ever.' 'Conquer death,' – and one can't. How can I put it? – Yes, when, as a child, one first tastes garlic one spits out the food containing it, one pulls a face, one simply cannot understand how anyone could ever want to use garlic. But an adult will use garlic in some dishes because they'd be incomplete without it. Not in all dishes, not always in large amounts, but it is an essential element in any well-stocked kitchen. I think the attitude of most doctors and lay people to pain and suffering today is like that of children towards garlic: it's childish. And then death – yes, death is like a good brandy. A child who sips brandy will spit it out, and complain that it burns his throat, and tastes horrid, and that he never wants even to smell it again. But an adult will take a sip of it, and another sip, and gain something from it – before finally draining the glass. So it should be with death. (*Pause*) Anyway, that is how I see it. Not so very long ago one's family and one's priest and one's neighbors – and yes, one's very own doctor – would help one to endure pain and anguish and death healthily: because there is a healthy way to deal with them. They aren't unhealthy. They're not 'out there': they're 'in here'. But now all we have is an impersonal doctor behind a mask who must kill the pain, blot out the anguish, and – this is the most absurd thing of all – he must kill death. I sit and hold my patient's hand when he is dying. There are three of us. One's God. (*Pause*) I'm sorry, judge, for rambling on and on.

HUNTER: You will recall, judge, when I was questioning Professor Weskoff, I indicated that high-technology medicine was now more productive of ill-health than of health, partly because it seemed powerless to deal with most of the diseases produced by high-technology affluence, but also because of certain negative effects it had, which I would detail later.

JUDGE: And you are about to say that Dr Aldam has detailed those negative effects for you?

HUNTER: Yes. It is my case that our newly developed attitudes to illness of any degree, pain, suffering, anguish, and death far outweigh any fresh gains high-technology medicine is now bringing us. Its big gains were all made 20 or 30 or more years ago. At some time in the last two or three decades we should have called a halt; or perhaps we should have done even better if high-technology medicine and all that led up to it had never got under way at all.

JUDGE: That last suggestion is to go a long way back, or a lot deeper even than today's evidence has gone.

HUNTER: In the two concluding sessions of this enquiry that is what will, I hope, be done. Thank you, Dr Aldam. (*Sits*)

JUDGE: Doctor, you are saying of suffering and pain and death that it is the patient who must deal with them. They are his responsibility. Accepting that makes him a true human being, a real person?

ALDAM: Yes, I'm just the patient's servant, his medical daily help.

JUDGE: But to turn the coin over: life in the country has its compensations?

ALDAM: Yes, of course, that is why I am in it. There is the windhover, the lark, the oak tree, the coppice, the fields, the streams, the patterns of hundreds of years. I think I could not now live in a city. I love the country. However, I have no illusions about it now. I used to: *et in Arcadia ego*. But I learnt. Anyway, it was the humans in the country, and their pain and death that I was talking about. If I may . . . I have reverence for life, but that does not mean I hate suffering and death, even though I try to make them as easy as possible for people. I love daylight, but I do not therefore want to destroy the night. I see the necessity, the beauty, of both. I like both. I hold my patient's hand when he is at death's door, just as I have often held his whole body in my hands when he entered life. And each time God holds me in a way.

JUDGE: The medical institution has many mansions, Mr Hunter? Any further questions? Then thank you, Dr Aldam. And this court is adjourned.

REFERENCES—SESSION TWELVE
1. Paulley, J. W., *Lancet*, July 24, 1976, p. 203.
2. *Priorities for Health and Personal Social Services in England*, Department of Health and Social Security, HMSO, London, 1976, fig 3, p. 21.

General Reading
Neeson, S., *JAMA*, April 28, 1975, p. 374. (A brief article, highly recommended, on modern American medicine.)
Editorial, *NEJM*, February 19, 1976, p. 442. (A trenchant attack on anti-doctor books by the distinguished editor of a most distinguished journal. He suggests their authors should 'compare the system of medical care in the United States . . . with alternatives such as are found in other countries', being perhaps unaware that this has been done to a great extent—see reference 21, Session 11—by the American firm of McKinsey and Co., Inc., the conclusions being on the whole highly unfavourable to the American system.)
Bradshaw, J. S., *BMJ*, March 27, 1976, p. 767.
Illich, I., *Medical Nemesis*, Pantheon Books, New York, 1976. (Published as *Limits to Medicine*, Marion Boyars, London, 1976; and published in an earlier version as *Medical Nemesis*, Calder and Boyars, London 1975.)
Spiro, H. M., and Mandell, H. N., *NEJM*, July 8, 1976, p. 90. (A short, perceptive piece on the right role for the older and the younger doctor.)
Steele, S. J., and Morton, D. J. B., *Lancet*, January 14, 1978, p. 85. (An excellent article by a doctor and a nurse on how patients should be treated during a ward round, with some examples of current defects.)
Pereira Gray, D. J., *Practitioner*, January 1978, p. 131. (Excellent account of what can be accomplished by family-doctor home visiting, and the drawbacks of home visiting by a variety of persons.)

PART III
What Doctors Might Be

FAMILY DOCTORS

Enter Dr Hector Roylance

JUDGE: Dr Hector Roylance? I have decided, doctor, to carry out the initial questioning of you and of the other witnesses in this third and last part of the enquiry myself. You are 35, you are board-certified in family practice here in the United States – that is, you are a specialist in family medicine – and you are just back from a one-year period of study of the workings of family medicine in England?

ROYLANCE: Correct, sir; and I greatly enjoyed my visit to your wonderful country.

JUDGE: Apart from the differences between the United Kingdom and the United States that have already been considered here with Sir Guy Chumley or with Dr Jaeger – in the methods of financing health care delivery, in the relative dearth of American family practitioners and their maldistribution, in their tendency to be perhaps more scientifically minded and less pastorally minded than their British counterparts, in the maldistribution of doctors in the United States, especially, and of resources in the United Kingdom – apart from all that would you say that the problems facing high-technology medicine in the two countries are identical? (*Roylance nods*) And the problems of our two countries are broadly those of the advanced countries of the west generally? (*Roylance nods again*) Then briefly, doctor, what are those problems, as you see them?

ROYLANCE: An over-emphasis, judge, on not-very-effective high-technology medicine, with too much specializing and sub-specializing; on hospital medicine as opposed to family practice; and in association with that, excessive prescribing, a failure always to appreciate the importance of psychosocial factors in the genesis of disease and of the whole person as distinct from the disease or diseased organ; a lack of emphasis on prevention, and on self-help; a failure to concentrate enough on caring for the old and the handicapped in society instead of trying to cure.

JUDGE: Yes, the problems we have heard about from other witnesses? And you see an answer to all or some of them in a renaissance of family medicine? (*Roylance nods*) Would you care to outline for us the likely nature, as you see it, of this renaissance and its effects?

ROYLANCE: Surely. In both our countries the main problem in my judgment is a lack of emphasis on the fact that family medicine is a specialty in its own right, a lack of prestige for it in relation to hospital-based medicine. However, if I may dwell on my own country for a moment: a recent development here is that as many as 40 percent of the students graduating at some medical schools now wish to enter family practise,[1] the average being about 20 percent.[2] There was a similar enthusiasm in your country a few years ago. Some young American doctors are going straight from their intern year – their first houseman job, as you would call it – into family practice.

JUDGE: Receiving no special training? (*Roylance nods*) You do not approve?

ROYLANCE: Of their enthusiasm, sir, I do: of their lack of specialized training, I do not. I might give it a qualified approval in only one circumstance – if they were mature students who had already worked for some time in the health field before entering medical school .

JUDGE: Is that type of entry common?

ROYLANCE: No, but it has been suggested in your country[3] and in mine – with the object of making medicine less of an exclusively middle-class profession.

JUDGE: These entrants would not be tempted to don the middle-class mantle?

ROYLANCE: I have a certain faith in the deep essential goodness of human nature, sir. However, this new interest in family medicine will enable us to remedy the maldistribution of family doctors.

JUDGE: In what ways exactly?

ROYLANCE: With a greater output of family doctors we could, as in your country, have areas in which such doctors are not allowed to settle because there are already enough; we could have other, under-doctored areas carrying financial incentives for settlement – and intermediate areas. One could improve the clinical facilities in under-doctored areas, or arrange for training in family practice to take place in them, especially in the ordinary community hospitals; or finance medical education for students from such areas, or for students who will agree to practice in them once their training is complete. One might even have to contemplate – it has been suggested – drafting young doctors into such areas.

JUDGE: Conscription? – In case the essential goodness proved not deep enough?

ROYLANCE: A very, very gentle form of conscription, sir. Somehow the American nation can and must and shall ensure high-quality care for all social classes. Certainly there is now no dearth of facilities for family practice training in the US. Funding is available in various forms,[4] including federal funding.

JUDGE: Money from central government?

ROYLANCE: That is correct, sir. Also there is now an American Academy of Family Practice just as you have for some years had your own Royal College of General Practitioners. Your College can award membership or fellowship of the college, indicating proficiency, but in the United States we have had the separate American Board of Family Practice as the certifying body since 1969. There has, in recent years, been a dramatic increase in the number of training programs and hospital residencies being offered for would-be family doctors: there are now more than 300 programs. When allied with a limitation on the number of residencies in other specialties, there is no doubt this will lead to a great outpouring of family doctors very shortly.

JUDGE: The patients in the hospitals are the same, and the doctors treating them, but the doctors have a different title?

ROYLANCE: That might be one way – perhaps, forgive me, a somewhat misleading way, sir – of characterizing the matter.

JUDGE: Mr Hunter presented evidence, while examining Sir Guy Chumley, that, although many young American doctors are now entering family practice training, there is evidence that they may, none the less, emerge as specialists of some kind.

ROYLANCE: Every innovatory move, judge, has its small teething troubles. However, to resume: the training of our American family doctors-to-be is sometimes in university teaching hospitals, sometimes in community hospitals. There is ano blind idolatory of a uniform approach.

JUDGE: What subjects are they taught, doctor?

ROYLANCE: The key subjects are internal medicine – general medicine, as you call it – pediatrics, and obstetrics and gynecology. Let me just emphasize that in the States for many years experts in these three fields have commonly provided primary care, have been the doctors of first contact, in other words. That has been a consequence of the lack of family doctors. People have to an extent decided for themselves what type of special doctor would be best for their complaints, and have gone to him. As in your country, various other subjects are also available to the family doctor in training – psychiatry, surgery, emergency medicine, geriatrics, community medicine, and so on. The permutations are endless, but the aim is always to avoid the divisiveness of hospital medicine, to train the young doctor to treat the whole person, face-to-face. And it is for that reason that some training in the behavioral sciences – social psychology, sociology, cultural anthropology, even economics – is now often given, either in the general medical student course or even during the specialized course I have just outlined for the budding family doctor.

JUDGE: There will be some training actually *in* a family practice, will there?

ROYLANCE: Oh, yes, indeed. Inadvertently I omitted that central element. It will be either of the kind encountered in the emergency room of the typical large American teaching hospital,[5, 6] or in the district associated with such a hospital,[3, 7] or in a community hospital;[8] otherwise the training will be in what we call a service practice – actually in the community.[7]

JUDGE: And this course will last for how long?

ROYLANCE: Normally three years, judge: that is, after a year of internship that comes immediately after the four years in medical school (which follow four years, occasionally two years, at the basic sciences). The times and the course-scheduling periods are now very similar in your country except that the medical-school period is usually five years. In your country two of the three specialist family-doctor training years are normally to be spent in a variety of house – or resident – posts, and one year in a general practice, and the three-year training is to be compulsory after 1980.

JUDGE: And on completion of their training how exactly will this new generation of family doctors operate, doctor?

ROYLANCE: Hopefully from what you would call a health center; that is, a building housing perhaps half a dozen doctors – keeping one another up-to-date – with full supporting staff: an administrator, secretaries, receptionists, nurses, social worker, and dispenser, and even a psychologist and a physiotherapist perhaps; and physician assistants, to which I will return later. Equipped with a laboratory, maybe with X-ray facilities, and so on. And computerized records, of course.

JUDGE: And the patients?

ROYLANCE: The whole complex will revolve round the patients, sir. Apart from diagnosis and treatment of most everyday complaints, and referral to appropriate specialists as necessary, there will be – I emphasize it again – a strong emphasis on whole-person rather than technical medicine, on prevention, on the pastoral and social aspects of medicine, and on the provision of care where cure is not possible. It has been suggested that here in the States there should be some measure of lay control of the centers, that each patient should have success to his or her medical records,[9] and that there should be complete openness by the doctors as to the training and experience they have had, the fees they charge, and so on.[9]

JUDGE: Perhaps a shade Utopian, doctor?

ROYLANCE: Agreed, judge; but one never knows . . . You see, consumer groups have started publishing details of doctors' fees, their training, and so on.

JUDGE: You mean that what you are suggesting is a defensive maneuver by the doctors?

ROYLANCE: Not defensive, judge. I would say responsive, which is not the same thing; or perhaps anti-unresponsive, which is subtly different again. There is even a suggestion coming from government that doctors should themselves advertise.[10] Consumer groups say it would stimulate true competition, throw health-care delivery open to ordinary market forces; but I personally find it repugnant.

JUDGE: Perhaps, of course, the consumer groups find the present position repugnant, doctor; but please go on.

ROYLANCE: These family doctors will have beds in the local community hospital,[11, 12] where they might even want to specialize in one branch or other of medicine, calling on full-time specialists for advice as needed. This would enable them to treat or manage – to care for – many patients with minor or moderately severe conditions much more cheaply than is done at present in the larger hospitals where, in any case, the emphasis is always on active treatment, which is often not possible in family-doctor cases. There would also, of course, still be *some* larger specialized regional hospitals (district hospitals, as you would call them) for grave emergencies, diagnostic problem cases, and so on. And then, at the top – as it were – some *very* highly specialized university hospitals providing tertiary care.[8]

JUDGE: Tertiary?

ROYLANCE: Medical jargon, sir. *Primary* care is, as its name suggests, the care a family doctor gives; secondary care is the kind one might get from a specialist in a community or a regional hospital; tertiary is the most highly specialized kind – say, from a subspecialty doctor in a university hospital. To resume: in this new type of family practice there would also be an emphasis on self-care by the individual, perhaps even with the aid of drugs off-prescription, and possibly self-monitoring of his condition – as, for instance, in the case of a raised blood pressure. And this self-help element would be particularly important in the preventive field which would include, as well as computerized immunization schedules and screening for various diseases or premonitory signs of disease, regular lectures on health matters for the man and woman in the street, to be given at the center or the community hospital; constant personal admonition of the public on health matters by all the health personnel involved; and attention by the family doctor to certain environmental health matters – involving housing, accidents, conditions at work, food, and so on. The health personnel would work as a health team,[13, 14] with the doctor as the coordinator; and finally, of course, there would have to be provision for continuing postgraduate education, and medical audit – for continuous monitoring of the effectiveness, including the cost-effectiveness, of the various procedures and personnel. (That is, if I may say, only one of various democratic ways we are devising in America to ensure a high quality of health-care delivery for all of our people at an economic rate.) And we shall also have built-in deterrents against excessive utilization of hospitalization.

JUDGE: You have made no specific mention, doctor, of care of the old and the handicapped in the community: a major problem, we have been told.

ROYLANCE: I have mentioned them but only by implication. They would, naturally, be given high priority in the caring process. They would be brought out of the hospitals or institutions – if they were in them in the first place and as far as was possible – and be housed instead in special old-person complexes or in hostels or . . . oh, there are many possible venues for the old and the handicapped.

JUDGE: And the physician assistants you did specifically mention?

ROYLANCE: Ah, yes, they act – the nurse-practitioner kind of assistant – as a sort of screen to determine which patients should see the doctor, which need no treatment, and which can safely be managed by the nurse practitioner herself or himself; or else they deal, with the aid of special protocols – formal printed guidelines, that is – with specific conditions, like diabetes or sore throat. Depending on what they do, these physician assistants may be fully trained nurses, or ex-army corpsmen, or ex-pharmacists, or even intelligent young people with only a few weeks' training. Naturally their knowledge and expertise and the amount of responsibility they can be given varies a lot, depending on their background and training.

JUDGE: The object being to take some of the strain off the doctor? And they have proved successful?

ROYLANCE: Quite successful. Indeed. There needs to be a physician in the background, naturally.

JUDGE: And in the areas you mentioned, Dr Roylance, where there is no physician? Are they used in such places?

ROYLANCE: Yes, judge, they are; and then, of course, they take on maximum responsibility, sending the patient off to the nearest doctor only when they feel quite out of their depth. They can prove useful in such circumstances, as a temporary measure, until family doctors can be provided.

JUDGE: Are they related in any way to the barefoot doctors one hears about?

ROYLANCE: Those with a minimum of training certainly are.

JUDGE: Physician assistants are common in the United States?

ROYLANCE: We have over 2000 of the nurse-practitioner type as of now, with many more being trained. The nurse-practitioner type of physician assistant is operating in one or two places in your country also, which, of course, has led the way in the use of nurses in more conventional roles in family practice – as maternity nurses, district nurses, health visitors, nurses in the doctor's surgery, or office as we call it; and so on.

JUDGE: Thank you, doctor. Mr Hunter?

HUNTER: (*rising*): Dr Roylance, are you aware that you have presented no evidence at all that this supposedly new type of family physician will achieve the objectives you mentioned?

ROYLANCE: The situation is open-ended, Mr Hunter. The family doctor will engineer solutions to the problems you yourself have so ably exposed in the past two weeks, and that I tried to summarize in my straightforward way.

HUNTER: I put it to you that this new family medicine of yours is an imaginative mishmash of items, some of which have already been operating for years, sometimes with success, sometimes not; others of which are recent and unproven innovations; while still others exist only as nebulous visions; and that the whole concept has come very largely from the temples of high-technology medicine that have produced the problems this new development purports to solve.

ROYLANCE: I assure you, Mr Hunter, that every single item is totally operational in one location or another.

HUNTER: Open access to medical records? 'Constant personal admonition of the public on health matters by all the health personnel involved' – that was, I think, the expression you used? Mature students entering medical school? In just how many locations?

ROYLANCE: Well, yes, you might say there is a visionary element – a genuine visionary element – to one or two of the peripheral components.

HUNTER: And how exactly does what you propose differ in the *end* from what a good family doctor achieves today? – Dr John Aldam, for instance.

ROYLANCE: I have not a word to say against Dr Aldam, but family doctors of the older generation, in your country and mine, had no special medical training, let alone in the behavioral sciences; such a doctor worked alone, or, like Dr Aldam, with one assistant; he had no clear objectives; he did not work from a health center, he did not have a range of ancillary support, he did not practice health education, he would not have tolerated lay control, he would not understand computerization or medical audit, he would not work as a member of a health team, he would not—

JUDGE: What Mr Hunter asked, doctor, was how your family doctor's achievements would differ from those of Dr Aldam.

ROYLANCE: It would be highly unethical of me to comment on his end results except to say that he achieved his success – and I feel sure, judged on certain parameters, he has been highly successful in some fields – *despite* his working conditions, not because of them.

HUNTER: You feel you should bring big medicine into the lives of doctors like Dr Aldam?

ROYLANCE: The good elements of modern medicine, yes.

JUDGE: Leaving the bad elements where, doctor? – In the hospital?

ROYLANCE: I like that, judge. I have always liked a good joke.

HUNTER: Dr Roylance, I want now to examine with you the relevance of the various elements in this new family-medicine of yours to the discovery of answers to the problems facing us. Your proposals fall under three heads: first, an escape from high-technology medicine and a giving of attention to the whole person; second, an emphasis on caring in the community and on psycho-social factors in illness; third, prevention, as manifested in self-care, health education, screening procedures, public health measures, and the like. That third element need not detain us as it is to be the subject of tomorrow's enquiry. Now, as to escaping from the world of high-technology medicine: are you not suggesting a move that is against the whole trend of our society towards more technology and more specialization, let alone the trend in the medical field? American lay people, you say, have been going to specialists for years as a first choice: to internists, to pediatricians, to obstetricians. What makes you think they will change? – Many American doctors approve of the practice, especially for your cities, do they not?[4] And are you aware that people in Britain are on the whole consulting their family doctors rather *less* than they used to? – That, unless it's a routine matter, they often regard a family doctor merely as a port of call on the way to the hospital?

ROYLANCE: These are the challenges we face, sir; from which we do not flinch.

HUNTER: Do you really think that after five years in a British medical school, a year in a pre-registration house job (internship, as you call it), and then three years of training in family medicine, two of them in hospital, any young British doctor has not been so brain-washed with the ideology of hospital medicine that he will never be able to escape it?

ROYLANCE: With respect, Mr Hunter, I escaped it in the USA after a similar apprenticeship.

HUNTER: The essence of my case, doctor, is that you have not; and that neither have most of the younger generation of family doctors; you are simply proposing to bring the ideas – sometimes incompetently and always inappropriately – the ideas of big medicine, hospital medicine, into the realm of family practice, where it already has a foothold anyway, as Dr Aldam said.

ROYLANCE: I look forward to hearing your evidence for that statement, Mr Hunter.

HUNTER: Very well. The essence of the new British scheme for training family doctors – and the American pattern, you said, is similar – is that the young doctor, aside from 12 months actually in family practice, will do four house jobs in hospital, each lasting six months. Correct?

ROYLANCE: Correct, Mr Hunter. Residencies, as we would call them.

HUNTER: I am now going to read you a list of the specialties or groups of specialties that, in one or other part of the United Kingdom, are offering such house jobs for budding family doctors. Stop me if you disagree that any one of these was on offer in 1976 – a year I chose at random. Any four – but only four, remember – to be studied, each for six months: general medicine; general medicine with infectious diseases; general medicine with neurology; general medicine with cardiology; general medicine with geriatrics; chest medicine; pediatrics; obstetrics and gynecology; pediatrics with obstetrics and gynecology; psychiatry and geriatrics; community child health; accident and emergency; ditto with orthopedics; accident and emergency with orthopedics and rheumatology; rehabilitation medicine; anesthetics; ear, nose, and throat – or ENT – surgery; ophthalmology; dermatology; infectious diseases with geriatrics; ENT surgery with ophthalmology; ENT surgery with dermatology; ENT surgery with ophthalmology, psychiatry, and dermatology.[15] As you yourself said, doctor, in relation to your country, the available permutations are almost endless: I could go on and on. At the end of it all there are at least four – perhaps five or six – exams the trainee can take. Some of the courses allow no time at all in hospital for general medicine; and yet here in your country, doctor, that subject – internal medicine – is looked upon as the cornerstone of family practice, is it not? – And in your country, by the way, the budding family doctor can also do community medicine, allergy, neurology, physical medicine – all kinds of subspecialties.

ROYLANCE: The list is a tribute to the wealth of experience being offered to your and our young graduates anxious to be properly equipped for the task that lies ahead of them.

HUNTER: For *whole*-person medicine? I put it to you, doctor, that the list indicates, first, confusion in the teaching staff as to exactly what the family doctor *does* need;[6] second, it indicates beyond a peradventure – because no course, naturally enough, offers anything like *every* option in the list – that no young doctor following a British course can, by the criteria that are implicit in the list, emerge fully equipped medically. He is *bound* to miss out on a number of subjects that it is thought elsewhere should be offered, or that are taken in his own hospital by some of his companions. And most important, of all, the budding whole-person doctor is being taught to divide his patients up, as hospitals do, by disease and system and organ, by sex, by age, by orifice – he is being taught all the time to hanker after the technical expertise such subdivision requires and encourages. The latter has been criticized in your own country.[16]

ROYLANCE: He is also taught, as you mentioned, Mr Hunter, in general practise, and it is that period of his training that will provide the cement to mould the separate elements together into a holistic living corpus of knowledge which will serve him well in the community.

HUNTER: Why then are departments of family medicine being established in university teaching hospitals? – A move that has been criticized here in the USA.[17, 18] Why is general practice called a *specialty* here? You say fewer specialties are needed, but you then invent a new one. *General* practice, doctor: a specialty? Is it not because hospital medicine, high-technology medicine, specialty medicine has an aura, and has the prestige and the status; and now family medicine has suddenly got a lot of the money – is that not why family medicine is being taught in university hospitals? Is it not a fact too that in the last 30 years the more prosperous people and the ordinary specialists and such family practitioners as there were in your country have moved to the outskirts of the big cities, where there are community hospitals, leaving behind the super-specialists in the big hospitals, often university hospitals, to provide tertiary care;[8] and that those university hospitals found, first, they had to provide primary care for the poor people left in the city centers[5, 18] because there was no one else to do it; and second, more recently, that the research money they had been receiving for many years were beginning to dry up?[4, 8] – The almighty dollar talking again. So that some of the highly specialized internists in those university hospitals (the consultant physicians, as we call them) have now taken to teaching what they call family medicine?[8] Is this not inappropriate? – Super-specialists teaching men to be family doctors? And are other less specialized American internists not very much afraid that, what with the *sub*-specialties of general medicine taking patients here and the new family doctors taking patients there, soon there will be no general medical patients left for themselves to handle?[6] – So that *they* disapprove strongly of the expansion of family medicine?

ROYLANCE: I agree that community hospitals are often on the whole better for the teaching of family medicine than a university hospital, though perhaps on the other hand the latter would do more to foster the spirit of scientific enquiry, of lifelong open-mindedness; but in a democratic country like mine we aim at diversity and richness, not a dull uniformity.

HUNTER: The same tendency, because of an inner-city dearth of family doctors, to the provision of primary care by teaching hospitals and by university departments of general practice is present in London, is it not?[19, 20] And isn't it a fact, doctor, that the professors of general practice and their lecturers wish to achieve high academic respectability? Want to be full members of the medical faculty? Is it not a fact too that some of your most able family doctors, men with many years of practical experience of family medicine, may be refused family-medicine teaching posts in the faculties because they lack a specialty qualification?[21] (*Pause*) When was the American Board of Family Practice set up?

ROYLANCE: In 1969.

HUNTER: So that any middle-aged family doctor could not reasonably be expected to have the board's bit of paper to wave at a university faculty? And yet is it not, on the other hand, also a fact that some of the *recognized* teachers of family medicine in your country are so involved with their teaching and administration and research that they run the risk of having no time left actually to practice family medicine?[7] – They may find themselves teaching what they are no longer involved in?

ROYLANCE: Very rarely, Mr Hunter. Hard cases make bad law.

JUDGE: They may sometimes indicate the way the wind is blowing, doctor.

HUNTER: (*to Roylance*): Family medicine, with its inappropriate hospital training—

ROYLANCE: You've got to have some hospital training, Mr Hunter.

HUNTER: I did not deny it. I said 'with its *inappropriate* hospital training' – implying there could be *some* hospital training, a limited amount, that was appropriate. Family medicine, I am suggesting, has become just another institutionalized specialty of high-technology medicine, with its own colleges and boards and academies, and its own jargon. And I put it to you what the judge put to Dr Batt: that the whole person medicine on which you lay such stress is incompatible with the fissiparous science that now dominates most hospitals, certainly most teaching hospitals; and that the objectivities of science, of medical audit, of trials and testing are *necessarily* incompatible with the subjectivity of person-to-person medicine, person-to-person contact. Each approach may have virtues, but the two cannot live together.

ROYLANCE: Each has its own role to play, Mr Hunter.

HUNTER: I am not digressing, but do you know that in one trial of the value of breast feeding the doctors told the mothers – this was in a poor country – to bring the babies along for weighing before and after the feeding, and that it just wouldn't work? – Because mostly the mothers could not *think* to bring the babies along before feeding them: their instinct to feed the baby who needed to be fed was so strong they did it at once, without any thought. The objectivity, the thought process, the idea of a schedule came to them only *after* they'd fed the baby.[22] Who were the wiser, the mothers or the doctors? – Objectivity and humanity cannot coexist more than a little, can they?

ROYLANCE: Forgive me, Mr Hunter, but I think you got a bad dose of science some place along the line.

HUNTER: I am sure you could prescribe a remedy.

ROYLANCE: Yes – go into any community hospital here or in your own country.

HUNTER: You know what I shall find in some of those in the United Kingdom? – I shall find general practitioners – *general* practitioners – working in a part-time capacity as specialists:[23] skin specialists, or eye specialists, or psychiatrists? You mentioned yourself the same process in this country. Does that not give the lie to your case? Why do you think those young American doctors you mentioned *choose* to go straight into family practice once they have finished their compulsory intern year? – I know why I think they do it: because they sense in their hearts that another few years in hospital, and all they would then be capable of doing, if they didn't specialize, would be to take the hospital out into the community. Electrocardiographs, and automated blood analyses, and prescriptions. Family medicine today, I suggest, Dr Roylance, means the hospitalization of society. You are making society into one big hospital ward.

JUDGE: No further comment, doctor? – I need hardly say that your silence is not to be construed as agreement. Mr Hunter?

HUNTER: So much for the first element in the new family medicine: escape from high-technology medicine with its specializing and sub-specializing; and an emphasis on the whole person. The second element again emphasized the whole person – in a concern for psychosocial factors in illness, and with caring in the community. You talked about the training of medical students in sociology, social psychology, cultural anthropology, and so on, all of it leading to better understanding of the whole person, of psychosocial factors in disease. I put it to you that such training has been discussed in your country for at least the last quarter of a century,[24] but that in practice what has mainly been taught has been more and more high-technology medicine, and little but lip service has been paid to these other, humanistic disciplines,[16, 24] whatever the effect of their teaching *might* have been.

ROYLANCE: Then I must say, Mr Hunter, you are not very well acquainted with the new direction of American thinking and practice in family medicine.

HUNTER: Health centers next, which you praised. It has been said of them by patients that they lack warmth and a feeling of confidentiality,[23] the very qualities that are needed for the person-to-person contact that is at the heart of your proposed holistic medicine. (*Pause*) And do you not think the use of your proposed health team, a whole conglomerate of people – perhaps strange people – to deal with one patient, could have the same effect, especially on older patients? (*Pause*) Next, doctor, I put it to you that the development of physician assistants, whether qualified or not, and all the other paramedical personnel you mentioned earlier suggests just one thing: that the family doctors have got themselves so up-stage, so far away from caring for the patient in the community, that other people, more simply trained people, have had to come in to take over a lot of the doctor's functions.

ROYLANCE: Oh, come now, Mr Hunter, you're joking. We've had nurses for many, many years in family practice. We've had receptionists for decades.

HUNTER: Nurse *practitioners* for many, many years, or only recently? Receptionists for decades who, when not acting as barriers the patients have to penetrate before they can get into direct contact with the doctors, may give advice and treatment? You said earlier that physician assistants had been 'quite successful'? (*Roylance nods*) That was an understatement, a conscious understatement? Doctors are doubtful about them on occasion, are they not?[25, 26, 27] – Could they even be jealous because the patients are very happy with them? – Because the patients find they can talk to the physician assistants about personal matters, psychosocial matters, in a way that is no longer possible with many doctors? – The doctors are too busy moving on to the next patient or reaching for the prescription pad or laboratory request form to sit and listen and talk and care. And yet sometimes they criticize the physician assistants for a lack of sympathy and warmth, which are the very qualities the patients say they very often lack themselves.

ROYLANCE: I think, Mr Hunter, you are taking isolated observations out of context and generalizing from them.

HUNTER: Then I will particularize for you instead. You are acquainted with the Burlington trial of the nurse practitioner?[28] (*Roylance nods*) Correct me if I am in error. It showed that, when assessment was made in accordance with a scheme worked out beforehand by doctors not involved in the trial, the nurse practitioners could deal satisfactorily with 69 percent of the sickness episodes they encountered and the participating doctors with 66 percent of such episodes. Those taking part did not know in respect of which episodes their management was to be judged, and the patients were not specially chosen for the nurse practitioners, or for the doctors.

ROYLANCE: Right. That's why, like I said, we need nurse practitioners in family practice.

HUNTER: You are acquainted with a Boston trial[29] of the routine follow-up management of patients with diabetes and raised blood pressure by physician assistants who had received only a few weeks of training, but who were chosen for their warmth, sensitivity, and intelligence – that is, ability to deal with psychosocial factors? These young people managed the blood pressure patients just as well as the doctors, did they not? And they managed the diabetic patients rather better than the doctors? – On a *technical* level? And they made no major errors, and, more important, the patients liked them and kept coming back for more, even bringing them presents.

ROYLANCE: Absolutely correct. They did a splendid job, those youngsters – always with the doctors in the background, of course, just in case anything did go wrong.

HUNTER: You are acquainted with a study – which Professor Hecht mentioned – that was conducted at the Health Services clinic of Duke University, North Carolina[30] – and showed that, if anything, the PAs and particularly the student PAs were superior to the doctors before a protocol for treatment of sore throats was introduced, and achieved at least as marked an improvement after it was introduced?

ROYLANCE: Like I say, we need more of these people in family medicine.

HUNTER: It could not be – could it, doctor? – that we want, not only more physician assistants, but fewer doctors, not the massive increase you mentioned earlier as being desirable. Why produce the inferior article?

ROYLANCE: I – I find this adulation of the physician assistant at the expense of the doctor most unfortunate.

HUNTER: I do not adulate them, doctor. I think they are open to all the corrupting influences that have already corrupted the doctors; and so are all their other paramedical colleagues: the laboratory assistant, the medical records' expert, the surgeon's assistant, and so on. I think they will all in due course, if they have time and as they are human, form their own colleges, have their own diplomas[31] – some of them have such things already – will institutionalize themselves, will demand the same financial rewards as doctors, will ask why they cannot *be* doctors . . . Like the doctors, they will hold society to ransom. This is the great advantage, you see, of self-reliance, of the love of one's family and friends, of the help of neighbors and of the priest and of the old-fashioned doctor, like Dr Aldam: you cannot make that into an institution, you cannot ever put a price upon true caring in the community. But any kind of professional substitute for that whole complex, whether it be a new-style family doctor or even a simple physician assistant or a nurse practitioner, will in the end submit to all those temptations. And yet where is our neighborliness today, our self-reliance, or our priest, our old-fashioned doctors, even our family very often? – Gone, destroyed; or watching the television, or too busy worshipping Mammon to bother with their neighbors or relatives. That is why we need those substitutes. But do not let us deceive ourselves that they are ever the real thing. Some are fresher than others, that is all. At the moment the PAs are fresher than the doctors.

ROYLANCE: Well, you're sure right out of my depth now, Mr Hunter.

HUNTER: I have here a leaflet about a new journal, established in early 1976. One passage reads, 'The journal is designed to provide a medium for the publication of scholarly papers . . . information of scientific, theoretical or philosophical importance . . .' It sounds very highbrow, does it not? But the title of the journal was to be the *Journal of Advanced Nursing*. If you were ill, should you like an advanced nurse looking after you, doctor? – Or just a plain, straightforward nurse? Finally, doctor, a ray of hope in that same physician-assistant field. Are you aware it has been said by a

Christian health worker[33] that the Chinese barefoot doctors have owed their success, not so much to their technical skills – although they possess some – but to the fact that they are in essence not technical workers but political workers in the widest sense? – That they typify the determination and ability of the community they serve to work out its own salvation so far as its health goes? – They typify the breaking of the medical monopoly of health matters. They represent, in other words, not communism necessarily, but radical social change of the kind that Professor Larkin told us was responsible for the improvement of health in western industrial countries from 1860 onwards. They are *not* seen as responsible to, or inferior to, doctors, though relying on them, of course, for technical expertise. Such physician assistants may perhaps never become professionalized. *They* may never form colleges or specialty boards. *They* may merely bring more health to the people, as they have done to a remarkable degree in China already: western doctors have said so. What those doctors missed was the heart of the matter – that health comes from a healthy society, not from doctors or any form of technical specialist. (*Pause*) No further questions.

JUDGE: You wish to comment, doctor?

ROYLANCE: I wish to say only that I simply do not follow all the convolutions of Mr Hunter's doubtless very subtle argument, judge.

JUDGE: I sympathize. It is an attempt that some of us, none the less, have to make for it is seriously intended and, I think, quite closely knit. Thank you, doctor. Thank you, Mr Hunter. The court is adjourned.

REFERENCES—SESSION THIRTEEN

1. Dunea, G., *BMJ*, September 20, 1975, p. 694.
2. Janeway, C. A., *NEJM*, August 15, 1975, p. 337.
3. Hart, J. Tudor, *Lancet*, November 16, 1974, p. 1191.
4. Stimmel, B., *NEJM*, July 10, 1975, p. 68.
5. Berarducci, A. A., Delbanco, T. L., and Rabkin, M. T., *NEJM*, March 20, 1975, p. 615.
6. Petersdorf, R. G., *NEJM*, August 14, 1975, p. 326.
7. McWhinney, I. R., *NEJM*, July 24, 1975, p. 176.
8. Spiro, H. M., *NEJM*, April 10, 1975, p. 792.
9. Boardman, D. W., *NEJM*, September 5, 1974, p. 497.
10. Editorial, *NEJM*, February 5, 1976, p. 334.
11. Weston Smith, J., and O'Donovan, J. B., *BMJ*, June 13, 1970, p. 653.
12. Kyle, D., *BMJ*, November 6, 1971, p. 348.
13. Garfield, S. R., *et al.*, *NEJM*, February 19, 1976, p. 426.
14. Marsh, G. N., and McNay, R. A., *BMJ*, February 23, 1974, p. 315.

15. Advertisements for General Practice Training Posts, *BMJ*, January 3, 1976–June 26, 1976, all issues inclusive
16. Ransom, D. C., and Vandervoort, H. E., *JAMA*, August 27, 1973, p. 1098.
17. Strauss, M. B., *NEJM*, September 12, 1974, p. 553.
18. Lathem, W., *NEJM*, July 1, 1976, p. 18.
19. Richardson, I. M., *BMJ*, December 27, 1975, p. 740.
20. Leading Article, *BMJ*, December 27, 1975, p. 724.
21. Draper, P., and Smits, H. L., *NEJM*, October 30, 1975, p. 903.
22. Morley, D., quoted in Muller, M., *The Baby Killer*, War on Want, London, 1974, p. 6.
23. Editorial, *Lancet*, November 10, 1973, p. 1069.
24. Middleton, W. S., *Annals of Internal Medicine*, June 1951, p. 1457.
25. Editorial, *Lancet*, April 6, 1974, p. 608.
26. Editorial, *Lancet*, April 12, 1975, p. 842.
27. Nelson, E. C., Jacobs, A. R., and Johnson, K. G., *JAMA*, April 1, 1974, p. 63.
28. Spitzer, W. O., *et al.*, *NEJM*, January 31, 1974, p. 251.
29. Komaroff, A. L., *et al.*, *NEJM*, February 7, 1974, p. 307.
30. Grimm, R. H., Jr, *et al.*, *NEJM*, March 6, 1975, p. 507.
31. Leading Article, *BMJ*, December 24–31, 1977, p. 1619.
32. Advertising leaflet for *Journal of Advanced Nursing*, vol. I, no. 1, Blackwell Scientific Publications, Oxford, 1976.
33. Rifkin, S. B., *Lancet*, January 7, 1978, p. 34.

Other Reading
The subject of family practice or family medicine or primary care (there are almost as many titles to it as there are professional attitudes towards it) is in a state of flux, particularly in the United States; almost every theory or mode of practice conceivable in this field exists, as does its exact opposite (by definition). This chapter has given an outline of the position, but further reading is needed to comprehend the subject fully.

General Reading
General Practice Today, Office of Health Economics, London, 1968.
The Work of Primary Medical Care, Office of Health Economics, 1974.
Cooper, J. K., and Heald, K., *JAMA*, March 25, 1974, p. 1410.
Massachusetts Department of Public Health, *NEJM*, March 13, 1975, p. 591.
Keith, J. F., *NEJM*, November 3, 1977, p. 1007.
Priorities for Health and Personal Social Services in England, Department of Health and Social Security, HMSO, London, 1976.
Butler, J. R., and Knight, R., *Health Trends*, February 1976, p. 8.
Cavenagh, S., *World Medicine*, February 25, 1976, p. 19.
Marsh, G. N., Wallace, R. B., and Whewell, J., *BMJ*, May 29, 1976, p. 1321.
Borus, J. F., *NEJM*, July 25, 1976, p. 140.
Robinson, D., *NEJM*, July 28, 1977, p. 188.
Older, J., *NEJM*, March 17, 1977, p. 627.
Brooks, D., *Lancet*, January 21, 1978, p. 140.
Editorial, *Lancet*, January 21, 1978, p. 134.

Training and Specialization
Josephs, C., *BMJ*, October 25, 1975, p. 224.
Chase, R. A., *NEJM*, February 26, 1976, p. 497.

Acheson, E. D., *BMJ*, July 3, 1976, p. 23.
Waters, W. E., Mercer, D., and Topliss, E., *BMJ*, July 10, 1975, p. 95.
Elstein, M., and Forbes, J. A., *BMJ*, July 10, 1976, p. 97.
Round the World, *Lancet*, October 29, 1977, p. 919.

Radical Mode of Delivery of Primary Health Care
Chamberlin, R. W., and Radebaugh, J. F., *NEJM*, March 18, 1976, p. 641.

Evaluation of Quality of Health Care
Kessmer, D. M., Calk, C. E., and Singer, J., *NEJM*, January 25, 1973, p. 189.

Medical Auxiliaries (in developed countries)
Sox, H. C., Jr, Sox, C. H., and Tompkins, R. K., *NEJM*, April 19, 1973, p. 818.
Merenstein, J. H., and Rogers, K. D., *JAMA*, March 18, 1974, p. 1278.
Bicknell, W. J., Walsh, D. G., and Tanner, M. M., *Lancet*, November 23, 1974, p. 1241.
Backett, E. M., and England, R., *Lancet*, December 6, 1975, p. 1137.
Perrin, E. C., and Goodman, H. C., *NEJM*, January 19, 1978, p. 130. (In a simulated 'telephone management' of acute illness in children nurse practitioners were significantly better than housemen or specialist pediatricians in history taking, interviewing skills, and advice given on management of the sick children: indeed, in all the aspects studied.)

PREVENTION

Enter Professor Gloria Dible

JUDGE: You are Dr Gloria Dible, an Associate Professor of Public Health in the United States? Your prime interest is in preventive medicine? We have already heard, professor, of the successes achieved in the past by means of improvements in housing, working conditions, nutrition, and education, and by means of sanitary and hygienic measures, and by the spacing of families; and as new challenges to health emerge, presumably new variations of this type of response may be expected?

DIBLE: Surely. Pollution of the environment, different in nature and scale from anything we have encountered before, the appearance of new carcinogens – cancer-producing substances – the hazards of processed foods: any of these may call for a fresh look at our chosen pathways for health maintenance. For most of the causes of premature death and of non-fatal disability in our day and age prevention provides the only hopeful approach. Coronary heart disease, lung cancer, emphysema, strokes – there's no cure. Add obesity, accidents, alcoholism, drug addiction, suicide attempts, dental decay – the list is endless: the rational approach for all these is prevention of one kind or another. Fluoridation alone will reduce dental decay by 50 percent – at minimal cost.

JUDGE: And am I right in thinking, professor, that one major element in prevention would be the screening of a seemingly well population, or certain sections of it, for the early signs of a disease, so that it could be prevented from developing?

DIBLE: Correct, in my view. But then I am an optimist. I am an American. You British tend to throw cold water on the screening of people,[1, 2] but in the States we do a lot of it.[3] The fetus who might be in some danger during pregnancy or labor, or have spina bifida; the newborn baby who might have things like phenylketonuria or a hip dislocation; adults with lung cancer, or breast cancer, or cancer of the cervix; or with bronchitis or a raised blood pressure; or having the risk factors for coronary heart disease; or a urinary tract infection, or diabetes, or anemia – screening in the case of all these is possible, and many more. We screen for some of these conditions pretty well everywhere in the States; and each of them is on the list some place or other. We also have a very open mind toward the idea of extending the process just as soon as it seems appropriate.

JUDGE: And what are the objections that you seem to be suggesting your British colleagues emphasize too strongly?

DIBLE: Please don't misunderstand me, judge. There *are* snags. There's not much point screening for a disease if you don't know for sure just how it would develop anyway – if you did not screen for it and treat it early. And it must be reasonably common and important to justify screening a *lot* of people. There must be factors present you can detect that indicate the disease *will* develop in time or is already present without symptoms. And if there are such factors, you must have tests that will pick up all or most of the people who have them (you don't want a lot of what we call 'false negatives' in other words), and also won't pick up a lot of people who just *seem* to have such factors but aren't actually going to develop the disease.

JUDGE: 'False positives'?

DIBLE: Correct. There's no point making people scary if there's nothing to be scary about. And then you must have people willing to come and be tested, and I think maybe Americans are better at this than you Britishers. And the tests mustn't be risky. Also, if the tests turn out positive, you must have all the facilities you need to go straight ahead and confirm the suspicion you've formed; and after that there must be some treatment available for whatever it is you've found – a treatment that will have a beneficial effect, better than if you just waited for symptoms to develop and *then* started treatment. You must have the ordinary doctors on your side, you must have people prepared to go on with treatment even when they have no symptoms. And you must work out what it all costs.[1] There's no good detecting a disease early if it's going to cost you ten thousand dollars a time to do it, and all you gain is an extra ten minutes of life – you get my point?

JUDGE: There seemed to be a number of points; it also seems as though the skeptical British doctors have been busy.

DIBLE: I don't want you to get me wrong, judge. We have skeptics here in the States; and you have some enthusiasts in the UK. The screening I personally favor most for adults is what we doctors call multiphasic screening – putting a seemingly well population through a whole battery of tests to detect any one of a range of diseases or features that might lead on to disease:[4, 5] some cancer or precancer cells, say, as in the Pap smear.

JUDGE: Just so. And battery in the sense of a large number? (*Dible nods*) Rather like the automatic carrying out of a range of laboratory tests?

DIBLE: That's right, judge – on blood or urine. The battery includes automated blood and urine tests, naturally; and a X-ray film of the chest, an electrical recording of the heart, blood pressure reading, breathing tests, eye and ear testing, psychological testing, examination of teeth, eyes, anus, rectum, examination of the breasts, and cervical smears – those last two in women only, of course. Which reminds me: the more you can narrow down the group you screen the better. In a way. Sometimes. Screening for specifics, that is; not multiphasics. I mean it costs less for a start if you have fewer people; and there's no point in screening whites for sickle cell disease because they don't get it.

JUDGE: No, of course not.

DIBLE: Or ten-year-olds for raised blood pressure because *they* don't get that. No, that's not true – actually they do now and again. Blood pressure readings should probably be a routine part of pediatric examinations.[6] Some people here and in your country are looking at blood pressure in new-born babies.[7, 8] Experimentally at this stage, of course. Now that really is something.

JUDGE: Yes, I suppose so.

DIBLE: Should you think big and get simply everyone into the net, or think mean and get a big catch for being choosy? – I confess I don't have the right answer right now.

JUDGE: You were telling us, professor, about the variety of tests available for the multiphasic work.

DIBLE: Yes, you name it, and someone includes it. Multiphasic screening can be very, very fruitful, especially if you have technicians and one or two computers around to do some of the donkey work before the doctor ever lays a hand on the patient. This pre-doctor work-up is called automated multiphasic health screening or health testing, and it can be very productive.[9]

JUDGE: And after conventional public health measures, professor, and screening what comes next in your list of preventive priorities?

DIBLE: Health education,[10, 11, 12] and its twin, self-care. Now here again you get the pessimists, and you get the optimists. I'm an optimist all along the line. There are three difficulties. First, does health education work? – Some people say doctors and lay folk are not interested in health, they're only interested in disease,[13] but I'm convinced, if you get at the children, the young people, the parents, the teachers, and the doctors and nurses, get at the politicians, and with every weapon you can lay your hands on – formal talks, open-ended talks, brain-storming, workshops, groups, Delphi, films, filmstrips, cassettes, television, radio, the newspapers, books, posters, the whole gamut of modern publicity – *then* you can get people to change, you can get them to do the things that will prevent disease developing. It's sometimes slow but it's always sure in the end.

JUDGE: And the second difficulty that is propounded?

DIBLE: Well, some people, judge – you know, the professional skeptics – say we don't yet know absolutely for certain what causes this disease or that. [14, 15] We think it's probably A or B, or X and Y and Z, but we're not absolutely sure. I think a strong probability's good enough for action myself. And they're reinforced by the people who go for the third difficulty [15, 16] – that it constitutes an infringement of people's freedom to go trying to change their life-style, it takes away their ability to decide for themselves. Well, what I say is what sort of freedom is it if people are going to use it to kill themselves? Other people have got to pick up the check when they get ill, for a start. Just what kind of freedom is it to smoke yourself to death? Anyway, that's my approach in a nutshell.

JUDGE: Thank you, professor. Mr Hunter?

HUNTER: (*rising*): Professor Dible, I want to reinforce what you said about those last two objections to health education that are sometimes raised. Was scurvy treated long before anyone knew its exact cause?

DIBLE: Surely – by your own James Lind with citrus fruits. It was 200 years before we discovered it was the vitamin C in the fruit that did the trick.

HUNTER: And John Snow discovered, decades before the cholera organism was identified, that cholera was transmitted in water, and that by changing the water supply it could be eradicated? (*Dible nods*) So a lack of full understanding of the whys and wherefores of a disease is not a bar to the curing or prevention of it?

DIBLE: Correct.

HUNTER: And in the case of many of the factors that are almost certainly responsible for today's main killing diseases – cigarettes, too much food, lack of exercise, and so on – no harm will be caused, as far as we know, if they are abandoned, and there may be very good reasons, quite aside from disease – economic or psychological reasons – for doing so?

DIBLE: I didn't think I'd have you so much on my side, Mr Hunter.

HUNTER: I am merely reinforcing *two* of your points, professor. Now, as to the second point: which would you say is the greater infringement of freedom – some anti-cigarette leaflets and posters and films, or some heavy pro-cigarette advertising?

DIBLE: The second, every time.

HUNTER: Well, now, I should like to ask in view of what you have said on those two points: have American doctors ever staged an all-medical march to the White House to protest against cigarette advertising or advertising for candy that makes you fat and makes your teeth decay? – That was one form of publicity you did not mention. Well, have they?

DIBLE: No, they have not done that up to now; but neither have your doctors marched to No. 10 Downing Street for that purpose.

HUNTER: Thank you for saving me the trouble of having to elicit from you that the medical malaise is transatlantic (*Pause*) Professor Dible, people do in the end have to die of something, do they not? You are not hoping so to control the environment, so to screen and educate people, so to immunize them that they will be immortal?

DIBLE: No, of course not. It is premature death, and unnecessary suffering prior to death that I want to see prevented.

HUNTER: You are sure it is just that? (*Dible nods*) Death is not to be conquered in the way you have indicated the environment is to be tamed and conquered and controlled in the interests purportedly of man's health?

DIBLE: If so, it's news to me. It'll certainly be in the dim distant future, if ever, that we get around to conquering death. Three-score years and ten, or a bit over – that's our span.

HUNTER: You don't read the London *Times*, of course?

DIBLE: Naturally not.

HUNTER: But it is a highly reputable paper? (*Dible nods*) What I have just been suggesting is not news to readers of *The Times*. I have here the issue of that newspaper for July 19, 1976, and on the very first page there is a piece[17] by the paper's science editor. It is headed, 'Genetic Find May Help to Explain Aging', and the body of the article explains that some workers for the British Medical Research Council feel that their research on chromosomes may before long lead to an understanding of the process of aging. Now, if they did understand that process, will you suggest to me what practical application it would have that would not imply at the least a deferment of death?

DIBLE: I think you're indulging in fantasy.

HUNTER: And *The Times* of London? *And* the Medical Research Council workers? (*Pause*) You are aware that work is proceeding in your own country on the use of a chemical allied to vitamin A, which would be taken regularly over a period of many years in order to prevent cancer developing?[18]

DIBLE: And why not?

HUNTER: Would you say the same if it was a chemical that would prevent death due to *any* cause developing?

DIBLE: Now I think you're being ridiculous.

HUNTER: Not merely giving expression to the dreams of some

medical scientists? (*Pause*) I suggest to you further that the implication of all your opening remarks was that you had in mind a very substantial deferment of death to be secured by preventive action, quite apart from its indefinite deferment by means of control of aging, cancer prevention, and so on; in the same way as your clinical colleagues believe now in conquering or controlling all dangers at a later stage, including – for as long as possible – death itself. (*Pause*) Do you not think one can have too much effort directed merely at some postponement of death? – That such effort may, if nothing else, diminish people's healthy power to adapt.

DIBLE: No, I do not see that at all. If I can do something good, I do it. I live in this day and age: if I have a computer, I use it.

HUNTER: To control all the records for immunization of a very large number of children, say? But suppose someone blows up the computer or it goes wrong; or a spare part is missing, and the supplier decides not to supply it or cannot because his workers are on strike? You are vulnerable, are you not? – Or rather, the children are. After a certain degree of complexity technological progress, so called, even the medical kind, becomes self-defeating, no? It invites defeat by its very complexity, it secures the opposite of what it is meant to secure.

DIBLE: I've never heard of a computer going . . . I mean who'd want to blow up a computer?

HUNTER: I think the court took the initial point you unwittingly made. (*Pause*) Do you think one can *ever* have an excess of hygiene?

DIBLE: No.

HUNTER: You know that the immunity of the people of poorer nations to poliomyelitis is commonly accepted as being due to their having been infected when quite young – as a result of relatively poor hygiene, so-called – and thus developing an immunity to the disease; whereas the young of rich countries are not so immunized, thanks to their perhaps over-hygienic surroundings; and so, before a vaccine was developed, *they* would become infected later in life when the results of infection are more serious, and they would often develop a paralysis and even die?

DIBLE: I am acquainted with that view. But then we developed a polio vaccine, and so now the disease is very uncommon.

HUNTER: For as long as the supplies of vaccine and the facilities for administering it remain intact? (*Pause*) You know that a similar factor has been suggested to explain the high prevalence of multiple sclerosis in colder countries, and its low prevalence in hot countries [19] – except that in that case the organism is perhaps what is known as a slow virus?

DIBLE: I am aware of the theory, which is not proven.

HUNTER: But it does look as though in one or two instances there *can* be an excess of hygiene, that after a certain point it becomes counter-productive?

DIBLE: It might seem so, if one took a very narrow view.

HUNTER: You do not? (*Pause*) You do not, for instance, agree with most of the relevant experts, that the true value of screening procedures has been proved for very few conditions – even in a selected population which is at special risk, let alone the general population?[2]

DIBLE: Now you're on the side of the professional skeptics.

HUNTER: No, Professor Dible, I am merely on the side of truth. I suggest to you that, if one asks for all the conditions you yourself put forward in relation to screening to be satisfied, then most of today's screening procedures would be dropped. Screening is useless against lung cancer, is it not?[1, 20] – Because there is no truly effective treatment for early or late lung cancer: by the time it is detectable it has usually spread elsewhere in the body. Undesirable against breast cancer except for certain special groups of women? – Because of the cost of mass screening, because women will not come back again and again for testing, because for every case that is found early – and perhaps helped somewhat – there are five women who have to be given a special examination before they can be reassured that they have an innocent condition, not cancer at all?[1, 21] And then regular X-ray mammography, which is one element in the breast-cancer screening process, may even *cause* cancer in a small proportion of women years after it has been used,[22, 23] may it not? And the value of screening even for cervical cancer is not absolutely proven?[1, 24]

DIBLE: But by your own argument, which you were using just now, that is no reason for not going ahead. What about scurvy, what about cholera?

HUNTER: I did not say that in the case of cervical cancer one should not screen. My understanding is that it is one of the few conditions for which one probably should. I was stating that its value was not absolutely certain; and yet it is presented as one of the great triumphs of screening, and as an argument for extending the screening process in all kinds of directions where such an extension is quite unjustified. (*Pause*) For instance, mass screening for a mildly or moderately raised blood pressure without symptoms has been suggested, has it not?

DIBLE: Yes. High blood pressure leads to strokes and helps to lead to coronary heart disease.

HUNTER: What proportion of the United Kingdom population is

thought to have a symptomless raised blood pressure, the treatment of which would be beneficial? (*Pause*) Will you accept the figure of 10 percent of the young and middle-aged[25] – the benefit for those over 65 being very doubtful?

DIBLE: All right. That 10 percent is still a lot of people. Let me see – about 4,000,000.

HUNTER: Yes, but it is known that people having high blood pressure without symptoms will very often not persist with drug treatment[26] – which is what would be needed to keep a raised blood pressure down. And you must be aware of one recent study[27] in your own country, which showed that 75 percent of a sample population had had a blood-pressure check in the previous twelve months, and yet half the people with a raised blood pressure didn't know it was raised. (I'm rounding off the figures.) Why didn't they? – Because the doctor didn't bother to tell them. Only three out of five people who had *ever* had their blood pressures checked said they were told anything about it. One half of all the people who knew they had a raised blood pressure were taking no treatment. One quarter of those who *were* once told they had a raised blood pressure were given no treatment. Most of those who had once been a treatment but had stopped it had done so because their doctors had told them to. A later and much bigger study[28] showed that as many as one in five of Americans have a raised blood pressure, and that of those with a known raised pressure more than one in four are getting no treatment or else inadequate treatment.

DIBLE: These figures are a challenge.

HUNTER: But you do not challenge their validity? (*Dible shakes her head*) And what do you think it would cost to track down those 4,000,000 out of a young and middle-aged population in the United Kingdom of around 40,000,000? Might the money not be better spent on finding ways to *prevent* high blood pressure?

DIBLE: Such as?

HUNTER: My dear professor, if I knew, should I ask the question? But you must know – and if not, you have only to wait until tomorrow to hear about it – of the value of simple relaxation techniques in the control of a raised blood pressure. A glimmer of hope for prevention perhaps? We need a new way of life? A better prospect perhaps than that of taking the blood pressures of new-born babies? Or designating a month as 'high blood-pressure month' as you designated May 1976 here in your country? One study,[6] to which you referred earlier, reported what the blood pressures were in those 55 children out of a total of 143 admitted to the hospital concerned who had *not* had it taken on admission. Sixteen of the 55 were found to have an abnormal blood pressure, but the rise was put down to stress – to the examination and so on – in eight of the 16 – in 50 percent, that is.

DIBLE: So?

HUNTER: Does it not strike you as odd that, in the case of an abnormal finding, it should be produced as often by the search for it as possibly by some real disease in the patient? Should one laugh or cry?

DIBLE: Neither – get on with treating the patients with a genuinely abnormal blood pressure.

HUNTER: It has also been suggested – has it not? – that people with a raised blood pressure should be trained to check it regularly at home.[25] (*Dible nods*) Do you know the cost of the machines needed for this? Will you accept that it is £15 to £100?[25] (*Dible nods*) So that, if we take, say, £30 per machine as a conservative estimate, we should be asked, if this particular proposal were to be implemented, to spend at least £120 millions on the machines needed simply to check control of this one condition in the United Kingdom. That leaves out of account the cost of drugs needed for control. (*Pause*) Now as to multiphasic screening: to what proportion of the population should you like to see it applied?

DIBLE: Way back in 1970 we had 750,000 Americans in multiphasic screening programs.[9] It must be many more than that now. Ideally one would like to see it applied to entire populations.

HUNTER: If it were performed annually and applied to everyone over the age of 15 in Great Britain, it would involve 42 million people. The costs per head of various multiphasic-screening programmes have been quoted[4] as $15, $21, $30, $60, $70, $79, and $93. That was in the 1969–73 period; so that, in view of inflation, the price today could safely be put at 100 dollars per head, or about £50. Whole-population multiphasic screening in Britain would therefore cost about £2000 millions a year – every year – which is a third of the total annual cost of the National Health Service.

DIBLE: If it keeps enough people out of hospital, your NHS might save that amount.

HUNTER: But all the properly planned studies of such screening have revealed little value in it.

DIBLE: Your authority being?

HUNTER: The reference I just quoted on cost, a *Lancet* article.

DIBLE: Oh well, you're always skeptical in the older countries.

HUNTER: The view it expressed, and that I have just mentioned, was, in fact, held in a young country: the article quoted an official Australian report to that effect. It suggested also that the cost of finding a single breast abnormality by means of multiphasic screening was £170, and of finding a single abnormal cervical smear was £5000. Perhaps you will also accept that, if you carry out one laboratory test on a number of individuals – as in multiphasic screening – 95 percent of them will be considered normal; but with five tests only 77 percent are normal; and as was mentioned to Dr Batt, when 20 tests are performed only about one third of people are found to be normal.

DIBLE: Well, so long as the doctor keeps his sense of proportion, checks the abnormal results, and treats those people whose results are genuinely abnormal . . .

HUNTER: But usually he doesn't do any of those things, does he? – We established that when Dr Batt was questioned. And you may recall a study[5] of the value of multiphasic screening in some 500 families here in the US. Just over 2000 abnormalities were found, and the patients' doctors were unaware of 57 percent of them.

DIBLE: I know the paper, Mr Hunter.

HUNTER: Then you will know that in the case of only 28 percent of the abnormalities found did the patients' doctors order a retesting to confirm what had been found (and incidentally the retesting, when it *was* performed, confirmed the original finding in only 35 percent of cases). And only 15 percent of the abnormalities were treated by the doctors.

DIBLE: There are snags to be ironed out in any genuine innovation.

HUNTER: Shall we turn back to health education? Having defended your case against two objections – absence of definitive proof of causation, and infringement of liberty – I have now with some regret to say that the first objection you mentioned does have some validity to it: health education does *not* always work.[14] If you want to induce people to go and have an inoculation against poliomyelitis, say, or get mothers to take their daughters for an inoculation against German measles, then health education will work: tell people of the benefits of a simple procedure like that, and they will take some action. But if you are wanting people to alter their life-style (to give up cigarette smoking, and to take plenty of exercise instead of sitting in automobiles and in front of television sets, and to eat less sugar and animal fat), then merely pointing out the benefits of one course and the dangers of the other will not induce most people to make a change. Most adults anyway.

DIBLE: We have had some success with cigarette smoking, as just one example. You must know we have.

HUNTER: A marginal effect in the United Kingdom, mostly in the top social classes; and a somewhat bigger one here in the USA in older people; but think of the years of heavy anti-cigarette propaganda there have been.

DIBLE: I did say to the judge that one must use every possible means and get at everybody; and I would now add 'over a period'. It's been shown[29] in California that fairly heavy use of the mass media will in time have a considerable effect on people's cigarette smoking habits, and on their consumption of animal fat, and even on their blood pressures – so that their risk of coronary heart disease is reduced.

HUNTER: But the high cost of using the mass media aside, does it not strike you as curious that one should use the very means to rid people of bad habits that are used to confirm them in those habits? – I mean, of course, the advertising in the mass media of cigarettes and so on.

DIBLE: We have to operate within the established behavior pattern of our society; and hopefully in the future our health educational activities will be backed up more and more by government action. However, you cannot transform society overnight, Mr Hunter.

HUNTER: But we could do a little more than wring our hands or issue pious exhortations about health and illness – which is about all that most governments do. People are dying now of preventable disease; and new threats to health are emerging all the time; and yet . . . You are aware that in 1977 a Committee of the House of Commons issued a long report[30] on preventive medicine? It ended with 58 proposals – not at all extreme – for improving people's health; but when the British government announced[31] in a White Paper some months later just what it proposed to *do* on the basis of the report very few of the main recommendations were to be translated into government action.

DIBLE: Carefully, slowly, and surely, is the way to tackle these very large problems, Mr Hunter.

HUNTER: Here in the United States the McGovern Senate Select Committee on Nutrition and Human Needs came out, also in 1977, with recommendations for widespread nutrition education, and for more informative food labelling.[32] Not very fundamental proposals, one would think; but again there is no guarantee that your Congress or your executive will act upon them. (*Pause*) And when it comes to genuinely radical action, professor, isn't the truth that no government could or would mount a really full-scale, all-out attack against the automobile, the TV set, cigarettes, sugar, white flour, fatty foods, and so on – because it would mean an alteration in our whole life-style? Any government that tried to do that would very soon be kicked out, would it not? – Because people are used to that life-style; they want it. And government would know in advance what its own fate would be, and the fate of any radical proposals it made?

DIBLE: But earlier you were criticizing doctors for not protesting to governments about advertising for cigarettes or candy, for not demonstrating on these issues. What would be the good?

HUNTER: I would hardly call a cut in the advertising of cigarettes or candy a radical alteration of our whole life-style, professor. As I just indicated in relation to those two Committees, a government perhaps *would* get away with cuts of that kind. And I was speaking earlier within the framework of – what did you call it? – the *established* behavior pattern of our society, and saying that doctors have not done what they might reasonably have been expected to do within it. I would not expect them to demonstrate for a very radical change – I doubt the desirability or the possibility of it would ever occur to them.

DIBLE: All right then, you tell me how we're going to secure this radical change in life-style.

HUNTER: It is not for me to propound solutions. However, since you ask – perhaps a radical change in life-style will follow a complete change of heart in the people. Nothing less will match the situation, will it?

DIBLE: And just how do you get a complete change of heart in people?

HUNTER: One or two of our later witnesses may address themselves to that topic, professor, much better than I could – even if it would not be improper of me to do so. No further questions. (*Sits*)

JUDGE: If it is any consolation to you, Professor Dible – not that you have made a complete convert of him – I think Mr Hunter felt less antipathy to your approach to the problems we are discussing than to the approaches of most of the other witnesses. Thank you for being with us; and this court is now adjourned.

REFERENCES—SESSION FOURTEEN

1. Whitby, L. G., *Lancet*, October 5, 1974, p. 819.
2. Holland, W. W., *Lancet*, December 21, 1974, p. 1494.
3. Marsh, G. N., Wallace, R. B., and Whewell, J., *BMJ*, May 29, 1976, p. 1321.
4. Knox, E. G., *Lancet*, December 14, 1974, p. 1434.
5. Olsen, D. M., Kane, R. L., and Procter, P. H., *NEJM*, April 22, 1976, p. 925.
6. Pazdral, P. T., et al., *JAMA*, May 24, 1976, p. 2320.
7. Medical News, *JAMA*, February 23, 1976, p. 785.
8. De Swiet, M., Fayers, P., and Shinebourne, E. A., *BMJ*, July 3, 1976, p. 9.
9. Howe, H. F., *JAMA*, February 14, 1972, p. 885.
10. *Prevention and Health : Everybody's Business*, Department of Health and Social Security, HMSO, London, 1976.
11. Editorial, *NEJM*, August 22, 1974, p. 415.

12. White, L. S., *NEJM*, October 9, 1975, p. 773.
13. Bluestone, N., *NEJM*, July 17, 1975, p. 148.
14. Meade, T. W., *Lancet*, November 29, 1975, p. 1053.
15. Meenan, R. F., *NEJM*, January 1, 1976, p. 45.
16. Harnes, J. R., *JAMA*, January 12, 1976, p. 157.
17. Wright, P., *The Times*, July 19, 1976, p. 1.
18. Medical News, *JAMA*, April 5, 1976, p. 1409.
19. Dean, G., *et al.*, *BMJ*, April 10, 1976, p. 861.
20. Colley, J. R. T., *Lancet*, November 9, 1974, p. 1125.
21. Irwig, L. M., *Lancet*, November 30, 1974, p. 1307.
22. Thier, S. O., *NEJM*, November 10, 1977, p. 1063.
23. Swartz, H. M., and Reichling, B. A., *JAMA*, March 7, 1977, p. 965.
24. Randall, K. J., *Lancet*, November 30, 1974, p. 1303.
25. Orme, M., *Prescribers' Journal*, April 1976, p. 31.
26. Sackett, D. L., *Lancet*, November 16, 1974, p. 1189.
27. Editorial, *NEJM*, December 20, 1973, p. 1369.
28. Stamler, J., *et al.*, *JAMA*, May 24, 1976, p. 2299.
29. Farquhar, J. W., *et al.*, *Lancet*, June 4, 1977, p. 1192.
30. First Report from the Expenditure Committee, *Preventive Medicine*, HMSO, London, 1977.
31. Department of Health and Social Security, Department of Education and Science, Scottish Office, Welsh Office, *Prevention and Health*, HMSO, London, 1977.
32. Select Committee on Nutrition and Human Needs, United States Senate, *Dietary Goals for the United States*, US Government Printing Office, Washington, 1977.

Screening and Treatment for Various Disease Risk Factors

Bailey, A., *Lancet*, December 14, 1974, p. 1436.
Editorial, *Lancet*, February 1, 1975, p. 259.
Anon., *JAMA*, February 23, 1976, p. 825.
Moser, M., and Wood, D., *JAMA*, May 24, 1976, p. 2297.
Levy, R. I., *JAMA*, May 24, 1976, p. 2334.

Life-Style Modification

Charrette, E. E., *NEJM*, March 25, 1976, p. 732. (The first of three letters in this issue of the journal, two critical of, and one favourable to the thesis concerning attempts to alter people's life-styles being an infringement of liberty, advanced in reference 15.)
Bradshaw, S., *BMJ*, February 10, 1973, p. 349.

ALTERNATIVE MEDICINE

Enter Dr Henry Spring

JUDGE: You are Dr Henry Spring? You are fully qualified in orthodox medicine? After nearly 30 years spent in the teaching of physiology to medical students you suddenly retired to devote yourself wholly to what is often called alternative medicine, which had interested you for many years? You are English? You have lived all your life in England?

SPRING: Oh, well, yes, you see, and at the same time, no. I mean only 21 years in teaching.

JUDGE: And what made you, a well-qualified allopathic doctor, turn to practices, most of which a majority of your colleagues despise?

SPRING: Well, again, it is not quite as simple as that. Some of them they do despise. They have no time for copper rings and radionics – you know, black boxes – and neither, I think, have I; or apple cider vinegar and honey, and neither have I most certainly. But they also despise the use of radiesthesia, which I do not; and Lakhovsky's oscillatory coils, and I am not so sure. After all, there is oscillation, isn't there? – I oscillate, you oscillate.

JUDGE: I hadn't noticed it, doctor.

SPRING: And then there are aspects of which they are more tolerant, though with varying degrees of skepticism: such as health foods, or herbal therapy, or special kinds of diet, or osteopathy, or faith healing. Now about all these I am less skeptical than my professional brethren. And let us remember that here in America osteopathy is officially recognized by orthodox medicine:[1] it has its own osteopathic physicians practicing side by side with allopathic physicians – ordinary doctors, that is. Osteopathy in America involves manipulation of various parts of the body; but chiropractic too – manipulating the spine, you know – is halfway to recognition here in the United States. It is recognized in all the individual states,[2] if not yet by the doctors; and chiropractic treatment is available under the government health schemes.[3] It seems chiropractic treatment includes attention to psychosocial factors in disease, to what the patients want,[4, 5] and is coming to be accepted by orthodox medical men.[4]

JUDGE: And are there some alternatives the doctors have accepted more or less completely?

SPRING: Oh, yes – relaxation techniques and yoga and transcendental meditation, all for control of a raised blood pressure; and hypnosis, and fasting for certain purposes, and homeopathy to quite an extent, and acupuncture[6] – all of them are now quite respectable. Acupuncture has been demonstrated at a British Medical Association annual scientific meeting[7] – you can't get more respectable than that, apart from being dead. There are a few skeptics in the profession still, but then there are some skeptics about most aspects even of orthodox medicine today; and there are just about as many people who are really enthusiastic about acupuncture and so on.

JUDGE: And yet acupuncture was more or less scorned by orthodox medicine only 10 years or so ago?

SPRING: It was, it was; and then all of a sudden we had a flood of people from the United States and our own and other countries visiting China, and coming back and saying it worked – they'd seen it work, they'd seen conscious patients undergoing operations with the help of acupuncture anesthesia. Some of them have sedative drugs, mind you, and some of them have pain-relieving drugs,[8] as well as the acupuncture; but many of the doctors who've seen it work are experts and were very skeptical beforehand. Isn't effective for everybody, mind you, and perhaps there's an element of suggestion in it, and in China everyone works together, everyone has confidence in everyone else, and there's premarital chastity. Of course, if you have confidence . . . Still, very remarkable.

JUDGE: Does anyone know how it works, doctor?

SPRING: No, judge, not for certain. Thank goodness, I say. If we start looking too closely, perhaps it will vanish before our eyes. That's the trouble with the conventional doctors. They always say, 'How does it work?' but often there isn't any neat little answer, complete with a diagram showing arrows pointing in all directions. Something simply works,[9] it's . . . it's like asking how a seed germinates. We don't *really* know how it does. We say we do. We know one or two things we can see and measure, but we don't know what goes on in the soul of a seed, do we?

JUDGE: I do not, doctor. But now control of a raised blood pressure, which you mentioned.

SPRING: Yes, you can get people to control it by teaching them how to relax properly: just simple relaxation will do,[10, 11] or you can use yoga,[12, 13, 14, 15] or transcendental meditation.[16] Some people have used what's called biofeedback, especially with yoga, to achieve control, either feedback of the blood pressure[15] or of the degree of relaxation.[12, 14]

JUDGE: Biofeedback, doctor, means what, in simple terms?

SPRING: Yes, well, in simple terms, judge, it simply means[17, 18, 19] letting the patient know – by means of a light or the pitch of a note, something of that kind – how the thing in his body that he's being trained to control is varying: usually some bodily function he's not normally conscious of. All it needs is one or two machines. For instance, while he's just lying down, perhaps trying to relax, he 'listens', in a manner of speaking, to his blood pressure, to a sound that is controlled by the level of it; and as the pressure's always going up or down a little, he soon discovers what things in him, if you follow me, make it go down and what things in him make it go up – and so he learns how, more or less, to make it go down or come up as he pleases, consciously. Biofeedback for the relaxation methods uses a recording of the skin resistance[12] – the more you relax the less you sweat, and so the greater your skin resistance to the passage of an electrical current – or else it uses a recording of actual muscle tension.[14] Mind you, simply teaching a person how to relax properly will bring down the blood pressure whether or not he gets any biofeedback – which simply makes it all a bit easier or quicker. Relaxing doesn't involve conscious control of the blood pressure, of course – it's unconscious. It's been shown that, when the blood pressure is brought down by meditation and relaxation, there are certain real biochemical changes occurring in the body too.[20] It's an absolutely genuine effect, in other words, by allopathic standards: it's been scientifically proved to occur; control patients were used, and so on and so forth. Perhaps it'll work only in early cases of high blood pressure.[21] Still, even that's an enormous advance.

JUDGE: And can this biofeedback technique be applied to many bodily functions?

SPRING: It has been, judge. Pulse rate,[18] electrical waves from the brain,[17, 18] undesirable extra heart beats,[22] some headaches,[17, 18, 19] all kinds of things can be controlled.[23] Biofeedback itself simply supplies information, of course: there must be *some* kind of reward as well – usually the patient probably gets satisfaction from learning to do a kind of trick with his body that he or the doctor wants him to learn to do. It is really a form of the behavioral therapy Dr McGilly was asked about the other day, the operant conditioning. But to have organic physical diseases that are normally treated with powerful drugs – to have them treated in this way is really, I think, a very great step forward to a new type of medicine, perhaps almost to a new way of life which Mr Hunter mentioned yesterday.

JUDGE: And now, what of the alternative medical approaches about which doctors are a shade dubious?

SPRING: Well, there are special diets, for instance, or health foods, or herbal remedies. Doctors prescribe diets often enough, or fasting – sometimes irrationally, if I may say – but they do seem to get hot under the collar if people put themselves on something like a macrobiotic diet or a Bircher-muesli diet. Oh, there are many diets. Mostly they go in for whole grains, and beans and lentils and brown rice, and fruit and vegetables and nuts, and no meat or sugar – that kind of thing. Does people no harm for a change, I'd say, at the worst.

JUDGE: Is there not a danger, doctor, that someone who is ignorant of dietetics might conceivably do himself a mischief by going too far with this kind of thing?

SPRING: Well, I think – if you'll forgive me, judge – the doctors have been at you. There's always a danger if you get a real crank, of course; but after what we've heard in the last couple of weeks about fats and sugar and white flour and cholesterol, the danger's pretty small relatively. And as for herbs: well, I ask you – where did digitalis come from? – Foxgloves. Where did aspirin come from? – The willow treee really. Where did penicillin come from? – Moulds. Where did opium come from? – The poppy. I mean I could go on for ever.

JUDGE: We won't put you to the test, doctor.

SPRING: But that list shows what medicine today is all about. Mr Hunter's said it's fissiparous, and it is. It gets hold of a perfectly good herb, and chops it up, and boils it, and distils it, and separates this from it, and extracts that from it . . . Well, you never know, perhaps there's something in the *whole* herb that's good for you [24] the way there's something in the whole wheat grain that's good for you. The *spirit* of the thing, the *élan vital.*

JUDGE: But even in the field of herbal remedies, doctor, you choose with discrimination?

SPRING: Oh, with great discrimination, I hope. I wouldn't be here today if I hadn't, would I? – I mean if you'd seen some of the things I've been offered, and not just in the way of herbal concoctions. I remember one one occasion I was given some blackeye beans and roast buckwheat – for yang, of course – and sprouting sunflower seeds, all with yoghurt and honey *and* a seaweed dressing on top. I said 'No'. I like seaweed. Don't misunderstand me. But not with all that yang.

JUDGE: Can you tell me, doctor, why you have such faith in this type of medicine as an alternative or a supplement to the orthodox kind?

SPRING: Well, because it works, you see, and very often when allopathic doctors have failed. I've seen it again and again, especially in chronic conditions. Obviously we couldn't manage without the allopaths; but let us have the homeopaths as well, and the osteopaths, and the ayuvedic remedies, and . . . and – well, everything else as well. I want people to be happy. When I was quite young there was a song 'I want to be happy, but I can't be happy if I can't make you happy too'. I've never forgotten it.

JUDGE: And you feel this leavening of the strong dough of orthodox medicine will remedy the defects in it that we have heard about in the past fortnight? (*Spring nods*) Mr Hunter?

HUNTER: (*rising*): Dr Spring: alchemy, anthroposophicalism, Bach's flower remedies, color healing, cupping, gravitonics, jewel therapy, moxibustion, naturopathy, phrenology, Reichian therapy, spiritual healing, telepathy, and water therapy – of the Kneipp, or Priessnitz, or ordinary spa kind: which of these, not to mention the other fifteen or twenty forms of alternative medicine you have yourself spoken about – which of them does one favor in the event that one falls ill? You agree one cannot apply forty or fifty *different* modes of treatment simultaneously?

SPRING: Oh, of course not. Some of those you mention I would never use. But of those I would use: sometimes one suits, sometimes another. You use whichever works, whichever happens to suit.

HUNTER: I put it to you that a lot of the attraction of these alternative forms of therapy is that people either understand fully how they work – or think they do, which is effectively the same thing – or else believe there is some mystery involved, in which they have enormous faith.

SPRING: I completely agree. That's what I just said. Or I meant to. An osteopath, for instance – a chiropractor, as he is called here in America – explains to his patient just which bit of his vertebral column is wrong, and just how it's causing symptoms, and just what he's going to do about it. (Mind you, he's often got a lot of manual skill too, far more than most doctors.) But with radiesthesia, say, it's pure faith that's involved.

HUNTER: And this attraction of alternative forms of therapy springs from the fact that allopathic medicine has destroyed mystery? – I do not mean that all patients of the allopathic doctor normally understand what is done to them and why, or that the doctor himself even bothers usually to try and explain, even if he understands himself. I mean that the patients have been led to believe that *somebody* – the family doctor, or the specialist, or the professor – somebody somewhere *does* understand it all, every last bit of it; and the patient could too if only he had enough time and intelligence to absorb the knowledge. He *doesn't* usually know, but he believes there's a package of complete rational knowledge just waiting to be opened by anyone who's quick enough with his mental fingers. It's all rational, all the mystery has been destroyed by the test-tube and the X-ray machine and the computer. There is no mystery to believe in, neither is there in most cases any true knowledge to rely on.

SPRING: I completely and absolutely agree.

HUNTER: On the other hand, if the patient really *does* understand, or thinks he understands, or if he has faith in some mysterious power – whichever it is, he will have confidence in the situation, will he not? He will feel he has, either in himself or from this mysterious power, the ability to get well? He does not feel helplessly dependent, puzzled, lost, as he very often does with the allopathic doctor?

SPRING: Yes, splendid.

HUNTER: But this situation is ripe for exploitation by any quack or cheap-jack cure-all who is cunning and glib enough?

SPRING: Oh, yes, I absolutely agree.

JUDGE: You are aware of what you are saying, doctor?

SPRING: Oh, yes, judge. There are plenty of quacks in this field. Fewer than you'd expect, though still plenty. But most of the alternative medicine healers aren't cunning enough to be charlatans. And anyway, why should they want to be? They believe in what they're doing: that's good enough for them. They're happy. They make other people happy. But there are quite a few charlatans.

HUNTER: So many that, whatever good there might be in this or that corner of the field, the whole of alternative medicine is suspect?

SPRING: No, there I would not agree with you.

HUNTER: Then let us consider certain elements that you felt were defensible. You implied you believed in radiesthesia. Correct me if I am wrong. Basically radiesthesia is a kind of dowsing for disease. Some practitioners even use a hazel twig, though most of them use a weight on the end of a string or thread – a pendulum, in other words. The theory is that the twig or pendulum moves in response to some kind of 'vibration' set up in the practitioner holding it, the 'vibration' being determined by the condition of the person who is being examined. There are many different types of movement, some practitioners hold the pendulum over a ruler, others make use of colored discs, and so on. The practitioner doesn't pretend to know how he does it, but he comes out with a kind of 'health profile' of the patient.

SPRING: A very reasonable description, Mr Hunter.

HUNTER: I put it to you that to any sensible being this is a lot of nonsense; and, even if there were some validity to it on occasion, it is clearly open to exploitation by the unscrupulous or even the hopeful ignorant.

SPRING: I accept that it might be exploited, but not that it is nonsense. It works, you see. Remember the psychosomatic disorders, Mr Hunter, about which you quizzed Mr Buck. Well, if the mind can affect the body and produce physical disease, why can't a physical disease affect the mind – someone else's mind? (*Pause*) You've no answer to that now, have you? (*Pause*) There, you see. It's the same with food allergies – we simply don't know what they mightn't be responsible for in the way of disease.

HUNTER: The same could be said of influences from outer space, could it not? Now health foods, doctor, for which you also had some kind words. As you rightly pointed out, much of our food today is not conducive to health, but that does not mean everything somebody chooses to label 'health food' will necessarily confer health.

SPRING: Oh, no, naturally it doesn't.

HUNTER: All it means is that the food carries that label? (*Pause*) It has been shown – has it not? – that some so-called compost-grown foods were not compost-grown at all, and neither were some free-range eggs laid by free-range hens. (*Spring nods*) They carried a label, that was all, and a premium price; otherwise they were identical with what could be bought more cheaply in the ordinary grocer's up the road?

SPRING: Yes, yes, I don't deny it.

HUNTER: And in fact, there is really no special virtue to compost-grown food as such, is there? – The benefit of using compost is mainly to the soil, and only in a minor degree to the crop it carries?

SPRING: With the greatest respect, Mr Hunter, I think you are now falling into the scientists' trap; and you have shown such insight into them otherwise. There may well be, and I believe there certainly is, something superior in compost-grown food; but it savors of that mystery you were talking about just now in connection with alternative medicine, and scientists will have nothing to do with mystery. They analyze the food, and say it's just the same, however it's grown, when what they should say is that they haven't yet devised – and maybe they never will devise, and I hope and believe they won't – an instrument to show the difference. That doesn't mean there isn't one, though. Oh, there's a lot of silly, half-baked science talked by the compost-grown, whole-food people. And they go on about pesticides and preservatives, many of which turn out to be quite harmless. And oh, yes, there are people profiteering from other people's gullibility. Not everything that's called 'fresh' is fresh, and not everything that's raw is good. But it is a bit deeper than that. There is something in it, I think. I may be wrong. Try a battery egg, then a free-range egg.

HUNTER: Let us instead move on to herbs, for which you also had a kind word. Aniseed, basil, chervil, dill, and mint have all been recommended as aphrodisiacs?

SPRING: I could give you a list of hundreds of things that have been called aphrodisiacs, from oysters to powdered rhinoceros horn.

HUNTER: And balm, basil, bergamot, catmint, chamomile, lemon verbena, and southernwood are all sedatives. What on earth do we need barbiturates and tranquilizers for?

SPRING: Lettuce too. Lettuce is a soporific.[24] I don't think any of those herbs are strong sedatives in the scientific sense, Mr Hunter. Mild sedatives perhaps, two or three of them. But I think if somebody takes one of them and thinks it *will* act as a sedative, then as often as not it will.

HUNTER: Now *you* are being very scientific, doctor. I wonder, therefore, if you will accept all the claims that have been made for sage, the herb we use in stuffing – that it is good for asthma, for the blood, for colds, colic, indigestion, coughs, as a gargle, for headaches, for the kidneys, the liver, and for rheumatism, as well as making a good cosmetic vapor, and a stimulant for hair growth.

SPRING: No, but it does have a nice smell, doesn't it? – I love sage.

HUNTER: To turn from nice smells back to the practitioners of alternative medicine, Dr Spring: I put it to you that, purely as practitioners, they owe much of their success, like the physician assistants we discussed with Dr Roylance the other day, to the fact that most allopathic doctors have distanced themselves from the patient, and simply don't understand and don't want to have to deal with the important psychosocial factors that often underlie an illness; and so when somebody comes along who does show some genuine interest, or what appears to be genuine interest, who doesn't say to the patient, 'You can't be ill because I've done all the tests and they're all normal,' and who offers to do *something* – it doesn't much matter what it is – then the patient is very impressed, and tells his friends, and so it goes on. Interest (or seeming interest) from the practitioner himself plus the mystery or knowledge (or seeming knowledge) of the procedure that I mentioned earlier – it is these that do the trick.

SPRING: Absolutely right. Mind you, I don't like that word, 'trick'.

HUNTER: But all of these people face, or soon will face, the same temptations as the physician assistants. Is that not so? – They will want to become as important as doctors, and to be paid like doctors, and to be recognized like doctors; have their own colleges and diplomas and annual conventions. They've started already, have they not? (*Spring nods repeatedly*) They will become institution-alized, in other words, just as the doctors have been – fossilized, inflexible, narrow.

SPRING: I pray not.

HUNTER: You mentioned that osteopaths are now accepted on level terms with allopathic doctors here in the States, and chiropractors are moving up the scale. Is it not a fact that the educational standards for entry into colleges of chiropractic in the United States are now quite high? – Often of university-degree standard?[2]

SPRING: That is true. I regret it.

HUNTER: And you yourself were obviously very proud of the fact that the value of relaxation techniques and of biofeedback in controlling blood pressure had been scientifically proved. The alternative medicine people – even those who are accepted by orthodox medicine – do hanker after *complete* scientific respectability, do they not?

SPRING: Yes, yes, I suppose we do all get bitten by the same bug; but that doesn't mean we must give up hope. I think it's just that we want everyone to be happy.

HUNTER: I put it to you finally that none of the many varieties of alternative medicine that have been mentioned have deep cultural roots in our society. All are revivals or new developments that have appeared, not because of any intrinsic virtue of their own, but because of the defects of high-technology medicine. They have no roots in our culture, and they will bear no worthwhile permanent fruits. They represent a cry of despair, mostly from cranks, not a shout of hope from the ordinary people.

SPRING: There is a measure of truth in what you say, Mr Hunter. I am a bit of a crank, yes. Not a full measure, I hope. However, having started, one has to go on in whatever seems the most promising direction, and that is how alternative medicine looked to me – and still looks to me.

HUNTER: Thank you, doctor. No further questions. (*Sits*)

JUDGE: Thank you, Dr Spring, for a most civilized testimony; and congratulations on very skilfully keeping Mr Hunter's ire at bay. The court is adjourned.

REFERENCES—SESSION FIFTEEN

1. 'Medical Education in the United States 1974–1975', *JAMA*, December 29, 1975, p. 1360.
2. Gibbons, R. W., *NEJM*, February 5, 1976, p. 344.
3. Editorial, *NEJM*, September 25, 1975, p. 662.
4. Firman, G. J., and Goldstein, M. S., *NEJM*, September 25, 1975, p. 639.

5. Rothenberg, R. C., *NEJM*, February 5, 1976, p. 345.
6. Bull, G. M., *Lancet*, August 25, 1973, p. 417.
7. 'Drug Treatment of Pain, How Others Do It', *BMJ*, August 3, 1974, p. 325.
8. Wall, P. D., *New Scientist*, October 3, 1974, p. 31.
9. Editorial, *NEJM*, August 21, 1975, p. 401.
10. Benson, H., *et al.*, *Lancet*, February 23, 1974, p. 289.
11. Benson, H., *NEJM*, May 19, 1977, p. 1152.
12. Patel, C. H., *Lancet*, November 10, 1973, p. 1053.
13. Patel, C., *Lancet*, January 11, 1975, p. 62.
14. Patel, C., and North, W. R. S., *Lancet*, July 19, 1975, p. 93.
15. Editorial, *Lancet*, May 31, 1975, p. 1230.
16. Blackwell, B., *et al.*, *Lancet*, January 31, 1976, p. 223.
17. Editorial, *NEJM*, March 21, 1974, p. 684.
18. Leading Article, *BMJ*, August 17, 1974, p. 427.
19. Segal, J., *JAMA*, April 14, 1975, p. 179.
20. Stone, R. A., and De Leo, J., *NEJM*, January 8, 1976, p. 80.
21. Editorial, *NEJM*, January 8, 1976, p. 107.
22. Benson, H., Alexander, S., and Feldman, C. L., *Lancet*, August 30, 1975, p. 380.
23. Miller, N. E., and Dworkin, B. R., *NEJM*, June 2, 1977, p. 1274.
24. Smith, A., *The Times*, October 13, 1976, p. 12.

General Reading
Law, D., *A Guide to Alternative Medicine*, Turnstone Books, London, 1974. (A simple panoramic guide to the whole field, strong in faith but not in science.)
The Catonsville Roadrunner, January 1975, p. 4–21 (Health Issue), 28 Brundretts Road, Manchester 21, England.
The Book of London, Time Out, London, 1973.
Alternative London, 4th edn, Nicholas Saunders and Wildwood House, London, 1974.
Alternative England and Wales, Nicholas Saunders, London, 1975.
(The last three references are not wholly or mainly concerned with alternative medicine. They do, however, contain the kind of information on it that is commonly available to young people, the group for which it has the greatest appeal in our society. The information is not especially authoritative, nor do these books claim it to be. However, if they are consulted under such heads as 'Acupuncture', 'Food', 'Health Food Shops', 'Herbalism', 'Herbal Medicine', 'Therapy', and 'Yoga', some knowledge and understanding of the alternative-medicine scene in the United Kingdom will be gained. They are very different in character from almost all the other references in this book—though no judgment of any kind is implied.)

Behavioral Therapy
Editorial, *JAMA*, May 8, 1972, p. 852.
Leading Article, *BMJ*, May 27, 1972, p. 478.
Editorial, *Lancet*, November 4, 1972, p. 962.
Editorial, *Lancet*, June 9, 1973, p. 1295.
Editorial, *NEJM*, March 21, 1974, p. 684.
Editorial, *JAMA*, April 15, 1974, p. 344.
Pomerleau, O., Bass, F., and Crown, V., *NEJM*, June 12, 1975, p. 1277.

SELF CARE

Enter Dr Stephen Blaik

JUDGE: You are Dr Stephen Blaik, you are aged 27, and you work in a part-time capacity in family practice in England?

BLAIK: Yes, to make enough money to live on.

JUDGE: And will you tell us what you do with the rest of your time?

BLAIK: I help, as unobtrusively as possible, in the provision of a health coloring to two community centers in England.

JUDGE: Unobtrusively? – Were you not instrumental in starting this operation?

BLAIK: In a sense. In another sense I think it arose merely as a response to a need that was already there in people. If I hadn't provided it, someone else would have in time. In any case, it's not meant to be an ego trip for me: the essence of it is that ordinary people shall as far as possible find out for themselves how to maintain their health, and how to deal with minor sickness or injury, and know when to see a doctor – which shouldn't be very often.

JUDGE: And this is because?

BLAIK: From my viewpoint – because I share most of the misgivings Mr Hunter has expressed or elicited from various doctor witnesses about the way modern medicine has developed. I see the crucial fault being the size, the centralization, the government connections of medicine – hence my work in a relatively small community; and the taking away from people the power and opportunity to find out for themselves and make their own decisions in the health field.

JUDGE: You see faults of this kind elsewhere?

BLAIK: Yes, in half a dozen fields – education, housing, transport, entertainment, welfare money, overseas aid . . . And always the result is the same: after a certain point people get less of the commodity the particular institution is meant to provide – less health, less truly useful knowledge (as distinct from a small encyclopedia in their heads), less relaxation and catharsis from the entertainment, less true benefit from the welfare money or the aid; and always – this is the crucial item – there is less of their own initiative. The institutions become huge and self-serving, they aggrandize themselves by feeding people all the time with a bigger and bigger spoon, which contains less of what is truly valuable, of what is needed.

JUDGE: So the people are to do it for themselves?

BLAIK: Yes. Above all, they must make their own decisions. Most people hate that, unless they are used to it. They like someone to make decisions for them. They have to be weaned very gradually from their dependence. I cannot stress too strongly that, in my view, this is the crucial point – crucial to the whole organization of our western societies, not just of medicine. People want to escape both the hard thinking needed before one takes a decision and the leap of faith that the actual taking of a decision always is. Our whole society is geared to the avoidance of the need for individual decision. Everything must be programed, everything foreseeable, everything certain and secure – and life means insecurity. Life means sickness, life means ignorance and remedies for it, life means responding to difficulties – with decisions and consequent actions; life means death and the decision involved in that. I cannot stress this point about decision-taking too strongly – I think it is the key to everything the court has been hearing about.

JUDGE: I understand; but now as to other elements in your thinking?

BLAIK: I feel we need less science and technology, of course, and also a less materialistic outlook, less avarice, greater concern for others, an acceptance – a glad acceptance – of what today would seem to some people near-poverty.

JUDGE: Why?

BLAIK: For two reasons. First, because our present selfish, materialistic outlook clearly does not make for happiness, for true health. Second, because equally clearly it results in damage to the environment, the using up of resources at a rate the world cannot sustain, pollution, and alienation – in huge factories, in relation to nature, in relation to one's fellow man.

JUDGE: This seems a long way from health, doctor.

BLAIK: No, you cannot separate health from the rest of life. Health comes from healthy living, it is a byproduct of a healthy society, not something separate, to be bought, sold, acquired.

JUDGE: And how is a healthy society recognizable?

BLAIK: In the same way as we recognize a healthy person. In the case of a society the best guide comes, I think, from its cultural artefacts – its architecture, its mode of agriculture, its paintings and plays and poetry, its machines, the clothes its people wear, its landscapes, its total atmosphere.

JUDGE: Our western society is unhealthy, judged by these criteria?

BLAIK: Profoundly unhealthy if you think of a typical factory, of Concorde, of motorways, of plastics, of the ridiculous fashions in clothes, changing wastefully every six months, of its energy-intensive factory farming, of most of its art; and of its atmosphere of alienation and violence and greed.

JUDGE: And so you favor restraint and smallness?

BLAIK: And an appropriate technology, a human technology, not this unrestrained religion of scientism that has added over-population to all our other troubles. We must not judge health by length of life merely, by its quantity, but by its quality also; and, of course, the quality of life, like almost everything else that matters greatly to human beings – love, compassion, friendship, brother-liness – the *quality* of life is not quantifiable. You cannot measure how much a person loves you. That is why – you said it yourself, judge, earlier and rather differently – why science and life are fundamentally at cross-purposes. I mean 'fundamentally'. Too much science, too much calm objectivity kills life, it must kill life. That is why it has to be restrained.

JUDGE: And now will you tell us something about the health coloring to these community centers in England?

BLAIK: Yes, it *is* a coloring only. It isn't something set aside, separate from all the rest. Each of the centers involved serves about five thousand people, and there are all kinds of facilities in them – for meetings, and games, and meals, baby-minding, quiet rooms, and so on. In one of the quiet rooms we have a small library on health matters: books, pamphlets, cassettes, filmstrips – that kind of thing – and people know by now that they can go there and try to find out for themselves whatever they may want to know.

JUDGE: And if they can't?

BLAIK: There's an ex-nurse, a woman, there who has a small office in one part of the building. She doesn't tell people what to do, but she suggests where they might look if they can't find some information they need; and now and again she'll nudge people into going to see their doctors.

JUDGE: You don't disapprove totally of modern medicine then, doctor?

BLAIK: Not at all. Obviously, as has been said already, if you have a bad injury, or a sudden very severe pain, or a difficult childbirth, or a severe fever, and you want a remedy, you should be in the care of the best doctor you can find – even though perhaps preven-tion would sometimes have been possible. If this nurse senses a person has some complaint that he or she really can't manage alone or with the help of a group, she suggests a visit to the doctor.

JUDGE: Group?

BLAIK: Yes, almost the most important element to the health coloring is that in the center people get to know one another and one another's difficulties during their ordinary social activities together; and those people with common problems – of being overweight, say, or wanting to give up cigarettes, or who have marital or work problems – are encouraged to form small groups of eight or ten people. The groups meet in the homes of members in sequence, and have discussions, exercises, confessional sessions, free-wheeling debates, meals, and so on – whatever they feel, after looking at the relevant information, is appropriate. Even doctors accept that most successful group or community health endeavors are lay-inspired or largely lay-managed. Alcoholics Anonymous, the Samaritans, psychoprophylaxis for childbirth, and so on. Even the religious charismatic groups.

JUDGE: And experts are not used at all?

BLAIK: The people who use the center are free to *ask* experts – doctors or psychologists or what-have-you – to come along and give a talk; and the groups can do the same, or even ask the expert to attend a series of meetings of a group. But *they*'re in charge, not the expert; and we find the groups don't use outside experts much, in fact.

JUDGE: You don't encourage them to?

BLAIK: I used it just now myself, but I don't think 'encourage' is the right word; or 'discourage'. They sound too paternalistic. I'm just a member of the centers, and happen to have a little specialized knowledge the other members can utilize if they wish; and – I don't know how to put this – I try by example, by silence, by establishing rapport, to help them and myself towards the right total situation out of which health will emerge.

JUDGE: And do you mean that these people look, and are, obviously healthy?

BLAIK: No, not too obviously. Health includes sickness, by definition, the way a painting can't be all black or all white. I mean they deal with life healthily, whether it happens to be pleasant or unpleasant.

JUDGE: Any other important aspects to this community-center effort, doctor?

BLAIK: Yes, just two I'd like to mention. We have some young people with jobs in the community, to whom I've given a quick course in hygiene, first aid, and so on, who act as eyes and ears – as well as helping hands – to the health scene outside.

JUDGE: Barefoot doctors?

BLAIK: Yes, a kind of imitation of them anyway. They keep an eye out to see if some group isn't being very successful, or some district in the community area seems very inactive.

JUDGE: And the second item?

BLAIK: Is that we've tried to stay on good terms with all the local doctors, and have succeeded so far, though we will not have clinics of any kind at the centers; and when the doctors do come they come by invitation and are treated pretty well the same as everyone else.

JUDGE: You have officials in connection with the health work at the centers?

BLAIK: Yes, though – forgive me – 'officials' is the wrong word. Various helpers, functionaries. And we have a change-around every few months.

JUDGE: To prevent people getting stale? (*Blaik nods*) And what do you call this medical presence in the community centers, doctor?

BLAIK: We don't have a name for it. We agreed on that. Giving a thing a name restricts it, makes it rigid, fossilizes it very often. We prefer to do rather than to say.

JUDGE: Mr Hunter?

HUNTER (*rising*): This may be a novel and well-intentioned development, doctor, but I query whether it is fruitful.

BLAIK: If you mean what evidence, measured evidence, have we of its effectiveness, the answer is 'none'. We have deliberately avoided trying to quantify any benefits. I said: those things in life that are most worthwhile are not quantifiable.

HUNTER: None the less, doctor, I thought I detected in your voice a hint of uncertainty as to whether what you have described does indeed represent the right path.

BLAIK: Yes, that is the case.

HUNTER: You think it won't succeed? Or perhaps wouldn't if applied on a large scale? – By means of the thousands of such centers that would be needed to serve the whole of England and Wales, say?

BLAIK: I don't know. I simply don't know. It's not the size of the total operation that worries me – so long as we stick to small autonomous units. It's whether this gradual, bit-by-bit approach is the right one – in the health and other community fields. The method's applicable to more than health. Obviously we could create new centers only slowly; and while we're doing that we might lose from one hand what we gain with the other. To put it in another way: I'm making a living out of conventional medicine, and yet doing this on the side. There's a contradiction. Conventional medicine and all that goes with it may increase their power faster than the centers could start to take effect.

HUNTER: The alternative to gradualism being? – Revolution?

BLAIK: Yes, widespread radical action, perhaps sparked off by a catastrophe of some kind, some ecological disaster, a major accident at a nuclear-energy power station, a new man-made disease. Various happenings might spark it off. And, you see, what is really being asked for in connection with these centers – beyond the health sphere, I mean – is a complete upturn in human nature; not merely being content with less, with a greater simplicity – though that's a big part of it – but, as I said, a constant preparedness to put other people before oneself.

HUNTER: And you are doubtful that this can be achieved?

BLAIK: Sometimes doubtful, sometimes hopeful.

HUNTER: You are suggesting an idealistic communist approach?

BLAIK: Yes, I suppose so. But not on the Russian model. All that the Russians do is to distribute the materialistic cake differently, among more people; they have no doubts that it's more cake that is needed. However it's distributed, there's a limit to the amount of cake that can be provided – because the cake comes from the earth, which is in every sense finite, as man is. Man on earth, I mean.

HUNTER: The Chinese model would be more accurate perhaps?

BLAIK: Yes and no. The spirit – yes, perhaps. But the details? – They have such a different culture, such a very different history and background from our own, their whole attitude to life is so different that I doubt the comparison is useful.

HUNTER: Do you think, if your present approach proves not to be feasible, that this revolution will come, and that, if it does, it will succeed?

BLAIK: I think that probably it will not come, not soon enough; or if it comes, that it will be in time corrupted, as all revolutions are in the end.

HUNTER: And in either event, what *then* will happen?

BLAIK: I think man will be finished. I think he will finish himself. He has the means. You can never destroy the various means, or at any rate the knowledge of how to produce them. If you did, man would soon acquire it again. So either you change men or man will destroy himself.

HUNTER: You mean thermonuclear war?

BLAIK: Yes, or any of the things I mentioned as possible sparks to a revolution, only bigger. Total death by mutant viruses; or by an irretrievable interference with the ecosphere. There are half a dozen ways in which it could happen. This is a unique feature of our time, and many people do not realize it: that for the first time in all of recorded history man has the power to wipe himself out. Genghis Khan, Attila, Hitler – none of these could destroy more than a few hundreds of thousands, or millions of people; perhaps tens of millions. They could not have destroyed all of mankind, all life. We can. It is like the main killing diseases we have: we are the first people in history, we of the west, to know pretty well what factors produce some of our main killing diseases, and yet do nothing or very little about getting rid of them. That is unique: the knowledge with the inaction.

HUNTER: You are saying that the uniqueness in these two spheres is not a coincidence?

BLAIK: I am saying modern western man is a new kind of creature. So much has appeared in the last 20 or 30 years that is unique, so much has altered radically that I think we are at a cross-roads.

HUNTER: Or the end of a cul-de-sac?

BLAIK: Yes, probably the latter.

HUNTER: You are very pessimistic, doctor.

BLAIK: No. Truthful. At least let us die – let some of us die – aware of the truth about ourselves, aware of our evil intentions, of our overweening greed and ambitions, of our guilt. We shouldn't die whispering lies to ourselves about why we're dying: we shall be dying because we are unfit to live.

HUNTER: No further questions. (*Sits*)

JUDGE: Dr Blaik, this has, without any doubt at all, been the quietest of all the sessions of the court. I wonder why this is. Are you religious?

BLAIK: I belong to no formal religion at present. But I reverence life. I practice meditation. I do not want death, but I am not afraid – I hope I am not afraid – of death: I mean, not just my own death, but that of the species. I am seeking to avoid it, but I will accept it without anger if it comes. It will not be the end. I believe there is something else. I don't think many doctors do. I am not blaming them.

JUDGE: Thank you kindly, doctor. And the court is now adjourned.

REFERENCES—SESSION SIXTEEN
General Reading

Illich, I., *Medical Nemesis*, Pantheon Books, New York, 1976. (See note to this reference in the bibliography to Session 12.)

Frank, A., and Frank, S., *The People's Handbook of Medical Care*, Vintage Books, New York, 1972. (A long list of titles of books on first aid, home medication, etc., could have been added, but it would have to be very long to be representative, and access to the relevant books—or cassettes, or filmstrips, or films—is not too difficult for the general public.)

Navarro, V., *International Journal of Health Services*, vol. 5, no. 3, 1975, p. 351. (A critique of the central hypothesis of Ivan Illich that the malaise of the medical and other institutions of the western world is due to industrialization. The use in an English-language text of words like 'problematique'— apparently meaning 'problem'—or 'fetishizing' or 'dehierarchicalization' is unusual; but the analysis in this critique is none the less acute. The author

sees the malaise of western institutions as arising from the capitalist nature
of the western societies in which the institutions occur; and the answer to
the various symptoms that he thinks Illich has quite accurately observed is to
be found, he believes, not in Illich's cultural proposals—which he regards as
conservative, and likely to become reactionary *chic*—but in a *democratic*,
decentralized, communist ordering of society after the Chinese/Cuban model.
He none the less accepts that Russian-style communism with its highly
centralized, non-democratic, *apparatchik* structure puts power in the hands
of the party, just as in capitalist countries it is in the hands of the owners and
managers of financial capital: there is a convergence of these two systems.

Western doctors, he thinks, although they may sometimes share power in
the health field by virtue of themselves coincidentally being on occasion
members of the upper-middle class, none the less do not *qua* doctors take any
major policy decisions in that field; and he cites the introduction, against
medical opposition, of health insurance and later of the National Health
Service in the United Kingdom as instances of this medical impotence in the
face of the covert capitalist manipulators of the health scene.

He does not, however, explain the apparent inability of *any* social order
having an industrial/scientific/technological base (whether politically it be
capitalist, or communist of either the centralized or the democratic type) to be
viable ecologically and health-wise. It is only right to add that it is not a
problem to which he here addresses himself, though no answer is conceivable
to the facts, for instance, that the Chinese seem to be very heavy cigarette
smokers and that lung cancer knows no ethnic boundaries; and that the
Chinese are members of the nuclear club, and the Cubans were once prepared
to have missiles with nuclear war-heads on their territory. The examples could
be multiplied.

Whatever one may think of this editor's analysis of the Illichian view of
medicine—which may merely reflect the fact of that view being out of tune
with the accepted canons of exegesis of the journal—the analysis does not
appear to be able to accommodate that fundamental ecological and health
objection; and it carries much less conviction in relation to Illich's evaluation
of the institutions of education or transport than in relation to his examination
of the medical institution.)

Bradshaw, J. S., *Royal Society of Health Journal*, August 1977, p. 159.

Dimond, E. G., *JAMA*, September 19, 1977, p. 1251.

Editorial, *Lancet*, November 26, 1977, p. 1114.

THE OTHER WORLD

Enter Dr Elizabeth Ojukbo

JUDGE: You are Dr Elizabeth Ojukbo? You are a graduate of an English medical school, and you have two extra postgraduate qualifications? You now live in your own country, which is a British Commonwealth country in West Africa? (*Ojukbo nods*) Tell us about yourself, doctor.

OJUKBO: I went to school in my country; and then because I was intelligent – though many girls were more intelligent – and, much more important, because my parents had money, I went to England to study medicine. Full of hope, I came back five years ago to my country. I was a stranger. Now my people have begun to accept me.

JUDGE: And your first position there?

OJUKBO: Was in a hospital, naturally. In our big new hospital, which cost £10,000,000. A beautiful hospital. Oh, so beautiful! And twenty miles away you cannot find even a hut with a few bandages in it.

JUDGE: So you left the hospital?

OJUKBO: I was not even scratching the surface of our real problems, I had not recognized them. That hospital was my glass-and-chromium ivory tower. So I went to a village to practice ordinary medicine, give some health education, advise on sanitation and nutrition, help the people. The dream of Dr Roylance and Professor Dible – though I did not have a health center, or an administrator, or even a single computer. But I was still half full of hope.

JUDGE: And you perhaps did not find fulfillment there either?

OJUKBO: Perhaps? – You are understanding me fast, judge. No, I did not find fulfillment. The people were helping me more than I was helping them.

JUDGE: But you must have done some good.

OJUKBO: Oh, yes, I removed some lumps, I cured a few diseases, I prevented others perhaps; but I also rediscovered my people and their thoughts, their religion, their way of life – which is more important for health than medicines or clean water or 'brush your teeth after every meal'. And I rediscovered something of myself. So I left the village.

JUDGE: And then?

OJUKBO: I was empty of hope, of the hope with which I had begun. I went to another ivory tower, one of our three medical research institutes, to study our native remedies, as you would call them. To study them by the very latest techniques: gas chromatography, fractionation and subsequent administration of the fractions to four different species of animal, the pharmacokinetics... And I found what I really knew I would find: that the more they were divided up, the closer you peered at them, the less effective, the less miraculous they became. As that nice Dr Spring said. They worked in the field with the ordinary people but not in the laboratory. Oh, extracts of some of them worked even there, sometimes they were much too strong; but mostly they did not – as you destroyed the mystery, the wholeness, you destroyed the miracle.

JUDGE: That was a disappointment to you?

OJUKBO: No, judge, it was an enlightenment, a joy to me. I suspected what would happen all the time deep-down. Anyway, why do you think I really went to that ivory tower? – Not for the experiments. No, I went to think. That research was just an excuse.

JUDGE: And your thinking bore fruit?

OJUKBO: Yes. I decided that western medicine, western society was wrong for my country, though I do not know just what is right. That is what I am now trying to find out. I am back in a village, though not as a doctor; helping a little, thinking a little, learning a lot. I am learning to be alive. A *new* hope is coming to me.

JUDGE: You say western medicine is wrong for your country, but the expectation of life has gone up in nearly all underdeveloped countries in the last 30 or 40 years.

OJUKBO: Oh, yes, by 10 years or so in my own country; thanks mainly to modern western medical technology – vaccination against smallpox, antimalarial drugs, 'death to the mosquito', and so on. And partly also thanks to a so-called improvement in social conditions – better sanitation, better housing, and the rest. All the factors that affected your country 100 years ago. Hospitals have not played a big part though.

JUDGE: You approve surely of the increased life expectancy?

OJUKBO: I approve of it less than I disapprove of the price my people are having to pay for it.

JUDGE: The price being?

OJUKBO: My society was a healthy society. It still is mostly a healthy society – except where it has been overwhelmed by your society, which is a sick society. Not sick with disease. Not just that. Much worse than that. It is sick in its soul, in the very bottom of its soul. And it has the strength of a man drowning. Yes, you have increased your expectation of life to 70, over 70, years; but as the quantity of your lives gets bigger the quality gets more than correspondingly less. We heard from Mr Hunter ten days ago that the top country in the world for health is Sweden.

JUDGE: You do not approve of its good health?

OJUKBO: Judge, do you know the price of its so-called health? – I will now quote to you from your own *Times* newspaper of May 11, 1972, which I have here. *The Times* of London. It was giving details [1] of a report on Swedish life prepared by a Swedish psychiatrist who was commissioned by the government to produce it when the number of people admitted to mental hospitals in Sweden jumped from 73,000 in 1969 to 83,000 in 1970. *The Times* said that the report 'has confirmed the image of a harsh, ruthless society which asks its citizens to sacrifice their mental well-being by working ever harder to pay for exorbitantly priced flats and consumer goods . . . More and more citizens cannot keep up as the planners demand even higher economic growth to pay for looking after those who have faltered along the way. But as the number of drop-outs increase more growth is needed, which results in more drop-outs.' Now just listen to this, judge: 'The typical young married couple make love on an average only twice a month, if the statistics are to be believed. They think this is because the women, and perhaps the men too, are simply too tired.' Too tired for love! The report also said, 'What we have managed to put together for our children is an extremely cold and anti-child society.' And it noted, according to *The Times*, that 'the growing mental health problem is not solely a Swedish phenomenon. It is happening in all industrialized societies.' Oh, yes! – Think, judge, of your new towns, look at your high-rise buildings. Think of the mentally sick, and the poor, and the unhappy, and the alienated patients, and the old people you have kept alive – all, all neglected by your society in England. It is happening faster in Sweden, that is all – that is what the report said.

JUDGE: And what relevance has this for your country, doctor, do you think?

OJUKBO: I will get around to that sideways, judge. *The Times* man goes on: 'It is axiomatic that perfectionism can be a psychologically disastrous goal for most people, but the Swedes nonetheless keep striving for it . . . For economic reasons Sweden continues to standardize . . . Few aspects of a Swede's life can be hidden from public scrutiny, from the time the state awards him his very own *personnumber* until the time he dies in one of the new computerized hospitals . . . A new style of writing is being introduced in comprehensive schools which will be easier for computers to scan . . . In the capital, high above the central square, roving television cameras monitor the movements of citizens.' And the report itself

said, 'We know that the style of life in the so-called super-indus-
trialized society leads to a prodigious, human-crushing process.'
No wonder the Swedes – so *The Times* article says – drink more
spirits per head than anyone else in the world. Television cameras,
computers, standardization, perfectionism, planning, ruthlessness,
no love, no time for children, drink – no, if that is the price of an
increased life expectancy, then I do not want it, judge, for my
country. I do not want to get rid of some sicknesses in people if the
price is to destroy them as persons, and to destroy the human
society they and their ancestors have built up.

JUDGE: You have not actually mentioned Swedish medicine yet,
doctor.

OJUKBO: Patience, judge. To that I am just now coming. A
Swedish doctor has said[2] that, whatever the expectation of life
and so on in Sweden, the medical system is alienating, it provides
assembly-line medicine: it is full of administrators, specialist care
is centralized and there are long waiting lists; if you telephone for a
doctor in an emergency you may find yourself listening to a taped
message telling you to phone a hospital, and when you do that a
nurse will say 'take an aspirin' and advise you to see the doctor
tomorrow. Personal friendly contact between you and a doctor
who really knows you hardly exists; and so on, and so on. Swedish
medicine, judge – a little replica of the Swedish society that
produces it. Do you remember what Dr Blaik said yesterday was
the crucial fault in our society: 'Everything must be programed,
everything foreseeable, everything certain and secure . . .' As in
Sweden. They are even proposing to have the multiphasic screening that Professor Dible talked about – to have it made compulsory
for everybody in Sweden.[3] For everybody every five years.

JUDGE: Are you saying, doctor, that, if one takes a broad view, your
society is healthier than that of the west?

OJUKBO: Yes, I do say it. Your wonderful western society is the
underdeveloped one: you reject God, and so you make western
man into a god; and his religion is technology and modern science,
including medicine; and this religion has its priests, called engineers
and biochemists and doctors, and so on. You covet trash – material
things, cars, food, planes, television sets, cigarettes, computers –
and you worship numbers; and you forget people. You set up
institutional churches for your religion, and each of them develops
a priesthood which serves itself, not the people; which positively
diminishes their health or satisfaction or delight – whatever it was
meant to provide. Dr Blaik told you. Man is the *measure* of all
things; and so you are losing all moral restraints, which means
you are becoming the worst slaves of all. And *your* sect of this

religion, which you call capitalist democracy, is ripe for take-over by another sect, more fanatical, called communism.

JUDGE: And western medicine more specifically, doctor?

OJUKBO: As Mr Hunter got from Sir Guy Chumley, it reinforces your western society in a dozen ways. It is a limb of that society. But your western life-style, which that society very deliberately chooses, includes the cars, the television sets, the too-much food – all those things I just said you adored – which cause your diseases; so your doctors will never really get rid of them, and particularly your coronary disease, till they get rid of your society. Which of them has suggested that? Of all the doctors who have given evidence the only two who sensed what was really needed were Dr Blaik and that American, Professor Brent, who talked about coronary heart disease. A total population approach, he said, was needed. But even he did not know just what that would mean, just how radical is radical. Dr Blaik knew it, though. But in the meantime, what do your doctors do for your self-caused diseases? They try to treat or prevent them either with the very things that caused them or with something similar; and so they prop up your sick society even more. Mr Hunter has made this point with many witnesses. I exclude Dr Aldam, from what I just said. He has never changed. The world has changed: he has not.

JUDGE: What you are saying, doctor, is that western medicine is an integral part of western high-technology society? Has sold out to it?

OJUKBO: I am saying that. Your western doctors are all the time carrying out research to find cures or vaccines, and at the same time their first cousins, the food technologists or the planning engineers or the polymer chemists, are working out new ways to cause new diseases. Not consciously – oh, goodness gracious me, no! – They are like doctors, they can't see beyond the ends of their noses. 'We didn't intend ... we didn't expect ...' They remind me of ants.

JUDGE: And is your indictment of the western ant-hill complete, doctor?

OJUKBO: Except to say there is one other important cousin to the doctors I have not mentioned – the physicist who makes atomic energy and thermonuclear weapons, and radioactive isotopes for the doctor to use on some of his patients. Never, never, never before has any civilization devised the means to destroy, not just itself, but all mankind, all life; but you in the west can do it with atomic weapons, or genetic engineering, or mutant viruses, or perhaps by destroying the ozone layer, or with some new chemical we shall not know about till we are dying of it. Dr Blaik told you this yesterday. And this civilization and its medicine I do not want in my country.

JUDGE: You think it inevitable that western high-technology will repeat in underdeveloped countries the mistakes it has made in the west?

OJUKBO: Of a similar kind – yes, I do. What has it *actually* done to my country? – It has thrown little bits of its technology into my country's very different culture, which is like watering a garden with oil or pruning a tree with an oxy-acetylene lamp. A culture is alive. It is strong in one way, delicate in another. A vine is strong, but what if you smother its roots with oil? What have you done to the poorer countries? – What have you not done? – Having poured your oil, having clumsily interfered by providing enough education and sanitation and vaccines and DDT to increase the life span by 10 years, but having so unfortunately failed to find ways of increasing the harvests of those countries as much as their populations, the west watches hunger and malnutrition getting worse, and famines occurring. Then what does the west do, the west that helped to keep the children alive? – Like Mr Hunter said, it first takes photographs of the starving children, and uses them to arouse pity in the west and to appeal for money. Second, with the money it provides aid – enough, assuming it ever gets to the starving people – to help them a little, keep them alive a little longer, miserably alive. But in helping them the west makes them dependent, takes away their need to try and be self-reliant. The more you *give* the more you need to give. It has been proved.[4] Third, it sends tourists to those countries; and in the colored advertisements for them where are the hungry children who figure in the appeal advertisements? – They have miraculously vanished, those countries have suddenly become 'romantic', 'picturesque', 'unspoiled'. Nothing must be real, must it? – Not for those nice clean tourists, fully inoculated, stepping off their jet planes, hoping they will be able to stick to their slimming diets, dying for a drink. What you do cries to heaven for vengeance.

JUDGE: And do you say, doctor – forgive me, I realize you feel strongly on these matters – that the impact of western *doctors* on such countries as yours has been *wholly* bad?

OJUKBO: Not wholly bad, judge. I do not say so. Obviously not. They save a few lives in the hospitals, and with public health measures they save far more who would have died from infectious diseases. But to what advantage if the children they save merely live a little longer to die more slowly of starvation, or of some *other* infection? And you cannot separate the doctors from the other people who come with them. The doctors come in a jet plane which also brings pilots, and businessmen, and engineers, and chemists, and university professors; and so cars and chemical fertilizers and pesticides and television sets and gadgets and throw-away items – and baby foods. The things that will destroy my people. It is not just the businessman selling his baby food who is responsible for the artificially-fed babies who die in my country: the doctors are responsible too, whether they know of what is happening or not, whether they are from your country or from this United States or native-born doctors come back, like me, or trained in their own western-style medical schools, whether they treat the babies or not. They are all infected with the same virus. The doctor is not the cure, the doctor is part of the disease. It is the doctors who want hospitals and research institutes instead of the simple health centers, or public health measures, or properly trained barefoot doctors who, even by western standards – by any standards – would do far more good: give first-aid, advise on hygiene and sanitation, advise on food, look after antenatal and postnatal care, give inoculations, treat some diseases, help with family planning, educate the people in health. I am preaching only what other doctors like myself have said,[5, 6] what your own best western doctors say themselves.[7, 8, 9] *If* we are to have western health activities, it is not more doctors we need: it is the ordinary simple worker in the field. If the doctors emigrate, let them: the country will be better off because they would keep the old system going, the old training, when what we need is a new training for new methods for new people.

JUDGE: If the west is to intervene at all, you mean?

OJUKBO: Yes, I am saying if – *if* we are to have western inter-ference, it should not give any kind of priority to doctors. Let us, *if* we are to have anything, have medical auxiliaries and prevention, and teachers, and those who will help and advise on simple indus-tries and simple agriculture – for these will do the least harm and the greatest good to health as well as to the economic and social life of a country like mine. But do I *want* the west? – No, I do not. I do *not*, judge. I am talking about softening the blow if a blow is to be landed. But it will not happen like that. We shall have *big* factories and *big* tractors and *big* hospitals – until the energy supplies run out. We shall have 'cultural adaptation', which means cultural destruction. We shall have the pill and the loop and vasectomy. The barefoot doctors will absorb it all, and yes, will form a college, and will want to become proper doctors. Think of the richer underdeveloped countries. What are they doing? – As fast as they can they are manufacturing the western froth.[10] And they are thinking of making themselves into carbon copies of the west. The sick west. So all right, *if* they do, they will increase their life span, they will maybe control their populations, they will produce the food, they will have nuclear energy,[11] they will have seven computers in every hospital, and a hospital in every town – and they will be like the Swedes. Mental disease is now increasing, even in the Middle East[12] – you told Dr Batt yourself. And the more the population growth comes under control the more the people will consume per head – more of oil and electricity and chemicals and paper and wood and plastics and minerals. They will simply join the west in destroying the earth to satisfy the lust the west has given them for those material things I told you about, taking what can never be replaced, taking and not even putting back when they can, polluting the seas and the rivers, wounding the land, damaging even the sky above us. It is the work of a devil.

JUDGE: You are basically opposed to *any* western intervention, doctor?

OJUKBO: Basically and completely. No World Health Organization, no other international organizations, no charities, no missionaries, no drugs, no pesticides. Let us choose for ourselves, find our own way out. Let us die if we must.

JUDGE: Mr Hunter?

HUNTER (*rising*): You will not be surprised to know that you have already made most of my points for me, doctor. China has steered clear of the worst excesses of the west, has she not? – Very few motor cars so that people do take exercise, enough food of the right kinds but no excess, population control through a combination of late marriage, and premarital chastity, and contraception; no venereal disease – compared with about a million new cases of gonorrhoea a year in the United States – no drug addiction; reasonable housing, good sanitation; and control, thanks largely to the barefoot doctors and appropriate training of doctors proper, of various diseases that used to kill a great many. And yet the people are seemingly content with their work, willing to help one another, not wanting our western rubbish?[13, 14, 15]

OJUKBO: Oh, yes, it is a kind of paradise compared with their past. But it is China's own solution to China's own problems. Like Dr Blaik, I do not believe one can export that kind of thing. One can export failure, corruption, but not success. And they have the bomb. And China is communist, so that man is worshipped, not God.

JUDGE: But any regimentation, any oppression that might be associated with the Chinese regime does not worry you, doctor?

OJUKBO: They were more heavily oppressed before the communists took over; and then they were also diseased and unhappy. I am not a communist, they would think I needed educating. But my objection goes deeper than just the regimentation.

HUNTER: Health, in your view, depends very largely on self-help,[9] on devolution of responsibility for health?[16]

OJUBKO: Yes, but not merely each individual helping himself. That certainly, but also families, communities, districts helping themselves. True health comes from healthy living, as Dr Blaik said. It *is* healthy living, which involves exercise as – what did Professor Brett call it? – yes, as a built-in element, a part of the life, not something added, like jogging; and it involves eating foods that give health, not eating foods that may give ill-health, and then taking something extra that will neutralize the badness in the food. And also one can have an illness healthily, as Dr Aldam told us. It is very unhealthy never to have an illness, and yet that is what the west would like: immunization, drugs, operations for everything – until death. And in time perhaps something for that too.

HUNTER: But healthy living: just what does that arise from?

OJUKBO: From the right culture, the culture that suits the people, that has grown up naturally in response to their needs. A healthy culture is always based upon a healthy religion involving mystery, and centered on God. One should not decrease the mystery in life, which is what science tries to do: one should try to increase it. One should develop rituals, customs, taboos that will be health-promoting. Oh, I do not mean one *should*, I am talking like a westerner: I mean that one *does* in a healthy society with a healthy culture. One does it without thinking. The health is in the culture, you cannot separate them. I agree with Dr Blaik: show me a society that makes beautiful churches or beautiful totem poles or beautiful kraals, and I will show you a healthy people – even though, in fact, very few of them may live to be 70.

HUNTER: And if I may summarize your objections to the western way, to so-called health, as applied to your own country: not being of indigenous growth and to judge from its effects so far, it may well continue to cause more harm than good for it is part of a larger way of life and of thought that will destroy your own culture and replace it with some kind of variant of the culture you described for Sweden, which provides a longer life but an unhappy one; that the whole western approach, of which medicine is a part, is ecologically destructive,[17] increases population faster than it can increase food supplies,[17, 18] consumes irreplaceable resources,[17] and uglifies the environment; and finally, that an integral part of it is the capacity in any one of half a dozen ways to destroy the human species, and perhaps all life on earth?

OJUKBO: You understand me, Mr Hunter.

HUNTER: No further questions. (*Sits*)

JUDGE: Dr Ojukbo, you are fully trained in western medicine. Suppose you were faced in Africa with an acute emergency condition, which you knew you could remedy by complex surgery that you were equipped to perform, and by no other means: would you operate?

OJUKBO: Yes, judge, of course. I cannot cast my knowledge away. I could not let that person die.

JUDGE: Parts of western medicine have some virtue?

OJUKBO: Yes, but they come from western high technology.

JUDGE: Nonetheless, you in particular cannot discard them, even if you would?

OJUKBO: You are right. I did not think you would be quite so understanding of my predicament. Yes, judge, I, a black woman, am branded for life by my training in science, in scientific medicine, by my years of living in England. Science means knowledge – of all the good and evil things I have talked about. I cannot escape but perhaps I may help my people to.

JUDGE: You mean?

OJUKBO: I mean, judge, that there is a child crying out to be born, and perhaps I can help to give it birth, perhaps even give some birth to it. I was so pleased – you do not know how pleased I was – to hear Mr Hunter put those good arguments against *all* births having to take place in hospital. Hospitals, hospitals! – I have here the *Lancet* of October 19, 1974. May I read from it, please?

JUDGE: By all means.

OJUKBO: There is a letter[19] from two English doctors, a man and wife, who had worked for some years in Africa. They said, 'The most lethal environment in Africa is not a village with the customary diet, but a well-scrubbed modern children's ward with an excellent supply of food.' They meant, if the child was ill, he needed his mother and home above everything else, and the food he was used to, and *then* perhaps some medicine – at home – for his illness. 'The modern acute general hospital,' they said, 'proved a disaster when imported into Africa. It destroyed more children than it saved, and provided a bottomless pit for misguided central Government expenditure . . . The gigantic mortality in hospitals is due to the hospital environment.' Well now, for women who are to have children . . .

JUDGE: Yes, doctor?

OJUKBO: How can I put it to you men? To the African woman as well as to the African child – and I think also to the white woman, no matter how much she may disguise it, even from herself – the hospital is threatening. It is cold, it is sterile, it is scientific, it is alienating. (*Pause*) Women are delivered of their babies lying on a bed or propped up on it. Sometimes, if there is any difficulty, if the doctor has to interfere, to use forceps, the woman's legs will be slung up by stirrups from metal poles at the end of the delivery bed; and so she is delivered. (*Pause*) In my country women stand or squat to have their babies.[20] What is more natural? Who wants to have her baby lying on her back? (*Pause*) You are men; but when you are to open your bowels, do you lie down, or do you squat on a lavatory seat?[21] (*Pause*) Forgive me, judge.

JUDGE: Not at all, dear lady. I squat. I am sure we all squat. I take your point.

OJUKBO: It is a symbol – of one's freedom. If there is to be a new birth, it must take place outside the hospital, away from the western doctors, away from their thinking and their forceps. That is why I live in a village, helping and being helped. Perhaps I will give birth only to one hair on the baby's head. You see how I am westernized? But if a million women like me are also giving birth, we shall all be together, and the baby will come together, and there will be a new living child, plump and shiny and laughing. It will make the pain seem like a nothing. There is some pain to having a baby, but it is a good pain, and after it there is the baby. And this baby is needed for your sakes too. Perhaps the good God will see the baby, and give us all his benediction. I have no more words to say.

JUDGE (*after a pause*): Thank you, doctor. And this court is now adjourned.

REFERENCES—SESSION SEVENTEEN

1. *The Times*, May 11, 1972, p. 5. (Reproduced from *The Times* by permission.)
2. Lofstead, S. J., *JAMA*, June 30, 1975, p. 1328.
3. Gotzsche, A.-L., *World Medicine*, October 19, 1977, p. 80.
4. Dass, K. K., *Lancet*, June 21, 1975, p. 1373.
5. Tavassoli, M., *JAMA*, December 16, 1974, p. 1527.
6. Mahloudji, M., *Lancet*, July 26, 1975, p. 175.
7. Croft Long, E., and Viau, A., *Lancet*, January 26, 1974, p. 127.
8. Essex, B. J., *BMJ*, July 5, 1975, p. 34.
9. Backett, E. M., and England, R., *Lancet*, December 6, 1975, p. 1137.
10. Tarbush, M., *The Times*, July 6, 1976, p. 15.
11. Leading Article, *The Times*, June 7, 1976, p. 13.
12. Grainge, A., *The Times*, November 24, 1977, p. 13.
13. Dimond, E. G., *JAMA*, December 6, 1971, p. 1552.
14. Sidel, V. W., *NEJM*, June 15, 1972, p. 1292.

15. Moser, R. H., *JAMA*, December 16, 1974, p. 1566.
16. Mahler, H., *Lancet*, November 1, 1975, p. 829.
17. Loraine, J. A., *World Medicine*, June 4, 1975, p. 51.
18. Bradshaw, S., *Lancet*, February 2, 1974, p. 177.
19. Lawless, J., and Lawless, M. M., *Lancet*, October 19, 1974, p. 947.
20. Dunn, P. M. *Lancet*, April 10, 1976, p. 790.
21. Editorial, *Lancet*, July 5, 1975, p. 18.

Delivery of Health Care in Non-Westernized Cultures
Chamberlin, R. W., and Radebaugh, J. F., *NEJM*, March 18, 1976, p. 641.

Use of Medical Auxiliaries, etc., in 'Underdeveloped' Countries
Health Manpower and the Medical Auxiliary, Intermediate Technology
    Development Group, London, 1971.
Medical Care in Developing Countries, Office of Health Economics, London,
    1972.
Dorozynski, A., *Doctors and Healers*, International Development Research
    Centre, Box 8500, Ottawa, Canada, K1G 3H9, 1975.
Elliott, K., *The Training of Auxiliaries in Health Care*, Intermediate
    Technology Publications, London, 1975.
Watts, G., *World Medicine*, April 23, 1975, p. 15.
Assignment Children, Alternative approaches to health care, January–March
    1976, Unicef, Geneva, p. 5–108.
The Doctor-Go-Round, Oxfam Public Affairs Unit, London, 1976.

THE JUDGE'S VERDICT

The judge speaks as follows:

I shall be as brief as possible. The purpose of this court was to determine whether western doctors today are more productive of ill-health than of health; and whenever I use the term 'doctors' it is to western doctors that I shall be referring.

I must preface my remarks by stating that, if any evidence on the matter was needed, we have heard a good deal in this court suggesting that most doctors are conscientious, hard-working, kind, and competent by their standards, and that they act in what they conceive to be the best interests of those they serve. Not even Mr Hunter would deny that.

To put the matter in another way: as various witnesses have said, nobody can dispute that, if a person has a sudden severe pain, if he has a fever, or if he breaks his arm, he would be very well advised to consult a doctor as soon as possible. And this is not greatly altered by the fact that a few doctors may be less than competent, that some may charge excessive fees or perform unnecessary operations, and that medicine can certainly be guilty of gross error, even in the purely clinical sphere.

What I have largely to determine, however, is whether the doctors' concept of what is in the best interests of the people they serve, or of the populace as a whole, is appropriate; whether on occasion, in other words, the sudden severe pain or the broken arm should ever have been allowed to occur, or should elicit the type of response the doctors favor; and whether other elements have not, in any case, to be put in the balance.

'Whether western doctors are more productive of ill-health than of health': in whom? – Only in individuals, or also in society generally, as Mr Hunter would clearly have us accept? Certainly doctors do not have the sole or the major responsibility in that regard; but being key members of society, and professional men to whom in our technological age people more than ever look for guidance, they must, I think, accept a good measure of responsibility.

Definitions of the health and the ill-health for which doctors carry varying degrees of responsibility are not easy to provide. Health, however, does not mean the complete absence of any disease or defect. If it did, the doctors would certainly be found guilty; but then so would a choir of angels. Even to a disease or defect there is a healthy way to respond, as Dr Aldam said; and doctors may be a help or a hindrance to such coping.

The health and ill-health of a society or culture are even less easily defined than those of an individual, but there is no doubt that a society is unhealthy when its life-style clearly cannot be sustained for more than a few decades. We can recognize health and ill-health much more readily than we can define them.

I shall first mention the salient points of the evidence the court has heard – salient in the light of the court's brief and of what I have just been saying. I shall present these points factually: I am not, I would stress, making any judgment at this stage.

In the first part of our inquiry (about the activities of doctors) Professor Mead, the American medical historian, gave us many examples of gross errors made by the medical profession in the past, some of them in the recent past. The implication of possible present or future error was clear. Even the 'conquest' of malaria seemed to have been a mixed blessing.

Obesity, Dr McGilly next told us, is due to a lack of exercise together with an excessive intake of food, and is treated by doctors, usually unsuccessfully, with tablets, the provision of diets, and, occasionally, fasting or operations of one kind or another. Doctors, we were told, do not pay enough attention to the psychological aspects of obesity, and are therefore not as successful with it as psychologists or lay groups.

Coronary heart disease, Professor Brent said, is the typical, and the most common, killing disease of western man, and is very probably due to some combination of a number of factors – cigarette smoking, a raised blood pressure, lack of vigorous exercise, lack of fiber in the diet, an excess of dietary fat, especially animal fat, and perhaps stress. He favored a preventive, total-population approach to it, but this has nowhere been attempted, although here in the United States the condition is becoming less common, probably because individuals are themselves taking preventive steps. Doctors in general treat coronary disease at a late stage by means of expensive, high-technology methods, such as coronary care units and bypass operations, which are not very effective. Much of their preventive effort – when there is any at all – consists merely of advising or exhorting their patients on the changes they should make in their life-style.

Various diseases, some minor, some major and even lethal, are almost certainly caused by a lack of dietary fiber (bran usually), and others may well be, Dr Hafod told us; and until recently some of them were misguidedly treated with a low-fiber diet. Again the late-stage treatments used by doctors for these conditions are the typical outcome of the western technological approach, which also, of course, produces the lack of dietary fiber. There is little in the way of a preventive approach. Like obesity and coronary heart disease, the dietary-fiber deficiency diseases are, we heard, typical products of our western life-style.

Next Professor Hecht told us of the heavy prescribing by doctors of the antibiotics, chloramphenicol and tetracyclines, after their dangers had been publicized; and the similar prescribing of amphetamines and barbiturates, both of the latter groups consisting of drugs of dependence. Mr Hunter produced even more recent instances of drugs with very serious side-effects, and some evidence, both of the size of the problem and of the fact that more education of doctors – of which there was little on this matter – would not alter the position. He said drugs were typical products of our western way of life, used to treat the ailments it caused.

Next Mr Buck, although admitting there were some forms of stress peculiar to our time, dismissed the idea that stress was particularly important in causing illness. He and other doctors dealt with developed disease, and it was not for them to be social reformers or to spend a lot of time on psychosocial factors that *might* lead to illness: tranquilizers and sedatives, which he agreed were characteristic of our age, were fairly effective. He could not accept either that doctors could have done more in combating cigarette smoking or abuse of alcohol.

Professor Larkin told us health was not to be equated with doctors. Most of the conquest of infectious diseases in the developed world was achieved by means that were not purely medical. Our modern killing diseases were largely a product of our way of life, and were preventable. Hospitals received a disproportionately high allocation of health money; but community work was more important, and he believed it would in time be undertaken without any preliminary major upheaval in society being necessary.

In the second part of our inquiry – about the nature of doctors and medicine – Dr Jaeger said he felt doctors deserved the high incomes, relative to those of others, that Mr Hunter established they received. The excellent motives Dr Jaeger ascribed to doctors appeared under questioning to be non-existent. He did not think that excessive, financially profitable surgery was practiced in North America: doctors in California and their spouses had more operations than equivalent groups. Doctors, he agreed, were very liable to have trouble with their marriages, and with drink, drugs, and mental illness. Dr Jaeger felt this was due to their hard work, despite Mr Hunter's evidence to the contrary. Until 1977 the USA had been taking in thousands of doctors every year from poor countries, although, as Mr Hunter established, the health of its citizens had not improved correspondingly. He also described work done by some idealistic young doctors in New York, and contrasted them with most British and American doctors who, Dr Jaeger agreed, were in the mainstream of our western high-technology society. He did not see why doctors should not travel the world, and combine business with pleasure.

Next Dr Batt agreed that western, high-technology medicine was an integral part of modern western society: they were not separable. He favored the gadgetry produced by high-technology medicine, and was not worried about the associated genetic engineering or ecological damage; and he approved of 100 percent hospital births, of the widespread use of computers in medicine, and of automated multiple laboratory testing. He was not concerned about the alleged cultural poverty of doctors. He agreed that science was fissiparous in its methods, and that measurement was of the essence of high-technology medicine; but he could not accept that this made for a fundamental incompatibility between it and the finer, non-measurable elements in life, normally thought to be involved in medical practice.

Professor Weskoff, the next witness, found it difficult to defend what seemed to be a combination of excessive investigation and inadequate treatment of certain patients in the USA suffering from high blood pressure, and the fright or terror induced in many patients by certain modern medical techniques. The fact that the lives of young people were saved by transplants of the kidneys from young people killed in automobile accidents did not trouble her. She could not accept that patients in a coronary care unit were treated with items similar to those that had caused their disease, or that scientific medicine made it impossible to treat the patient as a whole person. The modern management of spina bifida produced more benefits than drawbacks, she thought. However, she did accept that high-technology medicine had brought many ethical problems, and that doctors had certainly on occasion been guilty of ethical offences. Indeed, Mr Hunter established that the ethical safeguards she listed had seemed all to be ineffective. He yet again argued the close, unbreakable connection between modern western society and modern western medicine, and quoted a number of doctors who were themselves highly critical of the latter. Professor Weskoff denied there was such a close connection; but she could not bring herself to deny that the modern western doctor might be playing at being God.

Sir Guy Chumley was asked about the medical institution, the organized body of medicine, which Mr Hunter accused of being rigid, and over-concerned with itself and its interests. Among the evils for which it was responsible, he indicated, was a shortage of family doctors in the USA who, in any case, understood only high-technology medicine. The medical institution, he alleged, deprived people of more than it gave them; an accusation Sir Guy could not accept. In both the United States and the United Kingdom, Mr Hunter argued, an increased number of doctors had brought no corresponding increase of health. The medical institution worked hand in hand with government, helped to prevent radical social change, and connived at people's unhealthy life-style; but Sir Guy could not accept any of this, or that the institution had any defect other than being hierarchical, if that was indeed a defect.

The last witness in the second part of our inquiry was Dr Aldam. He runs an old-style family practice, and he felt that hospitals and the medicine that was practiced in them (and that had invaded general practice) were not compatible after a certain point with treating people as human beings. Nor were they successful against our major modern diseases. People now went to the doctor with every little worry, and were discouraged from handling their problems themselves, while social workers were no substitute for relations and friends. People had lost the power to face up to pain and suffering and death. They had lost belief in religion. The duration of life had increased, but its quality had diminished.

A different type of family doctor, Dr Roylance, was the first witness in the third part of our inquiry, which was concerned with possible remedies for defects in western medicine. He described the training and the proposed method of working of a new-style family doctor, but Mr Hunter said what was being suggested was a small-scale replica of high-technology medicine. Super-specialists were not suited to the training of family doctors, which often they undertook for the money involved. The emphasis Dr Roylance put on whole-person medicine and psychosocial factors in disease could not happen in practice – as far as doctors were concerned. Physician assistants were more successful in these matters but would become professionalized unless their true role was seen by them and by society to be political, not technical.

Preventive medicine was advocated by Professor Dible as the obvious answer to most of our modern diseases. Mr Hunter suggested that there could be too much hygiene, that the multiphasic screening suggested by Professor Dible was ineffective, and that health education was not successful when it had to try and accomplish a radical change in life-style. He did, however, seem to be less opposed to Professor Dible's approach than to those of any of the previous witnesses, other than Professors Brent and Larkin; and it is, of course, with Mr Hunter's case that I am very largely concerned.

Dr Spring talked about alternative medicine as a possible remedy to some of the defects of orthodox medicine. He found particularly impressive the ability of certain simple techniques to lower a raised blood pressure. He agreed with Mr Hunter that there were some charlatans in alternative medicine, and that it owed much of its success either to its mystery or to the fact that people felt they understood just how it worked. Moreover, its practitioners took an interest in their patients as people. Another element to its popularity was people's disenchantment with high-technology medicine.

Dr Blaik was an advocate of promoting a healthy life-style by various means inside lay-controlled community centers. He worked in two which offered information on health, the support of others in groups, and the help of young neighborhood health workers. Our whole way of life was unhealthy and non-viable; it made people selfish and materialistic, and took their powers of decision from them. He was not over-optimistic that the human species would not destroy itself before the total change that was needed in western society's life-style could occur.

Our final witness was Dr Ojukbo who, although well trained in western medicine, felt she was not best helping her people by carrying out research in her West African country, or by doing clinical work there in a hospital or in a village. The western way of life, and its medicine are, she thought, altogether wrong for her country and other underdeveloped countries. They had increased the life span of her people somewhat, but would in time destroy them and their culture, making the country into a replica of the western world, which, she felt, was not developed in the true sense. It rejected God, had science and technology as a religion, and lacked moral restraints on its material covetousness. Western medicine was an integral part of that society, and treated illnesses with analogues of the elements that had caused them. What her country needed were simple health workers, simple industries, simple agriculture (if they were to have anything from the west); but she did not think it would get them – it would ape the west and help to destroy the earth. The alternative was the birth of a quite new approach to life.

That was intended to be a factual summary of the evidence we have heard. I shall now briefly evaluate it, and make some comments on the witnesses before taking a wider view. We learned from the reliable first witness in the first part of our inquiry that doctors have made many grave mistakes in the past, and from the equally reliable last, and very helpful, witness in the first part that they have, perhaps unwittingly, greatly exaggerated their own importance in the achievement of our present control of infectious disease. In between we heard of five diseases or groups of diseases (if that term may be used in relation to the adverse effects of drugs) that are largely peculiar to our time, and against which doctors use, though with little success or understanding, and often with ill effects, the instruments of high-technology medicine, which are similar to the very factors in our western high-technology society that produce those and many of the other major diseases of our time. Doctors did not, as they might be expected to do, stand aside from the general trend of society. Special status should mean a correspondingly special virtue. Of the five witnesses concerned only Professor Brent seemed sufficiently seized of this point; and though I regret to have to say it, even he lacked that combination of knowledge, vision, fervor, and sense of urgency that would seem appropriate.

The first and last witnesses in the second part of our enquiry also complemented one another, Dr Jaeger unfortunately convincing me, as no other witness did, that today's doctors are often typical well-to-do and sometimes covetous – even unscrupulous – members of our modern western society; and Dr Aldam convincing me that they are very different, both as doctors and as persons, from doctors as we have known them in the past – and as, in my judgment, they should be. Sir Guy Chumley, who understood more than he admitted, gave details of the complex and influential power base doctors have, while Dr Batt and Professor Weskoff showed that modern medicine has become a technological science, bringing us, as well as various remarkable gadgets and some limited corresponding benefits, many problems, including ethical problems, with most of which doctors have not dealt satisfactorily. Dr Batt had no doubts of the rightness of his position (and so in a sense was the most frightening of all the witnesses). Dr Weskoff had some doubts about hers, and was, I think, much the wiser. High technology, then, is the key feature of the practice of modern western medicine, and money the key element in the social philosophy informing it. Medicine ought not to be like that. Neither should its practitioners ever imagine that they are, or ever will be, gods.

It may have been noticed that, in the third part of our inquiry, we moved in the matter of remedies from what was essentially the very conventional approach suggested by Dr Roylance through increasingly strong suggestions for radical change to the most sweeping contribution of all, that of Dr Ojukbo – who in essence felt we in the west were probably beyond redemption. Dr Roylance and Professor Dible, the one with a well-meant, if sometimes tempered and always wordy, honesty, the other with her misplaced hopefulness, convinced me that the official responses to the difficulties facing medicine are inadequate or inappropriate. Dr Spring presented us with an interesting case, and an engaging personality; but his remedy is probably a lightweight one in the present context. Dr Blaik was himself deeply impressive, and his solution had much to commend it; but Dr Blaiks are not two-a-penny, and, as he himself indicated, our society is racing to destruction very fast indeed, individuals' diseases aside. Dr Ojukbo, again a most impressive person, reinforced what Dr Blaik – and indeed most of the other witnesses – had said or implied. She showed us that her society and its people are healthy, and our society and we ourselves – and alas! our doctors – are not; but she gave us little hope. You cannot, she said, water a tree with oil; and you cannot create a new and healthy world by taking thought. None the less I have no doubt that, if there is to be a rebirth, she will be present.

What then must I conclude, taking into account *all* that has been said here, *all* the views that have been expressed. What synthesis can I produce? Western doctors, both personally and professionally, are central figures in our western high-technology society: they use its methods, they profit from its material well-being, they give it their support openly or tacitly, and they thus set an example to others.

The high-technology approach and its effects *must* be taken whole or not at all. In particular, one cannot choose to have the benefits of high-technology medicine without its drawbacks, or, more important, those of high-technology society generally; neither can doctors dissociate themselves from that society. Piecemeal solutions are therefore ruled out.

The life-style of that society, as doctors know much better than any other group of persons, is inimicable to health. It is responsible for various new, major causes of death (for example, coronary heart disease, lung cancer, road accidents, drugs), and of our new, major disabling diseases (for example, obesity, diverticular disease of the colon, dental decay, various psychosomatic and psychoneurotic conditions).

Do doctors respond either by denouncing that pathogenic life-style or the philosophy that has produced it, or by living their own lives in a radically different, healthier way? – With the doubtful exception of cigarette smoking the answer is a firm 'No': they are as much given to that unhealthy life-style as the next man. This is hypocrisy. It is, moreover, a unique situation that mankind should be knowledgeable about the causes of major diseases but do almost nothing worthwhile about them.

How *do* doctors respond to our self-inflicted lethal or disabling illnesses? – By treating them at a late stage and usually in hospital by high-technology means, indeed by analogues of the very factors that have produced the conditions; and on the whole with very little success. There are one or two exceptions; and it must be once again stressed that for, say, wounds or a difficult childbirth or most fevers or acute abdominal emergencies – which are often due to conditions or circumstances that have been with us for millennia – the hospital-medicine approach is fruitful. How for such states the use of that approach might, if necessary, be separated from the other elements of our high-technology society is not clear: it had posed a problem even for Dr Ojukbo.

It must, however, be added that some modern examples even of the states of ill-health or disability, just mentioned, would be better prevented, and *could* be prevented; as almost certainly could all the modern disabling or killing conditions that are produced by our life-style. Do western doctors preach prevention? – Many doctors give it lip service, which is worse than none at all. A few doctors preach it vehemently; but few practice it, and none has shown how prevention of the kind and scale needed can be achieved without a total change in our life-style and thus of the philosophy that informs it. I regret to have to differ from Professor Larkin on this point. The only major exception to the rule – and I am pleased to state it in this venue – is the moderate drop in coronary heart disease mortality in the United States during the last ten years. However, that is a relatively small element to put in the scales.

Doctors cannot plead that in the last 100 years *their* efforts have resulted in a massive conquest of disease and a greatly increased life expectancy in the western world for, contrary to popular impressions, both of these were secured only in part by them: other persons, other disciplines, other factors than the medical kind played a major role. If doctors did not produce great remedies in past decades, are they likely to do so for these new conditions in the future? In fact, life expectancy has for some groups of people in some countries been falling; not that I should wish it to be thought that the life expectancy of its members is in my view the only criterion of their health or that of the society that nurtures them.

It must be added also that the present very scientific medical approach to our diseases militates against the traditional compassion doctors have shown to their patients; and that it results in much damage in the shape of adverse effects of treatment, and also in the destruction of the individual's right to manage his own life and of a viable social group to manage its life and the lives of the individuals within it. Lastly and relatedly, the attitude to sickness, pain, suffering, and death fostered by doctors and the medicine they practice is an unhealthy one.

Two other, broader, and very grave effects produced by our society must be considered: effects the high-technology doctor would say were no special concern of his – thus stigmatizing himself as inadequate, not his critics as over-reaching themselves. That only Dr Blaik and Dr Ojukbo mentioned these effects is significant. First, our high-technology society has, albeit often with their connivance, introduced its thinking, its gadgets, its illnesses to the people of the so-called underdeveloped world, destroying their cultures and corrupting them – even if extending their life span – and has thereby helped to threaten its own continued existence. Second, it has made it possible for man in a number of ways to destroy or, at the least, decimate the species, and indeed threaten all life on earth. This capacity, like our inactivity in the face of known causes of disease, is a characteristic never seen before in man. We are unique in these two respects.

I exaggerate the threats to the species? – The world's sources of various crucial elements will be exhausted before this century is out. In this and other respects our society is simply non-viable. Shortages could lead to war – a nuclear war perhaps. Nuclear energy sources can be misused, or go awry. Genetic engineering poses another terrible kind of threat, overpopulation another, witting or unwitting pollution or other kind of interference with the biosphere yet another. Mankind is indeed at risk.

But what has this to do with doctors? – Doctors, more than any other group in our society, are supposedly concerned with life and its preservation. Is the life of the species not to be as important as that of individuals? Have the doctors said a word? – One that has had any influence, that has truly cost them anything? It is too big a problem for individuals to tackle? – There speaks Dr Faint-Heart. It is the problem of the politicians? – There speaks the fissiparous scientist, and yet the lives of himself and of his own wife and children may be at stake. Then too have doctors played no part in causing overpopulation? In genetic engineering? Are radioactive materials not used in medicine?

I will ask, as I am in the United States: do doctors not use energy wantonly, casting away their disposables, traveling by large automobile and fast jet plane, demanding bigger hospitals, intensive care units, research institutes – all of them profligate users of energy to no very good purpose? In their indifference to the energy crisis they are no worse than their fellow Americans? – No, but then they *are* doctors; and they will in my opinion share with their fellow Americans an unpleasant awakening before long.

I shall now summarize and pass judgment. Doctors are central and typical members of our high-technology society, and have a unique responsibility for health. That society is itself unhealthy to the point of knowingly threatening the survival of mankind, of destroying non-western cultures, and of knowingly causing much gross and even lethal disease among its own members. The response of doctors to the first two evils is almost non-existent. Their response to the third, the production of disease in individuals, consists of the late, largely unsuccessful and sometimes harmful application of high-technology remedies to the sick persons, the remedies being analogues of the causes. In the process doctors deprive people, sick or well, of their autonomy in those spheres where it might properly and beneficially operate, and give support to our unhealthy and disease-producing society.

High-technology medicine is incompatible to some extent with compassion, which is what is needed most in the face of pain and death, both of which high-technology medicine, significantly enough, seeks not to make bearable but to control completely and even to eliminate. Our high life expectancy in the west is due only in part to doctors, and is here and there now falling. Doctors neither condemn our present lifestyle vehemently nor show us an alternative. Above all, our society and its medicine being integrated, doctors cannot be absolved from a major responsibility for the state of that society, and they are not credible when seeking to separate the good that high-technology medicine does from the evils produced by it and by the society of which it and they are an integral part.

In view of all this, not to speak of many minor faults, I find western doctors today are certainly more productive, directly or indirectly, of ill-health, in every sense, than of health; and therefore in the terms of the brief of this court I have no hestitation at all in finding doctors 'Guilty'.

That most doctors – being often small-minded and of narrow vision – are perhaps unwittingly guilty may be pleaded in mitigation but hardly as a defense. We must look for hope, not to doctors, but to those, whether or not they are medically qualified, who see the need to create a new society, of which health will be an integral part (as ill-health is of ours); and who will search for the philosophy, the religion, needed for the establishment of such a society. I say 'religion' deliberately. Youth may find such a religion; its parents hardly. The alternative is that the ill-health of our present society, its terrible cancerous disease, will prove mortal to it, and to us and to our children; and will ensure that our children's children shall never be born.

INDEX